The Glaucomas

Volume 1   Pediatric Glaucomas

R. Sampaolesi · J. Zarate · J.R. Sampaolesi

The Glaucomas

Volume 1
Pediatric Glaucomas

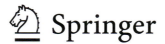

Springer

Roberto Sampaolesi, MD
Emeritus Professor
UBA (Universidad de Buenos Aires)
Faculty of Medicine
Department of Ophthalmology
and
Emeritus Professor
UCES (Universidad de Ciencias
Empresariales y Sociales)
Honorary Professor of the
Universidad del Salvador
Member of the Roman
Academy of Medicine
Parana 1239 1 A
1018 Buenos Aires
Argentina

Juan Roberto Sampaolesi, MD
Professor
UCES (Universidad de Ciencias
Empresariales y Sociales)
Faculty of Medicine
Department of Ophthalmology
Parana 1239 1er Piso
1018 Buenos Aires
Argentina

Jorge Zárate, MD
Professor
UBA (Universidad de Buenos Aires)
Faculty of Medicine
Department of Ophthalmology
Libertad 679
1770 Aldo Bonzi
Buenos Aires
Argentina

ISBN 978-3-540-69144-0   e-ISBN 978-3-540-69146-4
DOI 10.1007/978-3-540-69146-4

Library of Congress Control Number: 2008941263

Cover design: Frido Steinen-Broo, eStudio Calamar, Spain
Production & Typesetting: le-tex publishing services oHG, Leipzig, Germany

Printed on acid-free paper

9 8 7 6 5 4 3 2 1

springer.com

Dedication

This book is dedicated to my wife Erica. For the past 40 years she has attended all the anesthesias on children with congenital glaucoma, helped us during the examinations, and above all has supported the parents of the children with congenital glaucoma, whose experience is also difficult and emotional, requiring special care, as she has done with great tenderness and compassion. She also recorded each case in an index, which, in writing this book, was invaluable to consult the anatomical and functional results 12–40 years after the operations.

I also dedicate this book to my mother Angelita Bouzon Sampaolesi and to my father Dr. Juan Sampaolesi, from whom I learned the values of life and the ethics of our profession, which inspired me to write this book, and to my beloved children Anneliese, Juan Roberto, Mario, and Mariana. And also to my dear grandchildren, Lucas, Franco, Marina, Maximo, Camila and Santo, whose presence has brought joy to the last years of my life.

Foreword

Within the practice of glaucoma, indeed within the full spectrum of ophthalmic practice, there is no aspect more challenging than caring for the child with glaucoma. The childhood forms of glaucoma present unique challenges at every level of management. The examination to establish the diagnosis and monitor the progression of the disorder requires special skills. Medications are rarely effective or indicated, and surgical outcomes are often disappointing. Even when surgery is successful in lowering intraocular pressure, vision may be lost unless meticulous attention is paid to amblyopia therapy. And, on top of all these medical and surgical challenges, there is an added emotional burden. The stakes are especially high in these young patients, since failure could mean a life-time of visual impairment. The physician must also deal with anxious young parents, whose dreams of a healthy child have just been dashed, and who now look to their doctor to give their child a normal life.

For 57 years, Prof. Roberto Sampaolesi has faced these challenges. He has operated on over 800 children with glaucoma and has followed some for over 40 years. With exceptional skill and compassion, he has watched his fortunate, young patients achieve social integration and lead healthy, normal lives. Now we are the fortunate ones in having Dr. Sampaolesi share with us, in this volume, his vast knowledge and life-time of experience with the pediatric glaucomas.

As we know, children are not small adults. With regard to their eyes, they are unique both in the normal anatomical state and in many disease processes. In Chap. 12, Dr. Sampaolesi explains the appearance of the normal anterior ocular segment in newborns and children. A solid understanding of this normal anatomy is a prerequisite to recognizing disease states, and Dr. Sampaolesi's clear text and vivid illustrations provide the reader with an excellent starting point for the study of childhood glaucomas. He describes the gonioscopic appearance of the chamber angle in premature babies and newborns, as well as the biomicroscopic appearance of the iris, noting the variations of normal that can create confusion in distinguishing pathologic conditions. Finally, he provides helpful hints at the end of the chapter for performing these diagnostic procedures in children.

Having acquired an understanding of the normal anatomy, the physician must now become familiar with the range of pathologic findings in the child with glaucoma. In Chap. 13, Dr. Sampaolesi reviews the pathologic chamber angle in congenital glaucoma and its implications in indications for surgery. He describes the two basic types of pathologic chamber angles in children, which he clearly illustrates with schematic, gonioscopic, and histologic pictures. If the reader thinks that a person who has been practicing for 57 years might not be up on the latest technology, we have only to look further in this chapter and find a detailed treatise on the application of the slit lamp optical coherence tomograph in the diagnosis and follow-up of children with congenital glaucoma. Dr. Sampaolesi describes the use of this exciting new technology and provides many excellent illustrations.

One of the advantages of a life-time of experience in the practice of medicine is the individual stories that can be told, which provide guidance and encouragement for young physicians who are embarking on their careers. In Chap. 17, Dr. Sampaolesi presents several clinical cases from his years of practice. These cases highlight the difficulty of recognizing glaucoma in children, many of whom came to him after initial incorrect diagnoses. In addition, they illustrate, once again, his use of the latest technology, including confocal laser tomography and frequency-doubling technology, for those young people who are old enough for these studies. He also counsels ophthalmologists not to become discouraged by failure in surgeries and severe complications, noting that perseverance will often lead to a successful outcome even in situations that may seem hopeless. In support of this, he tells of his patients who have gone on to become successful athletes and dancers or simply able to lead normal lives.

Dr. Sampaolesi reminds us that the pediatric glaucomas are not limited to newborns and young children, but can appear at any age of childhood and even into young adulthood. In Chap. 20, he describes goniodysgenesis or late congenital glaucoma, as well as a form of pigmentary glaucoma. Once again, he turns to years of experience in describing the clinical findings, which he augments with illustrations from his practice and those of colleagues, as well as additional clinical cases.

What I believe is most valuable about this book is that it is almost like having a personal conversation with one of the giants of our profession. Dr. Sampaolesi shares with us his opinions and those of his respected colleagues. He also shares his experiences, not only of his successes, but of his heartaches and frustrations with difficult cases, and ultimately of his joy in seeing his young patients achieve success in their lives. This book then is not only a guide to the technical aspects of treating children with glaucoma, but it is also a guide as to how we, as physicians, should approach the challenges of our profession, with humility, compassion, and determination. On behalf of all the physicians and their patients and families who will profit from this guidance, I sincerely thank Dr. Sampaolesi for sharing it with us.

M. Bruce Shields

The 1994 edition of Roberto Sampaolesi's book on glaucoma was a handbook for glaucomatologists with knowledge of Spanish. With this English edition, this long hidden treasure becomes available to all English-speaking ophthalmologists. The extensively updated edition is the result of a lifelong work dedicated to ophthalmology and glaucoma by an exceptionally talented and efficient person, tireless in patient care, research, and teaching, always ready to reach out for new concepts and to turn ideas into action. The book is extraordinary in many regards. It is old-fashioned while being at the height of modernity: old-fashioned, because it is a book summarizing 60 years of experience in every field of glaucoma; modern because it is at the forefront in evaluating and using new technologies and new therapeutics; old-fashioned, because it quotes publications in many languages as far back as the times of von Graefe; modern because it makes use of new research techniques and databases such as Medline and others.

That this book could reach this level of excellence has its roots in the way Roberto Sampaolesi has accumulated knowledge and skills since his youth. After finishing medical school in 1951, he acquired a background in basic sciences – physics, chemistry, anatomy, histology and especially in physiology – spending years with Bernardo Hussay, the Nobel laureate of 1947. Then he trained in ophthalmology in a way that today has become impossible, becoming a fellow for varying periods of time with some of the best-known ophthalmologists of the time: H.K. Müller and G. Meyer-Schwikerath in Bonn, W. Leydhecker in Würzburg, C. Cüppers in Giessen, for surgery with Leornardi and Bietti in Rome, Paufique in Lyon, and Schepens in Boston, not to mention that this training period began under Marc Amsler in Zurich in 1955, as documented in "Remembrances of Things Past" in Survey of Ophthalmology [1]. He became the most prominent fellow that the Eye Department of Zurich had ever had and also one of its best friends. When later he became Professor of Ophthalmology and department head in Buenos Aires, he continued broadening his network of knowledge sources, localizing with a particularly sharp instinct the new ideas and techniques of younger

and older colleagues throughout the world. With this background, he documented with painstaking accuracy what he observed in more than 8000 glaucoma patients.

A few highlights in his skills may be pointed out:

The first is Sampaolesis's experience with pediatric glaucomas. He is an excellent teacher in care for newborns and infants in daily practice and measuring intraocular pressure without anesthesia in infants. In 1969, he taught us that normal newborns, infants, and children have much lower intraocular pressure than what had been assumed until that time and that this had to be considered in glaucoma control in infants. In 1973, he showed that the most reliable tool to check glaucoma in newborns and infants was the measurement of the length of the globe using echometry as long as intraocular pressure had to be measured under general anesthesia with all its sources for errors. He has been teaching since 1972 that trabeculotomy combined with -ectomy was the surgical procedure of choice in refractory congenital glaucomas.

The second is gonioscopy. Highlighted by his drawings, he stresses the undeniable importance of gonioscopy for glaucoma classification. He demonstrates how to differentiate normal findings and true dysgenetic changes in the developing angle. Gonioscopic findings are complemented by histology and electron microscopy of trabeculectomy specimens in an exemplary way.

The third regards the role of intraocular pressure and its level in open-angle glaucoma. Since his beginnings in ophthalmology, Roberto Sampaolesi has puzzled over so-called normal or low-pressure glaucoma. In 1961, in his publication on 24-h pressure curves – pressures taken when most ophthalmologists are still sleeping! – he had unveiled pressure peaks in most of these normal and low tension glaucomas. His growing experience let him withstand the wave that came around every 20 years attempting to downgrade intraocular pressure to a simple risk factor among others. The evaluation of the follow-up of approximately 7000 glaucoma patients 47 years later confirmed his 1961 findings and the recent placebo-controlled prospective multicenter studies prove what may have been considered a hypothesis; namely that for the single eye, overly high intraocular pressure is the main cause of glaucomatous damage.

Springer Verlag deserves thanks for publishing a book that will become a landmark of both past and future knowledge. The book may become an excellent companion and a source of knowledge for every ophthalmologist caring for glaucoma patients for many years.

Zurich
August 2008

BALDER P. GLOOR
Prof. emer. Dr. med.

Reference

1. Jay B, Sampaolesi R (1996) Rembrance of things past. Surv Ophthalmol 40:400–404

Prolog

GLAUCOMA was Roberto Sampaolesi's first book dealing with all aspects of the most important and difficult disease of ophthalmology. In 1974 this book in Spanish language (2nd edition 1994) with its 904 pages was the most complete description of all aspects of glaucoma.

Having dealt with the problem of congenital glaucoma for a great deal of his life, Roberto Sampaolesi was one of the very few ophthalmologists to not only describe all aspects of its diagnosis, but also show the results of the greatest number of surgically treated patients. He was the one who finally demonstrated the enormous importance of the "Curva diaria", which had already been mentioned by Hans Goldmann and Wolfgang Leydhecker. Roberto Sampaolesi evaluated the importance of this symptom for very early diagnosis and the precise follow up of glaucomas. This and many other aspects have already been described in the two books, which so far comprise the most complete description of this disease.

In the Spanish speaking world these classics on glaucoma are recognized as standard text books on the topic. Those of us not quite fluent in Spanish must be grateful that these texts have now been translated into English. Furthermore, the present edition gives the most complete overview of this topic – evaluating the world literature published 15 years after the last book and also summarizing the author's own wide experience.

Looking at this collection of a life devoted to studies of glaucomas by one of the great masters of ophthalmology of our time, I think that it confirms the statement by my/our great-grandfather in ophthalmology, Theodor Axenfeldt, who summarized his wisdom in 1929 at the 13th International Congress of Ophthalmology in Amsterdam: "Science and the art of medicine can develop their highest bloom only if all people collaborate for the great tree of life. The various branches alternate in producing flowers and fruits within the family of people. The spirit shows up here and there unpredictably. Everybody of us is responsible that he includes everything for the care of his patient regardless where it originates. So the joint cooperation and effort from all of us is essential and an indispensable duty."

Roberto Sampaolesi, his coauthors, and the publisher deserve praise for making the publication of this summa of a lifetime of work in ophthalmology and particularly in glaucomas possible.

May this study remind us that ophthalmological originality and creativity does not only arise in the English-speaking world, although we realize that English today has become the *lingua franca* of science everywhere.

Hamburg

PROF. JÖRG DRAEGER
MD, FRC Ophth

Erlangen

PROF. G.O.H. NAUMANN
MD, ML. FRC Ophth (hon.)
Immediate Past President International Council
of Ophthalmology (1998–2006)

Congenital glaucoma is a complex problem that in the past was a frequent cause of blindness. The poor prognosis that Anderson (senior) attributed to this condition in 1939 has improved extraordinarily:

- Manzitti was the first in Argentina to examine children under general anesthesia (1965) [1]. Sampaolesi (1967) [2] and Dr. Adneris Carro developed a method of anesthesia through inhalation with a mask on the mouth and nose of the child, at that time with Penthrane and today with Sevorane, which made it possible to measure the ocular pressure in the slit lamp, perform an anterior segment examination, and most particularly gonioscopy and measurement of the axial length with echometry..
- The study that demonstrated normal intraocular pressure in children from birth to 5 years of age confirmed that it is 5 mm less than in adults, with a mean of 10 mmHg, using both clinical measurement methods [2] and experimental methods [1]. These values have also been confirmed in numerous clinical studies.

Knowledge of the influence of different anesthetics on intraocular pressure [2–4]:

- Measuring the axial length of the eye with echometry provided a new parameter in early diagnosis, which is not affected by general anesthesia (Gernet 1969 [5]; Sampaolesi 1972 [6]; Buschmann 1974 [7]). This parameter was also shown to be very important for follow-up and for the indication of reoperation when necessary.
- Barkan's introduction of the goniotomy surgical technique in 1936 [8] was one of the greatest advances, regulating intraocular pressure in at least 40% of cases.

- The description of the surgical technique of trabeculotomy by Burian in 1960 [9] was highly effective after Cairns (1968) [10] introduced the scleral flap, which reduced the thickness of the sclera so that the Schlemm canal could be located more easily. Harms (1970) [11] and Paufique (1970) [12] developed its definitive application.
- Excellent knowledge of refractory congenital glaucoma, the angle of congenital glaucoma type II, enabled the combined technique: trabeculotomy and trabeculectomy applied in a single session (Sampaolesi 1988 [13]).
- Kozlov's technique [14], nonpenetrating deep sclerectomy (NPDS), improved the disclosure of the Schlemm canal (Sampaolesi et al. 2006 [15]).
- During 55 years at the Clinical Hospital of the chair of Ophthalmology of the University of Buenos Aires, my collaborators and I have operated 800 cases, 400 of which have at least 3 years' follow-up and 128 patients a much longer follow-up: between 5 and 40 years. In the latter group, we studied the optic nerve with confocal tomography (HRT) and the visual field with the conventional and nonconventional techniques, enabling us to evaluate the results much more accurately.
- The possibility of studying the trabeculectomy and the combined operation specimens with a great variety of histological techniques enabled us to understand the gonioscopic findings much better, focusing especially on the pretrabecular tissue, which provided a better understanding of the physiopathogenesis of this disease.

Buenos Aires   R. Sampaolesi

Acknowledgments

My co-authors and I would like to thank above all my teachers in medical school who guided me toward research: Dr. M. Varela, professor of histology; Dr. De Robertis, professor of histology; Dr. Bernardo Hussey, professor of physiology and Nobel Prize-winner for Physiology, and Dr. Juan M. Muñoz, professor of physiology, in whose departments I was an assistant for several years.

I wish to thank each of the colleagues who taught me, through practice or theory, about congenital glaucoma. I extend special thanks to:

- Dr. Edgardo Manzitti, who between 1950 and 1953 let me spend time in his pediatrics department in the Hospital de Niños where I learned his technique for examining newborn infants. The child was placed face up in a raised stretcher and examined under general anesthesia, using the Schiötz tonometer to take the intraocular pressure and carrying out the exam with a slit-lamp [16]. This required removing the chin-rest from the lamp. He performed the anterior segment exam in this way and gonioscopy with a contact lens. When Goldmann's applanation tonometer appeared, he took the pressure with this device in the slit-lamp. He also showed me how to perform the first goniotomies and allowed me do them on several patients.
- Dr. Robert Schaffer with whom I spent 1 month living in his house in Sausalito and attending his consulting room in San Francisco every day. I perfected my goniotomy technique but fundamentally I learned that congenital glaucoma was the acutest of the glaucomas and had to be operated immediately. Before performing the examination under general anesthesia, he requested permission from the parents to operate immediately after the examination, if it proved to be positive.
- The American Academy of Ophthalmology, which invited me for 12 consecutive years to give the course titled "Chamber angle anatomy, histology and surgery."
- Dr. J. Ytterborg. When I started to work on ocular pressure with applanation in the child under anesthesia, I found that the mean was 10 mmHg, and not 15 mmHg, as found in adults. I went to Oslo to visit Dr. Ytterborg, who had written a paper [1] on a study in the eyes of children who had died in the first 6 months of life, and discovered that their scleral rigidity was completely different from that of the adult, concluding that ocular pressure in children from birth to 6 months of age should be 5 mmHg less than in adults, i.e., 10 mmHg.
- Dr. Archimedes Busacca (Fig. 2, in the middle). For an entire year he allowed me go to São Paulo once a month where we examined the chamber angle in adult patients. He taught me all the normal histology and pathology of the anterior segment in terms of the chamber angle, showed me his original histological preparations under the microscope, and gave me a copy of his marvelous book, *Éléments de Gonioscopie* [17]. As I was already examining many children with congenital glaucoma under general anesthesia with the slit-lamp, Busacca traveled several times to Buenos Aires to examine five or six children at a time (Fig. 2).

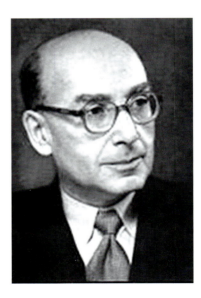

Fig. 1 Hans Goldmann, 1899–1991

– Dr. Jean Kluyskens, whom I met in 1960 and who gave me a copy of his wonderful book *Le glaucome congénital* [18]. From him I learned that the apparent high insertion of the iris in refractory congenital glaucoma was not what it appeared to be, as he explains in his book. The iris root is always inserted in the inner face of the ciliary muscle, in all classes of congenital glaucomas. I also learned this idea from Busacca and above all from the correspondence he held on this subject with Dr. Purscher.

– Dr. Johanes W. Rohen and Lutchen Decroll, with whom I spent a month at the Institute of Anatomy in Erlangen, Germany. I discussed the problems of the normal histology and pathology of the angle in congenital glaucoma, but above all I was able to read Rohen's irreplaceable book, *Das Auge und Seine Hilfsorgane* [19], particularly Chaps. 4–8, 146 pages devoted to the anterior segment in the zone of the chamber angle, which I can recommend highly.

– Dr. O.M. Calasans (from São Paulo) [20], from whom I learned the structure of the ciliary muscle through his microdissections, which led him to consider it as a ciliary quadriceps in order to explain its various actions.

– Dr. Tord Jerndal [21], with whom I had the pleasure of sharing the only world symposium on congenital glaucoma held in Venice and later exchanging knowledge through numerous letters. He gave me his book, *Goniodysgenesis*, which he wrote with Hans Arne Hansson and Anders Bill in 1978. This book is a most extraordinary work and I recommend reading it several times to anyone interested in this subject.

– Dr. J.G.F. Worst, whom I visited in his clinic in the Netherlands, attending his surgery practice. Worst visited us in Argentina and we had 3 days of meetings with several colleagues to discuss the etiopathogeny and pathology of the eye with congenital glaucoma. His 1966 book on congenital glaucoma [22] is extremely useful.

– Dr. P.P.H. Alkemade [23] whose book *Dysgenesis Mesodermalis of the Iris and the Cornea* (a study of Rieger's syndrome and Peter's anomaly) is one of the best books on the subject.

– Dr. Hans Goldmann (Fig.1), who gave me the first hand applanation tonometer to be marketed, designed by him and manufactured by Haag Streit, which enabled me to take the pressure of children lying down with or without general anesthesia after the age of 8. In 1969, I dedicated to Dr. Goldmann's 70th birthday an article titled "La pression oculaire et le sinus camerulaire chez l'enfant normal et dans le glaucome congénital au-dessous de l'âge de cinq ans" [5]. It was the first time that I had published my new findings on ocular pressure and echometry in the normal infant, and congenital glaucoma. As a result of this article, Goldmann invited me for 1 week to his house on Lake Maggiore, in Switzerland, to discuss the topic together with Dr. Reca, and for all the knowledge he transmitted to me on glaucoma, for having taken an interest in the daily pressure curve and for all that he contributed to world ophthalmology with all the apparatus he created that we ophthalmologists use all round the world (Fig. 2, at the left side).

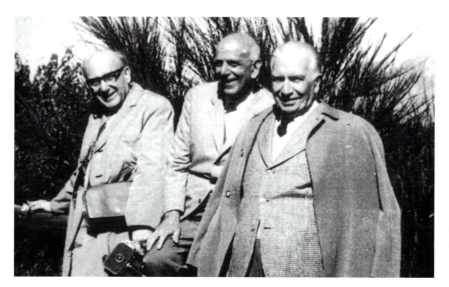

Fig. 2 Goldmann, Busacca and Malbran. First South American Glaucoma Symposium, Bariloche, Argentina, 1966

- Dr. Draeger, [24] whom I visited several times in his clinic to discuss the topic and attend the congenital glaucoma operations that he performed. In the world congress in Munich in 1966, he gave me the first hand-held applanation tonometer to be sold in the world, manufactured by Mueller. Dr. Draeger gave the hand-held tonometer to the parents of children operated for congenital glaucoma and showed them how to make periodic ocular pressure checks and for the self-tonometer.
- Dr. Sohan Hayreth, who, with his profound knowledge of physiopathology of glaucomatous optic neuropathy, made me apply HRF for the study of open angle glaucomas with arterial hypotension and with whom I worked in Buenos Aires.
- Dr. Burian, who sent the first trabeculotome in the world to me in Argentina with Dr. Ferrer Arata and Dr. Gomez Morales. Delaporta, first a pathologist and then professor of ophthalmology, told Burian that many of the cyclodialyses that he did penetrated into the Schlemm canal and then into the anterior chamber, resulting in what was actually a trabeculotomy. From this the idea first arose of performing a trabeculotomy. As Cairns had not yet published the first trabeculectomy, the scleral flap, which reduces the thickness of the sclera by half, was not known. Consequently, the incision to find the Schlemm canal was very deep (through all the thicknesses of the sclera) and it was very difficult to find it.
- Professor Harms of Tübingen, Germany, who showed me how to perform the trabeculectomy, which he was the first to introduce, almost simultaneously with Professor Paufique of Lyon, France. Dr. José Barrraquer and I spent 2 weeks together in his care and he allowed us to perform several trabeculotomies.
- Dr. Fankhauser [25] and the firm Haag Streit, who gave me the new lens designed by Roussel and Fankhauser, which enabled us to photograph the chamber angle with extraordinary resolution. All the gonioscopies presented in this book were made with this lens. Prof. Dr. Fankhauser taught me and Dr. Reca about computerized perimetry with the Octopus 200 in Bern.
- Dr. Ludmila Koslowa and Dr. André Mermoud, who helped me to complete my knowledge of deep non-perforating sclerectomy. Years later, I replaced the Harms method of trabeculotomy with deep sclerectomy to find the Schlemm canal.
- Dr. Jorge Malbran [12] (Fig. 2, at the right side), who, as well as everything I learned in his theory and practice classes at the Hospital Italiano, taught me that the chamber angle in pigmentary glaucoma is actually a late congenital glaucoma (goniodysgenesis).

- Prof. Nassim Calixto, who helped me correct the first edition of my book on glaucoma and with whom I worked on research on the daily pressure curve and congenital glaucoma.
- Prof. Naumann and Prof. Gloor, to whom I gave copies of the second edition of my book, *Glaucoma*, in Spanish, for having asked and encouraged me to write the present edition in English.
- Prof. Naumann, for all I learned from his publications and for his great contribution in recent years to the knowledge of pseudoexfoliation and his discovery of pseudoexfoliative corneal dystrophy.
- Prof. Balder Gloor [13], for all the ophthalmological knowledge he gave me on goniodysgenesis in adults and for his conference "The site of glaucoma" [27]. For "Differential diagnosis of the cup disc: the pseudoglaucomatous optic disc," which he wrote with Prof. Dr. Landau [28].
- Prof. Michele Virno [29, 30], with whom we worked on his magnificent Ibopamine provocative test. We tested its worth by comparing it with the diurnal pressure curve, obtaining the same result and making the latter unnecessary for early diagnosis. But above all, his finding of how a congenital alteration of the pathways of aqueous humor outflow is revealed is accepted worldwide. When there is a family with goniodysgenesis (dominant inheritance), it is extremely useful to perform the test in the children and predict which of them will be affected by glaucoma in the future, and in a case of low-tension glaucoma, if the Ibopamine test gives positive results, the diagnosis changes to pseudoglaucoma.
- Drs. V.P. DeLuise and D.R. Anderson [31] for their wonderful review: "Primary infantile glaucoma (congenital glaucoma)", in *Survey of Ophthalmology* (1983). They said, "In 1939 J. Ringland Anderson [32] stated that the future of children with 'hydrophthalmia (primary infantile glaucoma) is bleak … little hope of preserving sufficient sight to permit the earning of a livelihood can be held out to them.' Today, a much more optimistic outlook has been achieved. Pivotal to the new philosophy about primary infantile glaucoma is accurate and early diagnosis."
- Dr. Lotmar, Goldmann's collaborator in Berne, Switzerland, who taught me to perform optic disk stereochronoscopy and made me construct the original equipment in Zurich, to be added to the Zeiss retinoscope. This method enabled me to check whether or not there was progression in the optic nerve of the children I had operated. With Mr. Faita, whom I want to thank for his extraordinary collaboration, we performed more than 500 stereochronoscopies in operated children.

- My good friend, Prof. Dr. Andre Lobstein, who taught me ophthalmodynamometry, which enabled me to write the chapter in the second volume of this book on low-tension glaucoma and with whom we shared many hours listening to music.
- Prof. Dr. Demailly, my great friend, because he was the one who initiated me to the Kozlov's deep non-penetrating sclerectomy surgery.
- Prof. Epimaco Leonardi, in Rome, who trained me for 2 years in ocular surgery, not only of the anterior segment, cataract, and glaucoma, but also taught me all the techniques in palpebral plastics and during that time let me operate numerous patients in his clinic.
- Dr. Paolo Brusini, one of the best ophthalmological surgeons I have known, I thank for introducing me to nonconventional perimetry. He developed the Glaucoma Staging System in 1995, now used throughout the world. I express my great affection to him for having operated on me for cataracts and for writing the chapters in Volume II on visual field in glaucoma.
- Dr. Jorge Zarate, co-author of this book in everything related to the histology and pathological anatomy of the subject. He started working as a pathologist in 1972 in the Instituto Lagleyze, as head of the pathology department, then in the Hospital Italiano with the same position, and finally as head of the pathology department in the Institute of Ophthalmology, Universidad de Buenos Aires. We have been working together since then, for the past 37 years, in the hospital and in private practice. He carried out the studies of trabeculectomy specimens in more than 2000 open-angle and secondary glaucomas. When we started with combined surgery in congenital glaucoma, he analyzed more than 80 specimens of these cases. He applied a variety of histological techniques that confirmed the gonioscopic findings and thus provided a more complete knowledge of the physiopathology of this disease. Our interest was especially focused on pretrabecular tissue, which we believed to be the most important in the study of congenital glaucoma. We began to better understand the physiopathology of the disease. Over all these years, Jorge Zarate has also become one of my greatest friends.
- My son Juan who started working in my consulting room beginning at the age of 12, first learning the techniques of campimetry and other examinations. When I decided to import the first HRT for studying the optic nerve (this was the first equipment in Central and South America, in 1992), Juan spent 2 months with Dr. Burk, in the ophthalmology department of the Heidelberg ophthalmology clinic in Germany, where he studied in depth how to work the machine, and then took charge of the section in that clinic. He continued expanding his knowledge with me in Buenos Aires, and in 1996 he was co-author of the annual work that I presented in the Ophthalmology Society entitled "Confocal tomography of the retina and the optic nerve" [33–35]. This report was later published by the Ophthalmology Society in a 210-page book and then translated into English in 1999 and published in Germany. In this work, Juan performed the standardization of the optic nerve in normal subjects, in five developmental stages, but he especially studied the optic nerve in children that I had operated in the first 6 months of life. He conducted the study between 10 and 15 years after the operations. He was thus able to trace the profile of the optic nerve and to know what lesions had occurred, in pure congenital, refractory, and late congenital glaucomas. He made up a control group of 50 normal eyes in young people between 10 and 15 years of age. He is also particularly responsible in this book for the presentation of new clinical cases and for the chapter on congenital glaucoma surgery with valves. In addition, he covers topic of the chamber angle before and after surgery and comparing the SL-OCT equipment with gonioscopy.
- Joss Heywood, who has translated this book into English.

I do not want to finish without thanking my secretary, Miryam Tencha, for her enormous help, and the draftsmen, Francisco Revelli and Mario Gomez, who gave the finishing touches to many of my original drawings and illustrations.

Finally, I want to extend my sincerest thanks to Mariano Gaiazzi for making the lay-out and for all computer-related tasks.

References

1. Manzitti E (1963) Técnica de examen en el glaucoma infantil. Arch Oftal B Aires 38:345
2. Sampaolesi R, Reca R, Carro A (1967) Presión ocular en el niño hasta los 5 años bajo anestesia con Pentrane (Metoxifluorane). Arch Oftal B Aires XLII:180–185
3. Ytterborg J (1960) On scleral rigidity. Oslo University Press, Oslo
4. Sampaolesi R (1969) La pression oculaire et le sinus camérulaire chez l'enfant normal et dans le glaucome congénital au-dessous de l'âge de cinq ans. Documenta Ophthalmologica. Adv Ophthalmol 26:497–515
5. Gernet H, Hollwich F (1969) Oculometrie des kindlichen Glaukoms. Zusammenkunft Dtsch Ophthalmol Ges 69:341–348

6. Sampaolesi R, Reca R, Armando E (1974) Normaler intraocularer Druck bei Kindern bis zu 5 Jahren mit und ohne Allgemeinnarkose. Seine Wichtigkeit für die Frühdiagnose des angeborenen Glaukoms. Glaucoma Symposium. Würzburg, Germany, pp 278–289

7. Buschmann W, Bluth K (1974) Ultrasonographic follow-up examination of congenital glaucoma. Graefes Arch Ophthalmol 192:313

8. Barkan O (1936) New operation for chronic glaucoma: restoration of physiological function by opening Schlemm's canal under direct magnified vision. Am J Ophthalmol 19:951–966

9. Burian HM (1960) A case of Marfan's syndrome with bilateral glaucoma. With description of a new type of operation for developmental glaucoma (trabeculotomy ab externo). Am J Ophthalmol 50:1187–1192

10. Cairns JE (1968) Trabeculectomy: preliminary report of a new method. Am J Ophthalmol 66:673

11. Harms H, Dannheim R (1970) Trabeculotomy – results and problems. Adv Ophthalmol 22:121–213

12. Paufique L, Sourdille PH, Ortiz-Olmedo AH (1969) Technique et résultats de la trabeculotomie ab externo dans le traitement du glaucome congénital. Bull Soc Ophthalmol Fr 54–65, Masson, Paris

13. Sampaolesi R (1988) Congenital glaucoma. Long-term results after surgery. Fortschr Ophthalmol 85:626–631

14. Kozlov VI et al (1990) Non-penetrating deep sclerectomy with collagen. IRTC Eye Microsurgery. RSFSR Ministry of Public Health, Moscow 4:62–66

15. Sampaolesi R, Sampaolesi JR, Zarate J (2006) Non-penetrating deep sclerectomy (NPDS) Anatomic landmarks. In: Shaarawy T, Mermoud A (eds) Atlas of glaucoma surgery. Jaypee Brothers, New Delhi pp 112–130

16. Manzitti E, Damel A (1964) Valores de la tonometría aplanática en el lactante normal. Arch Oftal B Aires 39:360–362

17. Busacca A (1945) Éléments de gonioscopie normale pathologique et expérimentale. Tipografia Rossolillo, Sao Paulo

18. Kluyskens J (1950) Le glaucome congénital. Rapport présenté à la Societé Belge d'Ophtalmologie

19. Rohen JW (1964) Das Auge und Seine Hilfsorgane Springer, Berlin Heidelberg New York

20. Calasans OM (1953) Arquitettura do musculo ciliar no homem. Ann Fac Med Univ S Paulo 27:3–98

21. Jerndal T, Hansson HA, Bill A (1978) Goniodysgenesis: a new perspective on glaucoma. Scriptor, Copenhagen

22. Worst JGF (1966) The pathogenesis of congenital glaucoma. PhD dissertation, Royal Van Gorcum, Assen, The Netherlands

23. Alkemade PPH (1969) Dysgenesis mesodermalis of the iris and the cornea. A study of Rieger's syndrome and Peter's anomaly. Van Gorcum, Assen, the Netherlands

24. Draeger J (1992) Neue Wege zur Fruhdiagnose und Verlauskontrolle des Glaukoms. Spektrum Augenheilkd 6:267–272

25. Roussell P, Fankhauser F (1983) Contac glass for use with high power lasers –geometrical and optical aspects. Act Ophthalmol 6:183–190

26. Malbran J (1957) Le glaucome pigmentaire, ses relations avec le glaucome congénital. Probl Act Ophtal 1:132–146, Karger, Basel

27. Kniestedt C, Kammann MTT, Sturmer J, Gloor BP (2000) Dysgenetische Kammerwinkelveränderungen bei Patienten mit Glaukom oder Verdacht auf Glaukom aufgetreten vor dem 40. Lebensjahr. Klin Monatsbl Augenheilkd 216:377–387

28. Landau K, Gloor BP (1997) Differential diagnose der glaukomatösen Optikusneuropathic. In: Das Glaukom in der praxis, Glaucoma Meeting, Basel, 22–23 March 1996, Karger, Basel, pp 32–38

29. Virno M, Taverniti L, Motolese E, Taloni M, Bruni P, Pecori Giraldi J, Ibopamina (1986) Nuovo midriatico non cicloplegico (nota preliminare). Boll Ocul 65:1135–1146

30. Virno M, Pecori Giraldi J, Taverniti L, Taloni M, Bruni P (1987) Effetti ipertensivi oculari dell'ibopamina somministrata per via locale in soggetti con turbe idrodinamiche endovulari (Nuovo test di provocazione). Boll Ocul 66:833–845

31. Anderson JR (1939) Hydrophthalmia or congenital glaucoma. Cambridge University Press, London, pp 14–16

32. De Luise VP, Anderson DR (1983) Primary infantile glaucoma (congenital glaucoma). Surv Ophthalmol 28:1–19

33. Sampaolesi R, Sampaolesi JR (1995) Tomografía confocal del nervio óptico y de la retina. Relato Anual 1995. Arch Oftalmol B Aires 76

34. Zarate J (1995) Correlacion entre anatomia patólica y tomografía computada del nervio óptico. Redefinición de la nomenclatura hitológica.In: Sampaolesi R, Sampaolesi JR (eds) Tomografía confocal del nervio óptico y de la retina. Relato Anual 1995. Arch Oftalmol B Aires 76:423–441

35. Ebner R (1995) Aplicación de la tomografia confocal en neurooftalmologia. In: Sampaolesi R, Sampaolesi JR (eds) Tomografia confocal del nervio óptico y de la retina. Relato Anual 1995. Arch. Oftalmol B Aires 76:553–566

Contents

Primary Congenital Glaucoma

Contents

History

Hippocrates, 400 years before Christ, and Celsus and Galen, 100 years after Christ, noted the phenomenon of buphthalmos but did not relate it to glaucoma.

In 1561, Ambroise Paré wrote: "Oeil de boeuf est une maladie d'oeil quand il est gros et éminent, sortant hors de la tête, comme voits les bœufs les aboir," which is one of the first descriptions of buphthalmia. The observations of Schiess-Gemuseus in 1863 and 1884 [1, 2] are also important, but in fact it was Von Muralt [3] who related this alteration to a type of glaucoma. These observations were later confirmed by Von Hippel, Parsons, and especially by Seefelder [4] and Seefelder and Wolfrum [5], who demonstrated the true pathogeny of this disease.

Taylor [6, 7] was the first to publish Carlo De Vincentiis's surgical technique for the treatment of glaucoma [8, 9]. Designed in Naples and known as the "incision of the angle formed by the iris and the cornea" or internal sclerotomy, this technique had the same requirements as goniotomy, since it was performed with a small sickle-shaped knife (the De Vincentiis knife), specially manufactured to prevent aqueous humor from overflowing. Ocular fixation was good and the incision was nontraumatic and superficial to prevent damage to other structures of the chamber angle. He used the technique for all sorts of glaucomas and it

was the first blind goniotomy, though it is actually an ab interno trabeculotomy. It was then abandoned for 30 years, perhaps because it was reported only in a local Italian journal and because its author died too soon. In 1900, Scalinci [10] presented 13 cases of congenital glaucoma successfully operated using this technique.

The technique was forgotten until Otto Barkan [11] revived it as an operation for congenital glaucoma and called it goniotomy (cutting the angle).

Among those who studied the anatomopathological aspects of this disease are Kluysken [12], Shaffer [13], and Allen et al. [14]. One step forward was the introduction of trabeculotomy by Burian, Harms, and Paufique, which improved the prognosis of congenital glaucomas greatly. For the first time in 1987, R. Sampaolesi [15] introduced combined surgery: trabeculotomy and trabeculectomy in a single surgical session for refractory congenital glaucomas. In 2005, he applied Koslov's technique of nonpenetrating deep sclerectomy to find the Schlemm, changing Harms's operation for the latter (see Chap. 15).

Concept

Congenital glaucoma is an infrequent disease, an inherited developmental defect, occurring within the 1st year of life and referred to the ophthalmologist within the first 24 months.

It is characterized by a congenital anomaly of the chamber angle at the level of the trabecular meshwork, which obstructs the aqueous humor outflow pathways, leading to high intraocular pressure (IOP) and to an early elongation of the eyeball, corneal enlargement, and corneal edema. If immediate and proper surgical treatment is not provided, it produces progressive impairment leading to serious damage of the entire eye, particularly in the optic nerve.

Congenital glaucoma is a complex disease. It is completely different from simple adult glaucoma, due to the anatomical and physiological features of the eyes of newborns. From its clinical manifestations, its pathophysiology, and anatomopathological findings, its immediate cause has been suggested to lie with goniodysgenesis caused by arrested development of the chamber angle.

In this chapter, only cases in which the disease presents from birth to 24 months of age will be discussed. These are pure congenital glaucomas, with definite clinical features, progression, and anatomopathology. They have been named primary congenital glaucomas, primary infantile glaucomas, or developmental glaucomas.

Goniodysgenesis may develop more mildly than is seen in congenital glaucoma and, in this case, ocular hypertension will occur progressively and later, because of factors that remain unknown. These cases belong to completely different clinical forms known as juvenile glaucoma, late congenital glaucoma, or goniodysgenesis, which manifest at 5, 10, or 18 years and are even more frequent in adults until the age of 40 years.

In our experience [15–17] and in that of Kwitko [18] and Walton [19], a dividing line between infantile congenital glaucomas and late congenital glaucomas can be drawn at the age of 4 years, because from this age, the axial length can no longer grow as a consequence of elevated IOP. Glaucomas associated with ocular and systemic malformations belong to an independent group (see Chap. 22).

Infantile congenital glaucoma is the most severe of glaucomas, which means that just as in the acute glaucomas in adults, surgery has to be performed immediately, without losing time. Shaffer did the examination under general anesthesia in the same room where surgery would be performed. Before the examination under general anesthesia, he asked the parents for their approval to proceed with surgery if the diagnosis was positive.

The degree of ocular damage depends on the length of the period between the appearance of the first clinical manifestations and surgery, or on the failure of surgery to regulate IOP. Damage may include glaucomatous optic disc cupping; visual field loss; ocular distension with acquired refractive errors and macular disorders; Descemet membrane and endothelium tears, which, if located centrally, cause severe visual loss (in this case a corneal graft is needed immediately); peripheral retinal disorders; anisometropia; amblyopia with or without strabismus, etc.

Since perimetry, visual acuity, and macular function tests are useless for diagnosis and monitoring the progression of this disease so early in life, echometry, applanation tonometry with paquimetry, or better yet with Pascal tonometer measurements, and gonioscopy have become the most valuable tools for these purposes.

In addition to all the postoperative checks, visual acuity must be constantly monitored with the preferential looking test.

These advances developed during the last two decades have changed the attitude of ophthalmologists, who are now optimistic when they encounter this disease, since early diagnosis can be made with family education and the cooperation of the pediatrician.

Epidemiology

The prevalence in the population is 8:100,000 children [20] (congenital glaucoma occurs in 1 out of 10,000 births). In 80% of cases, it is bilateral. It affects males in 70% of cases. It is the most frequent cause of early blindness of congenital origin: 50% of cases with blindness from glaucoma.

The most complete papers on the subject are those authored by Anderson [21]; Westerlund [22]; Kluyskens [12]; Gallenga and Mateucci [23]; Van der Helm [24]; Carvalho and Calixto [25]; Shaffer [26]; Kwitko [18]; Jerndal et al [27], and De Luise and Anderson [28] (Table 1.1).

Heredity

Most cases are sporadic, nonhereditary, and nonfamilial. From 10% to 12% have a family tendency and an autosomal recessive heredity pattern as reported by François [34] and Duke Elder (1964) [35].

It is striking that in family cases, father and son are the members affected, an uncommon trend in autosomal recessive heredity. In 1972, Merin and Morin [36] studied 64 families and concluded that heredity is multifactorial both in congenital and in open-angle glaucoma.

This is consistent with the results obtained by Demanais in 1981 [37]. In identical twins, both are affected by congenital glaucoma [38], though Fried et al. [39] described the case of a pair of monozygotic twins where only one was glaucomatous; this suggests a role of nongenetic factors.

Kluyskens [12] was the first to create genetic maps according to goniodysgenesis.

The cases studied by Jerndal et al. from 1970 to 1974 [27] demonstrated that goniodysgenesis is a dominant disease in congenital glaucoma. When the disease runs in the family, cases of congenital glaucoma, late congenital glaucoma (juvenile glaucoma), and adulthood congenital glaucoma occur. Manifestations are varied, as shown by one family studied by Jerndal et al., in which the father married twice: from one marriage, he had one son with congenital glaucoma and from the other, one with late congenital glaucoma. The father, aged 46 years, has glaucoma with severe goniodysgen-

Table 1.1 Frequency, bilaterality and gender

Frequency	0.01%–0.07% of ocular diseases	Anderson 1939 [21]	
	0.008% ± 0.0012% of the population	Westerlund 1947 [22]	
	0.0056% of the population	Van der Helm 1963 [24] with Sturge-Weber and Krause syndrome not included	
Bilaterality	Gros 1987 [29]	116 cases	64% bilateral
	Seefelder 1906 [30, 31]	47 cases	67% bilateral
	Brons 1937 [32]	127 cases	81.4% bilateral
	Anderson 1939 [21]	94 cases	86% bilateral
	Van der Helm 1963 [24]	630 cases	75.3% bilateral
	Sampaolesi 1991 [33]	875 cases	78% bilateral
Gender	Van der Helm 1963 [24]	425 males (68%)	202 females (32%)
	Sampaolesi 1991 [33]	595 males (68%)	280 females (32%)

esis. This chapter and the others on pediatric glaucomas, will describe several families whose family trees are consistent with those studied by Jerndal et al.

From a practical point of view, when their first child is diagnosed with congenital glaucoma, parents want to know the risk of having another child with the same disease. The answer is that one out of four children is affected, though this is not actually predictable (See Chap. 7) and the chance of a second child having the disease is small: 1% – 3%.

Prevalence

Primary congenital glaucoma occurs in all ethnic groups. The birth prevalence, however, varies worldwide:

- 1:5,000–22,000 in Western countries;
- 1:2,500 in the Middle East;
- 1:1,250 in the Rom (Gypsy) population of Slovakia [40];
- 1:3,300 in the Indian state of Andhra Pradesh, where the disease accounts for approximately 4.2% of all childhood blindness [41].

In Saudi Arabia and the Rom population of Slovakia, primary congenital glaucoma is the most common cause of childhood blindness [40, 42].

Etiopathogenesis

The study of etiopathogenesis is based on the clinicopathological correlation of gonioscopic findings in relation to the pathological anatomy of specimens obtained during surgery (when combined surgery was required). We were pioneers in the study of trabeculectomy specimens and the French authors followed.

Proper interpretation of the pathology and etiopathogenesis of pediatric congenital glaucomas is based on:

1. Knowledge of the embryological development of the chamber angle;
2. Knowledge of the normal chamber angle in children, its gonioscopic appearance, and its variations within normality;
3. Pathological gonioscopic findings in pediatric congenital glaucoma;
4. Pathological anatomy of the specimens obtained from combined surgery procedures performed in cases of refractory glaucoma;
5. Correlation between the gonioscopic picture and the pathological anatomy.

In addition to the items above, it should be remembered that trabeculectomy specimens always belong to very severe or advanced cases within the first 24 months of age, since either goniotomy or trabeculotomy are performed in mild cases. In this large group of patients, anatomopathological verification is therefore impossible.

Another factor also leading to misinterpretations is disagreement as to the nomenclature used: wholly different words are used to refer to the same element, when they are actually synonyms. All the following terms refer to the anomalous tissue obstructing the trabecular meshwork and preventing the aqueous humor from reaching its natural outflow pathways:

1. Pectinate ligament: a term adopted by comparison with the structure located at the chamber angle in ungulates (horses).
2. Anterior iris insertion (or high insertion of the iris). This is a misinterpretation, since this anomalous tissue overlaps with the iris root, reaching the scleral spur and covering the ciliary body band or, even further, it extends up to the Schwalbe line and covers the trabecular meshwork. It should be kept in mind that the iris root never shifts and, even in congenital glaucomas, it inserts at the usual place at the ciliary body band, which is made up of the inner surface of the ciliary muscle. It is simply an apparent high insertion of the iris.
3. Fetal mesoderm.
4. Pathological mesodermal remnants. From now on we will use this term here and the reason for our choice will be explained later.

A review of useful literature with a summary of the findings of each author follows:

- Raab [43] reported the first demonstration of an obstruction of the iridocorneal angle in a congenital glaucoma case.
- Taylor [44, 45] was the first to publish the surgical technique conceived by Carlo De Vincentiis, from Naples, designated by the author as *l'incisione dell'angolo irideo* (incision of the iridic angle). This was the first blind goniotomy.
- Scalinci [46] presented 13 cases of pediatric congenital glaucoma operated on with this method, with successful results. This technique was not actually put into practice until 1938, by Barkan.
- Barkan [47–49] proposed a goniotomy with visual guidance by means of a gonioscopic contact lens he designed, in order to remove "an imperforated membrane covering the angle of the anterior chamber, and preventing the aqueous humor from outflowing, thus leading to ocular hypertension."
- Barkan [50] described a "transparent or semitransparent membrane in a vertical position from Schwalbe's line to the iris in the angle. The vertical position of this tissue is in contrast with the horizontal position of the iris. After goniotomy, the iris falls backwards, as if it had had a high insertion, and uncovers Schlemm's canal with its normal anatomic relationships with the other structures. Therefore, the angle, free from any obstructing tissue, is available for the aqueous humor."
- Barkan [51] described the pathological anatomy in order to correlate it with the gonioscopic findings. He describes "a membrane lining the inside of the angle from Schwalbe's line to the iris," and he reports the presence of mesodermal remnants inside or under this membrane.
- Maumenee [52] described the absence or aplasia of the spur, but this is one of the rare quotations in the literature that has not been verified by other authors. We have always found the spur in more than 300 specimens studied.
- Shaffer [53] described an "abnormal mesodermal reticulum" in a case with apparent high insertion of the iris.
- Hansson and Jerndal [54] demonstrated that the chamber angle in congenital glaucoma resembles that of a normal fetus at stage 200–240 mm, 7 months of gestation.
- Sampaolesi et al. [17] conducted a study with light microscopy and surface electron microscopy, where they described what they called pathological mesodermal remnants obstructing the trabecular meshwork covered by a membrane, which are stained with dark silver colorants (Gomori's stain) due to the large amount of reticulin fibers contained in them, which are the same as those on the tissue obstructing the chamber angle in normal fetuses at month 7 of gestation (200–240 mm). This morphology of the chamber angle in primary or pure congenital glaucomas resembles the morphology of the normal developing chamber angle.
- Anderson [55–57] makes one of the most interesting contributions: his explanation of the movement of the different components of the chamber angle during its formation and, fundamentally, the mechanism causing the ciliary muscle to shift frontward in congenital glaucoma, which will be discussed later.
- Allen et al. [58] hypothesized that the formation of the chamber angle may be due to what they termed cleavages (separation between mesodermal layers) caused by an uneven growth of the structures of the chamber angle from the 5th month. But Kupfer and Kaisser-Kupfer [59], some years later, demonstrated that this theory was based on a critical mistake, thus invalidating it.

The theory of migration of neural crest cells has been considered [56], but Alvarado has reported otherwise [60, 61].

There are other important papers in the literature, such as those by Smelser and Ozanics [62]; Mann [63]; Holmberg) [64], and Maul et al. [65], confirming the findings detailed above.

A very important paper has been specially reserved for the end of this chapter because of its great value: in 1906, Seefelder [4] and Seefelder and Wolfrum [66], for the first time described the pathology of congenital glaucoma as a detention in development at the 7th month of gestation; they presented the pathological anatomy of congenital glaucoma and compared it with the histology of a normal fetus at the 7th month of gestation in order to show their similarity. More recently, Worst [67] published a similar image in his book; it is a specimen published by Castelli [68] and interpreted by himself. Finally, according to Jerndal and colleagues [27], of the different theories – cleavage, atrophy, and resorption – postulating a detention in development is the most consistent with the way of thinking of current authors.

The original papers on the pathological anatomy of our specimens will be discussed in Chap. 15.

Our research into congenital glaucoma was conducted following the following steps:
- 1960–1970: IOP (normal and pathological);
- 1970–1980: echometry in the diagnosis and follow-up;
- 1980–1990: functional results in operated primary congenital glaucomas;
- 1982–1983: optic disc changes in congenital glaucoma;
- 1990–2006: confocal tomography of the optic nerve head;
- 1983–2006: surgical methods to apply according to the type of chamber angle: type I, type II, refractory glaucoma, and according to the echometric values. New evaluation of the anatomical and functional results of surgery 12–35 years after surgery.

References

1. Schiess-Gemuseus HV (1863) Zur pathologischen Anatomie des Keratoglobus. Graefes Arch Ophthalmol 9:171–198

2. Schiess-Gemuseus HV (1884) Vier Fälle angeborener Anomalie des Auges. Graefes Arch Ophthalmol 30:191–195

3. von Muralt (1869) Ueber Hydrophthalmus cangenitus PhD dissertation, Zurich

4. Seefelder R (1920) Hydrophthalmus als Folge einer Entwicklungsanomalie der Kammerbucht. Graefes Arch Ophthalmol 103:1–13

5. Seefelder R, Wolfrum H (1906) Zur Entwicklung der Vorderen Kammer und des Kammerwinkels beim Menschen nebst Bemerkungen ueber ihre Entstehung bei Tieren. Grafes Arch Ophthlmol 63:430–451

6. Taylor U (1891) Sull'incizione dell'angolo irideo, contribuzione all cura del glaucoma. Lav Clin Ocul Napoli 3:125

7. Taylor U (1894) Sull'incizione dell'angolo irideo. Lav Clin Ocul Napoli 4:197

8. De Vincentiis C (1894) Incisione dell'angolo irideo nel glaucoma. Ann Ottal 22:540–555

9. De Vincentiis C (1895) Sulla Cosidetto "sclérotomie interne". Lav dell Clinical Ocul di Napoli VI:227

10. Scalinci N (1900) La incisione del tessuto dell'angolo irideo nell'idroftalmo. Ann Ott 29:324

11. Barkan O (1936) New operation for chronic glaucoma: restoration of physiological function by opening Schlemm's canal under direct magnified vision. Am J Ophthalmol 19:951–966

12. Kluyskens J (1950) Le glaucome congénital. Bull Soc Belge Ophtalmol 94:3–248

13. Shaffer R (1955) Pathogenesis of congenital glaucoma gonioscopic and microscopic anatomy. Trans Am Acad Ophthalmol 59:297

14. Allen L, Burian HM, Braley AE (1955) A new concept of the development of the anterior chamber angle. Its relationship to developmental glaucoma and other structural anomalies. Arch Ophthalmol 53:783–798

15. Sampaolesi R (1987) Congenital glaucoma. Long-term results of surgery. In: Krieglstein GK (ed) Glaucoma update III. Springer, Berlin Heidelberg New York, pp 154–161

16. Sampaolesi R, Argento C (1977) Scanning electron microscopy of the trabecular meshwork in normal and glaucomatous eyes. Invest Ophthalmol Vis Sci 16:302–314

17. Sampaolesi R, Zarate JO, Caruso R (1979) Congenital glaucoma. Light and scanning electron microscopy of trabeculotomy specimens. In:Krieglstein GK, Leydhecker W (eds) International glaucoma symposium, Nara, Japan, 1978: Glaucoma update. Springer, Berlin Heidelberg New York, pp 39–51

18. Kwitko ML (1973) Glaucomas in infants and children. Appleton-Century-Crofts, New York

19. Walton DS (1979) Primary congenital open-angle glaucoma. In: Chandler PA, Grant WM (eds) Glaucoma. Lea and Febiger, Philadelphia, pp 329–343

20. Miller SJ (1962) Genetic aspect of glaucoma. Trans Ophthalmol Soc UK 425–434

21. Anderson RJ (1939) Hydrophthalmia or congenital glaucoma. Cambridge University Press, London

22. Westerlund E (1947) Clinical and genetic studies on the primary glaucoma diseases. PhD dissertation, Vol. XII, Opera ex domo biologiae heredit. hum. Univ. Hafmensis. E. Munksgaard, Copenhagen

23. Gallenga R, Matteucci P (1952) Hidroftalmi. Relazione al 39 Congreso della Societá Italiana di Oftalmologia, Torino

24. Van der Helm FGM (1963) Hydrophthalmia and its treatment. A general study based on 630 cases in the Netherlands. Bibl Ophthalmol 61:1–63

25. Carvalho CA, Calixto N (1969) Semiologia do glaucoma congénito. In: XV Cong Brasil Oftal Porto Alegre, pp 105–174

26. Shaffer RN, Weiss DI (1970) Congenital and pediatric glaucomas. Mosby, St. Louis, p 37

27. Jerndal T, Hansson HA, Bill A (1978) Goniodysgenesis. A new perspective on glaucoma. Scriptor, Cophenhagen

28. De Luise VP, Anderson DR (1983) Primary infantile glaucoma (congenital glaucoma). Surv Ophthalmol 28:1–19

29. Gros EL (1897) Etude sur l'hydrophtalmie ou glaucome infantile. Thèse de doctorat en médecine, Paris

30. Seefelder R (1906) Klinische und anatomische Untersuchungen zur Pathologie und Therapie des Hydrophthalmus congenitus. I. Teil Graefes Arch Ophthalmol 63:205–280

31. Seefelder J (1906) Klinische und anatomische Untersuchungen zur Pathologie und Therapie des Hydrophthalmus congenitus. II. Teil Anatomisches Graefes Arch Ophthalmol 63:481–556

32. Brons H (1937) Uber die Vererbung des Hydrophthalmus congenitus. Inaung. disseration Tübingen, Germany

33. Sampaolesi R (1991) Glaucoma, 2nd edn. Medica Panamericana, Buenos Aires, Argentina

34. Francois J (1961) Heredity in ophthalmology. Mosby, St. Louis

35. Duke-Elder S (1964) System of ophthalmology, Vol. 3. Klimpton, London, pp 548–565

36. Merin S, Morin D (1972) Heredity of congenital glaucoma. Br J Ophthalmol 56:414–417

37. Demenais F, Elston RC, Bonaiti C, Briard ML, Kaplan EB, Namboodiri KK (1981) Segregation analysis of congenital glaucoma. Approach by two different models. Am J Hum Genet 33:300–306

38. Rasmussen DH, Ellis PP (1970) Congenital glaucoma in identical twins. Arch Ophthalmol 84:827–830

39. Fried K, Sachs R, Krakowsky D (1977) Congenital glaucoma in only one of identical twins. Ophthalmologica 174:185–187

40. Plasilova M, Ferakova E, Kadasi L, Polakova H, Gerinec A, Ott J, Ferak V (1998) Linkage of autosomal recessive primary congenital glaucoma to the GLC3A locus in Roms (Gypsies) from Slovakia. Hum Hered 48:30–33

41. Dandona L, Dandona R, Srinivas M, Giridhar P, Vilas K, Prasad MN, John RK, McCarty CA, Rao GN (2001) Blindness in the Indian state of Andhra Pradesh. Invest Ophthalmol Vis Sci 42:908–916

42. Bejjani BA, Stockton DW, Lewis RA, Tomey KF, Dueker DK, Jabak M, Astle WF, Lupski JR (2000) Multiple CYP1B1 mutations and incomplete penetrance in an inbred population segregating primary congenital glaucoma suggest frequent de novo events and a dominant modifier locus. Hum Mol Genet 9:367–374

43. Raab F (1876) Beiträge zur Pathologischen Anatomie des Auges. Buphthalmus congenitus. Klin Mbl Augenheilk 14:22

44. Taylor U (1891) Sull'incisione del tessuto dell'angolo irideo, contribuzione alla cura del glaucoma. Lav Clin Ocul Napoli 3:125

45. Taylor U (1894) Sull'incisione dell'anglo irideo. Lav Clin Ocul Napoli 4:197

46. Scalinci M (1900) La incisione del tessuto dell'angolo irideo nell idrottalmo. Ann Ott 29:324

47. Barkan O (1938) Technique of goniotomy. Arch Ophthalmol 19:217–221

48. Barkan O (1942) Operation for congenital glaucoma. Am J Ophthalmol 25:552–568

49. Barkan O (1948) Goniotomy for the relief of congenital glaucoma. Br J Ophthalmol 32:701–728

50. Barkan O (1953) Surgery of congenital glaucoma. Review of 196 eyes operated by goniotomy. Am J Ophthalmol 36:1523–1534

51. Barkan O (1955) Pathogenesis of congenital glaucoma. Gonioscopic and anatomic observation of the angle of the anterior chamber in the normal eye and in congenital glaucoma. Am J Ophthalmol 40:1–11

52. Maumenee AE (1958) The pathogenesis of congenital glaucoma: a new theory. Trans Am Ophthalmol Soc 56:507–570

53. Shaffer RN (1967) Genetics and the congenital glaucomas. Am J Ophthalmol 2:243–247

54. Hansson HA, Jerndal T (1971) Scanning electron microscopic studies of the development of the iridocorneal angle in human eyes. Invest Ophthalmol Vis Sci 10:252–265

55. Anderson DR (1972) Pathology of the glaucomas. Br J Ophthalmol 56:146–157

56. Anderson DR (1979) The pathogenesis of primary congenital glaucoma. Third Meeting of Pan-American Glaucoma Society, Miami, FL, 29 Feb 1979

57. Anderson DR (1982) Discussion of Quigley HA in Childhood glaucoma. Ophthalmology 89:225–226

58. Allen L, Burian HM, Braley AE (1955) A new concept of the development of the anterior chamber angle. Its relationship to developmental glaucoma and other structural anomalies. Arch Ophthalmol 53:783–798

59. Kupfer C, Kaisser-Kupfer MI (1979) Observations on the development of the anterior chamber angle with references to the pathogenesis of congenital glaucomas. Am J Ophthalmol 88:424–426

60. Alvarado JA, Murphy CG, Maglio M, Hetherington J Jr (1986) Pathogenesis of Chandler's syndrome, essential iris atrophy and the Cogan-Reese syndrome. I. Alterations of the corneal endothelium. Invest Ophthalmol Vis Sci 27:853–872

61. Alvarado JA, Murphy CD, Juster RP, Hetherington J (1986) Pathogenesis of Chandler's syndrome, essential iris atrophy

and the Cogan-Reese syndrome. II. Estimated age of disease onset. Invest Ophthalmol Vis Sci 27:873–882

62. Smelser GK, Ozanics V (1981) The development of the trabecular meshwork in primate eyes. Am J Ophthalmol 71:366–385

63. Mann I (1957) Developmental abnormalities of the eye. Lippincott, Philadelphia

64. Holmberg AS (1965) Schlemm's canal and the trabecular meshwork. An electron microscopic study of the normal structure in man and monkey (*Cereopithecus ethiops*). Doc Ophthalmol 19:339–344

65. Maul E, Strozzi L, Muñoz C, Reyes C (1980) The outflow pathway in congenital glaucoma. Am J Ophthalmol 89:667–673

66. Seefelder R, Wolfrum C (1906) Zur Entwicklung der vorderen Kammer und des Kammerwinkels beim Menschen nebst Bemerkungen über ihre Entstehung bei Tieren. Arch Ophthalmol 63:430–451

67. Worst JGF (1966) The pathogenesis of congenital glaucoma. Royal Van Gorcum Publishers, Assen, Netherlands

68. Castelli A (1940) Contributo alla conoscenza della anatomia patologica e della eziologia dell'idroftalmo congenito. Ann Ottalmol Clin Ocul 11:801–824

Hereditary congenital glaucoma	*Primary congenital glaucoma*	
	Pure congenital glaucoma	
	Refractory congenital glaucoma	
	Secondary congenital glaucoma	
	Associated with ocular malformations	I. Rieger syndrome (Ad)
		II. Peter syndrome (Ar)
		III. Aniridia (Ad)
	Associated with ocular and somatic malformations	*Phakomatoses*
		I. Von Recklinghauser neurofibrosis (Ad)
		II. Sturge–Weber–Krabbe (Ad)
		III. Otta nevus
	Associated with congenital metabolism errors	I. Hyperaminoaciduria: Löwe oculo-cerebrorenal syndrome (Xlr)
		II. Homocystinuria (Ar)
		II. Hurler syndrome: Pfaundler–Hurler disease
		IV. Endogenous ochronosis (alkaptonuria); glaucoma secondary to luxation of the lens
	Congenital mesodermal dystrophies	I. Marfan syndrome (Ad)
		II. Marchesani syndrome (Ar)
	Late congenital glaucoma or goniodysgenesis	Pigmentary glaucoma (Ad)
Nonhereditary congenital glaucoma	Embryopathies	Rubeola
	Leukokorias	I. Persistent hyperplasic primary vitreous (fetopathies)
		II. Trisomy 13-15 or Bartholin–Patau syndrome
		III. Reese's Dysplasia
		IV. Norrie Disease
	Secondary pediatric glaucoma	I. Retrolental fibroplasias
		II. Tumors
		III. Injury
		IV. Glaucoma secondary to congenital cataract surgery
	Other syndromes associated with glaucoma	I. Rubinstein–Tabai syndrome
		II. Pierre Robin syndrome

Ad Autosomal dominant; *Ar* Autosomal recessive; *Xlr* X linked recessive

Clinical Features

Contents

Congenital glaucoma cases may be referred to the ophthalmologist by the obstetrician, the neonatologist, the pediatrician, or the child's parents. This occurs either at birth, immediately after it, or during the first weeks of life.

The first signs and symptoms which are commonly observed are photophobia, tearing, or whitish or gray corneas. When the disease is unilateral, consultation is often made rather later because one eye "is larger than the other one."

If both eyes are involved and the these signs do not appear, then parents think their child has large, pretty eyes since both eyes enlarge simultaneously, and the child may be taken for consultation much later.

In some cases, the ophthalmologist is visited because of a sudden corneal haziness produced by a tear in the endothelium and the Descemet membrane. Finally, there are a very few cases in which there is a complete absence of signs or symptoms, and they are diagnosed later when optic nerve damage is detected.

Symptoms

The main symptoms of congenital glaucoma are the following: photophobia (hypersensibility to light), epiphora (excessive tearing) without secretion, and blepharospasm (during the day, especially in full daylight). Frequent sneezing is sometimes added. Blinking is very frequent due to photophobia and sometimes there is ocular redness. These symptoms are secondary to the corneal irritation that accompanies corneal epithelial edema, caused by elevated intraocular pressure.

It should be borne in mind that epiphora might erroneously be attributed to an imperforation of the lacrimal points or to a dacryocystitis of the newborn, and pediatricians in training should be made especially aware of this. If there is redness, this can also be mistakenly attributed to conjunctivitis of the newborn.

When mistakes like these are made, and the supposed disorders are being treated, precious time is lost. Surgery is delayed until the correct diagnosis is made and during this time, irreversible damage occurs in the child's eye.

Signs

Cornea

The corneal diameter is measured by means of strabismus callipers. This is always done at the horizontal meridian, but it can also be measured by means of the scaled eyepiece of the slit lamp. The vertical corneal diameter can also be measured, but we feel this measurement is less significant, mainly because of the anterior embryotoxon, which makes this measurement inaccurate and difficult to take.

According to Kaiser's statistics [1], the normal corneal diameter in the newborn is $X = 9.44$ mm, while, according to Horven [2], it is $X = 9.8$ mm with extremes between 8.5 and 11 mm.

Our experience is consistent with these authors' reports: the corneal diameter in children up to the 2nd month of age may range from 9–9.5 mm to almost 10 mm, but between the 5th and 6th month of age, the lowest diameter we have measured in normal children is 11 mm. Any horizontal corneal diameter above 11.5 mm may be indicative of anomalies in the eye.

In the absence of other signs, the child's parents say that their baby has large, pretty eyes (Figs. 3.1 and 3.2).

Corneal edema can be intermittent at first, with the cornea turning from transparent to translucent. It is the child's mother who typically notices this. These changes correlate with intraocular pressure fluctuations. Sometimes, during crying episodes, the cornea becomes hazy. Carvalho and Calixto (1969) [3] described successive stages of edema: (a) superficial edema involving the epithelium of the entire cornea; (b) central edema

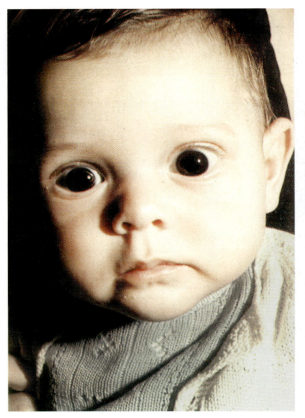

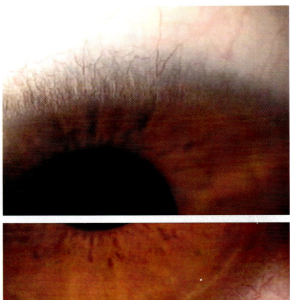

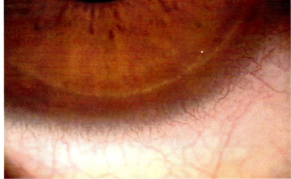

Fig. 3.1 Eight-month-old boy with congenital glaucoma. Appearance of large and "pretty" eyes

Fig. 3.2 Anterior embryotoxon makes the measurements of the corneal diameter more difficult to measure in the vertical axis

involving both parenchyma and epithelium; and (c) total diffuse edema. The child may be born with a corneal edema such that the iris parenchyma cannot be seen. Proper surgical treatment will both reduce intraocular pressure and eliminate the corneal edema. The cornea will recover its normal transparency and the iris will appear clearly.

When tears appear in the endothelium and Descemet membrane, there is a strong aqueous infiltration of the cornea, which suddenly becomes hazy. The parents usually notice this sign and bring the child to consultation because they can no longer see the color of their child's eyes, as the cornea becomes almost completely white after these tears.

Failure to quickly regulate intraocular pressure by means of surgery leads to tears in the endothelium and Descemet membrane (Fig. 3.3). These tears usually occur near the limbus and, secondarily, in the central area. With time, and even if intraocular pressure has been regulated, these tears in the Descemet membrane can opacify (at 4–6 years of age) and lead to leukoma of

similar features. The first description of these tears can be traced back to Haab (reported in [4]) (Haab striae).

Tears in the endothelium and the Descemet membrane can be central or peripheral. When they cross the pupil, there is a considerable reduction in visual acuity. At other times, they are peripheral and concentric with the limbus, and then they do not hamper vision.

Sometimes, the first three symptoms we mentioned – photophobia, tearing, and blepharospasm – appear suddenly, after a tear in the Descemet membrane.

The later the development of glaucoma after birth, the less likely tears of the Descemet membrane will occur; the symptoms are also less severe.

Tears in the endothelium and Descemet membrane are caused by increased intraocular pressure, provided that the cornea has enlarged beyond the elasticity of the membrane. When this happens, the endothelium also tears and corneal edema appears immediately in the epithelium around the area of the tear.

Timely surgery can successfully regulate intraocular pressure; the endothelium heals and covers the dam-

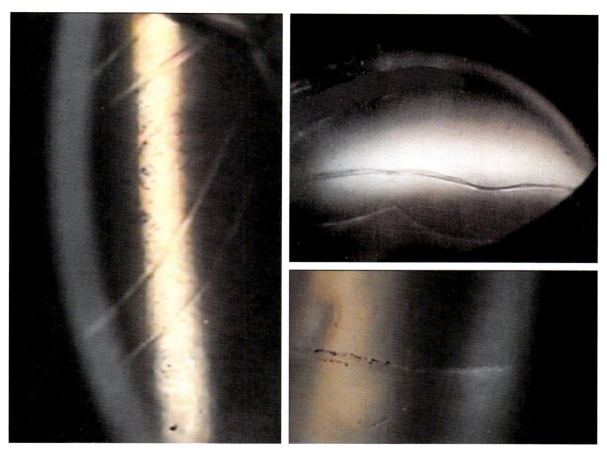

Fig. 3.3 Tears in the Descemet membrane and endothelium

aged area. Corneal edema disappears but the Descemet membrane always remains torn. This can be seen as two parallel curved lines corresponding to the edges of the Descemet tear, drawn back because of the membrane's elasticity.

Children with no congenital glaucoma may still have tears of the endothelium and the Descemet membrane caused by injury from the use of forceps during birth. In these cases, the chamber angle is normal. A study of these tears can be found in the study by Angell et al. [5].

The band-shaped structures typical of corneal posterior polymorphous dystrophy [6] are similar to endothelium and Descemet membrane tears and they are often misdiagnosed as such.

When surgery regulates intraocular pressure, corneal edema improves immediately. Figure 3.4a, b shows this very well, with two echograms: one preoperative and the other postoperative.

When hypertension is not reversed quickly or if the child is taken too late for consultation, both sclera and cornea enlarge because they are both elastic. In this case, congenital glaucoma has led to buphthalmus (hydrophthalmus). This term was coined by Ambroise Paré in 1561: "it is an ocular disease, where the eye is big, standing out of the head like an ox's: ox-eye"(Fig. 3.5).

Enlargement is bigger in the anterior segment (deep anterior chamber) but it also involves part of the posterior segment. This is the reason why children between 4 and 6 years of age have myopia and need the proper optical correction.

After surgery, echometry confirms that the axial length is reduced immediately by between 0.5 and 1 mm. This reduction is greater in children who have hereditary myopia in addition to glaucoma. Nevertheless, the eye never recovers its normal size.

Ocular enlargement, either due to unsuccessful surgery or to late consultation, can lead to leukoma, myopia, and regular astigmatism. Robin et al. [7], demonstrated that two-thirds of cases have a myopia of 3 diopters (D) and an astigmatism of 3 D. Myopia and astigmatism have a good correlation.

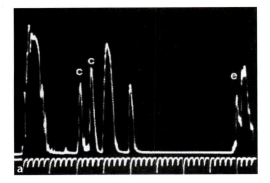

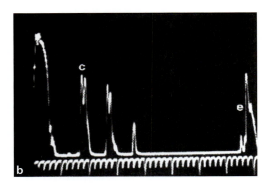

Presurgery   C 1,94 + AC 2,68 = 4,62

C	AC	Lens	V	AL		$\dfrac{AC}{AL}$	$\dfrac{AS}{V}$	$\dfrac{C+AC}{V}$
1.94	2.68	3.28	15.32	23.57	0.12	0.52	0.30	
0.78	3.83	3.28	15.32	23.56	0.17	0.51	0.30	

Postsurgery   C 0.78 + CA 3.83 = 4.61

Fig. 3.4a,b Echogram **a** shows a corneal edema separating the spikes representing the anterior and posterior surfaces of the cornea, *c* and *c*. The anterior chamber is very depressed. The following spike represents the anterior lens surface and the fourth spike, its posterior surface; the fifth spike, *e*, represents the posterior wall of the eyeball. Echogram **b** is postoperative. The spikes of the anterior and posterior corneal surfaces, which were separated before, have become separated in a bifid spike, *c*. The anterior chamber has enlarged substantially. The total value C + AC is identical both in the preoperative and in the postoperative period; the corneal edema has disappeared and the anterior chamber has enlarged. As the corneas were completely hazy, this is a very valuable sign for the surgeon, since this can be known beforehand and all the necessary precautions can be taken to perform surgery on an almost nonexistent flat chamber. *C* cornea, *AC* anterior chamber, lens, *V* vitreous, *AL* axial length, *AC* anterior chamber over axial length, *AS/V* anterior segment over vitreous, *C+AC/V* cornea plus anterior chamber over vitreous

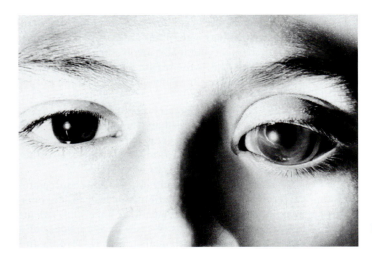

Fig. 3.5 Buphthalmus in an untreated unilateral congenital glaucomatous eye

When there is bulbar enlargement, however slight it may be, the so-called diffuse sclerocorneal limbus is observed. This condition has been known since 1920, when Axenfeld [8] termed it anterior embryotoxon. It is present in all the cases with enlarged corneas and particularly in congenital glaucoma (Fig. 3.2). Its morphology is that of a pale crescent, mainly visible at the superior limbus, as the inferior limbus is generally poorly developed. This pallor is mainly attributable to its scarcity of vessels. The crescent's edge near the cornea is definite and nacreous, and the edge near the conjunctiva gradually disappears. Inside the crescent, the vessels are fine, parallel, and enlarged. Sometimes there are whitish striae. This condition shows overall peripheral corneal thinning, offset by a greater development of episcleral and conjunctival tissue. Upon gonioscopic examination, the presence of the embryotoxon is evidenced by a white tissue, which shows through the cornea and goes beyond the level of the Schwalbe line. This condition occurs very frequently in congenital glaucoma, in the superior part of the limbus. Radial vessels are seen through this tissue. The image can be seen better using the 59° mirror of the Goldmann three-mirror lens. In 1967, Busacca [9] made a magnificent description of the anterior embryotoxon.

Chapter 15 explains the importance of studying this area, with transillumination or back illumination, in order to find the iris root behind the opacity and properly place the surgical incision.

The Optic Nerve

The optic nerve becomes rapidly cupped, which can be reversed if intraocular pressure is regulated in time. Chandler and Grant [10], stressed this phenomenon, and later, Shaffer [11–13] and Anderson [14] also covered this topic.

In many cases, it is difficult to examine the optic nerve because of the condition of the cornea. Moreover, it is important to bear in mind that this reversion does not occur in all cases because when the optic nerve fibers are damaged, optic disc and visual field damage is irreversible.

As regards optic nerve cupping in congenital glaucoma, it is important to summarize the studies conducted by Robin et al. [7]. He studied normal embryological development in embryos and fetuses of 5, 7, and 8 months of gestation, in infants aged 1 month, in children aged 12 years, and in adults aged 49 years, showing with microscopy, histochemistry, and electron microscopy that the development of the connective tissue of the lamina cribrosa is incomplete at birth (Fig. 3.6).

Robin et al. [7] also exposed the eyes of newborns and adults to intraocular pressures above 60 mmHg and found that disc cupping in newborns reacts with substantial increases, while in adults, it remains unchanged. Therefore, it is the lack of connective tissue at the level of the disc that allows disc cupping and its reversal in children.

The ophthalmologist also needs to know that after surgery for pediatric congenital glaucoma, postoperative hypotension can result in disc edema with swelling of the optic nerve vessels. This condition, which I have observed in several cases, can also be present in young adults, as demonstrated by Robin et al. [7]. Despite the congenital glaucoma, the pupil is hardly ever mydriatic, but generally miotic.

When measuring intraocular pressure, the pupil must never be dilated to see the fundus, because this might modify the intraocular pressure. The disc can be easily observed by means of an ophthalmoscope with a small-range diaphragm, with its illumination axis very close to the visual axis, or with a gonioscope. If pupil dilation is necessary, tropicamide, but only at 0.5%, must be used, because at 1% concentrations, it has cycloplegic effects. This examination can be performed on another occasion, without general anesthesia and with drug-induced pupil dilation.

At the beginning of congenital glaucoma, the disc is normal. If intraocular pressure is not regulated, the disc rapidly becomes cupped and it has the appearance of a glaucomatous disc. The main feature is that disc cupping is reversible if there is timely intraocular pressure regulation.

The appearance of papillary and retinal vessels should be carefully monitored after surgical operations intended to regulate intraocular pressure. In these cases, and to a greater extent, the younger the child, the more significant vessel dilation will be, and this dilation will lead to the consideration of the presence of aneurysms or congenital vascular diseases. But in a short time, they revert to their normal appearance.

The Eyelids

In large eyes, with or without hypertension, there is a venous remora shown by the dilation of upper eyelid veins. This is a typical sign, illustrated in Fig. 3.7.

Chronology of Symptoms

In bilateral congenital glaucomas, the symptoms and signs mentioned above do not occur with the same se-

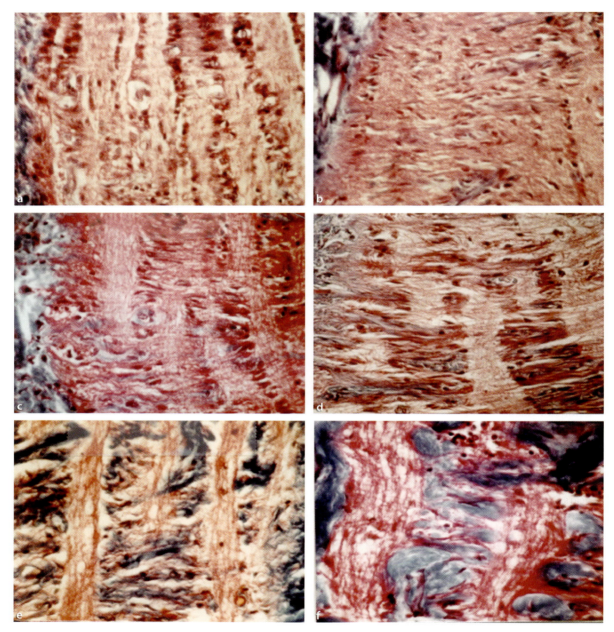

Fig. 3.6a–f Variation of the optic nerve structure between the 5th month of gestation and 49 years of age (Courtesy of H.A. Quigley). These microphotographs show preparations of the area of the lamina cribrosa and the optic nerve head, stained according to Mallory's trichromic technique. The connective tissue is stained with *blue*, the nerve fibres and astrocytes with *red*. The sclera can be seen on the *left* in all cases, except in **e** and **f**. The photographs are arranged according to age, so the youngest (fetal) eye is on the *top left-hand side* and the oldest (adult) eye is on the *bottom right-hand side*: **a** 5 months of gestation; **b** 7 months of gestation; **c** 8 months of gestation; **d** 1 month of age; **e** 12 years of age; **f** 49 years of age. In the two first photographs taken from fetal life, there is no connective tissue stained with blue in the optic nerve head; in the newborn (**d**) some *blue coloration* is starting to appear, but much less than in the optic nerve of the 12-year-old patient (**e**). The connective tissue is very dense at 49 years of age (×250). This accounts for the fact that optic disc cupping in children with congenital glaucoma is generally reversible when IOP is regulated with surgery

Fig. 3.7 Dilation of upper eyelid veins

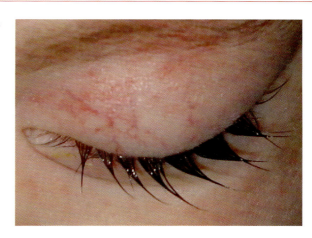

verity in both eyes. They are stronger in the eye with more anatomical and functional disorders.

Signs and symptoms combine in a different way, but as Costenbader and Kwitko [15] showed, when glaucoma has its onset at birth, the signs appear in the following chronological order: hazy cornea, photophobia, eye enlargement, and epiphora. When the onset is between the 6th and 12th month of age, the order changes to eye enlargement, hazy cornea, photophobia, and epiphora. In glaucomas with an onset after the 1st year of age, photophobia is rare. As a symptom of congenital glaucoma, photophobia presumably originates in the stimulation of the sensory trigeminal branches by corneal alterations [16].

Hypertension can cause eye enlargement when it appears within the first 4 or 5 years. After this age, late diagnosis of congenital glaucoma is only possible by means of gonioscopy. This topic has been discussed by Cardia and Reibaldi [17].

References

1. Kaiser B, cited by Kluyskens J (1950) Le glaucome congénital. Rapport présenté à la Societé Belge d'Ophtalmologie
2. Horven I (1961) Tonometry in infants. Acta Ophthalmol Kbh, 39:911–918
3. Carvalho CA, Calixto N (1969) Semiología do glaucoma congenito. XV Cong Bras Oftal Porto Alegre, pp 105–174
4. Shaffer RN, Weiss DI (1973) Congenital and pediatric glaucomas. Mosby, St. Louis
5. Angell LK, Robb RM, Berson FG (1981) Visual prognosis in patients with ruptures in Descemet's membrane due to forceps injuries. Arch Ophthalmol 99:2137–2139
6. Cibis GW, Tripathi RC (1982) The differential diagnosis of Descemet's tears (Haab's striae) and posterior polymorphous dystrophy bands. A clinicopathologic study. Ophthalmology 89:614–620
7. Robin AL, Quigley HA, Pollack IP, Maumenee IH (1979) An analysis of visual acuity, visual fields and disk cupping in childhood glaucoma. Am J Ophthalmol 88:847–858
8. Axenfeld T (1920) Embryotoxon corneal posterior. Ber Dtsch Ophthal Ges 38:301–302
9. Busacca A (1967) Le tableau biomicroscopique de l'embryotoxon. Ophthalmologica 153:1–5.
10. Chandler PA, Grant MW (1965) Lectures on glaucoma. Lea and Febiger, Philadelphia
11. Shaffer RN, Hetherington J Jr (1960) The glaucomatous disc in infants. A suggested hypothesis for disc cupping. Trans Am Acad Ophthalmol Otol 73:929–935
12. Shaffer RN (1967) New concepts in infantile glaucoma. Can J Ophthal 2:243–248
13. Shaffer RN (1955) Pathogenesis of congenital glaucoma, gonioscopic and microscopic anatomy. Trans Am Acad Ophth 59:297–308
14. Anderson DR (1975) Pathogenesis of glaucomatous cupping. A new hypothesis. In: Symposium on glaucoma. Transactions of the New Orleans Academy of Ophthalmology. Mosby, St. Louis, pp 81–94
15. Costenbader FD, Kwitko ML (1967) Congenital glaucoma. An analysis of seventy seven consecutive eyes. J Pediat Ophthalmol 4:9–15
16 Offret G (1960) La photophobie et son traitement. L'Année Thérapeutique et Clinique en Ophtalmologie. XI:303–317
17. Cardia LE, Reibaldi A (1985) Sulla diagnosi e trattamento del glaucoma congenito. Malattie congenite dell'apparato oculare. Verduci, Roma, pp 225–254

Examination of the Newborn Under General Anesthesia

Contents

Examination of newborn infants under general anesthesia, to assess whether they have congenital glaucoma, takes 7–10 min and is extremely safe if assisted by a pediatric anesthesiologist. In the last 54 years, we have performed more than 4,000 examinations under general anaesthesia on infants from 5 days to 2 years of age.

To obtain the normal IOP and axial length values, we take chamber angle photographs and perform funduscopy in all cases studied. For the study of normality, examinations were also conducted on infants undergoing general anesthesia for suspected diseases other than glaucoma.

It should be stressed that general anesthesia influences IOP values, either raising or lowering them, and this hinders accurate diagnosis of hypertension in children from 1 to 2 years of age with primary congenital glaucoma. However, fortunately, it does not affect axial length as measured with echometry. Children's eyes are distensible up to the age of 5 years, and in the presence of raised IOP, the axial length also increases, and the measurements are not influenced by general anesthesia.

Effects of Anesthetic Agents on Intraocular Pressure

Finding the proper anesthetic agent was difficult and long. In children, anesthesia should be simple, quick, and superficial, and it should not influence intraocular pressure readings. Only if these requirements are met will the intraocular pressure readings be valid and give the right information on the state of the child's eye.

We have tested different anesthetics with the following results:

- Ether: this increases bronchial secretion and produces bronchospasms. It gives the effect of a Valsalva manoeuvre and intraocular pressure increases.
- Barbiturates: dosing is inaccurate. In the case of insufficient doses, the child awakens and becomes defensive, with a consequent rise in intraocular pressure. If the dose is excessive, there is respiratory depression, the blood pressure drops, and therefore intraocular pressure also decreases.
- Anesthesia with intubation: we no longer recommend this practice because it requires deep anesthesia, causing blood pressure to drop, with a consequent IOP decrease, or, when succinylcholine is used, it produces paralysis of respiratory movement, causing venous pressure to rise to nearly 30 cm H_2O, and intraocular pressure consequently rises. It also causes blood pressure to increase, and therefore raises intraocular pressure.
- Halothane (Fluothane) compared to Methoxyflurane (Penthrane): both induction and recovery times are shorter with Halothane and slightly longer with Methoxyflurane, but Halothane induces strong blood pressure reductions [5], and therefore a substantial drop in intraocular pressure. We checked brachial blood pressure in all the children by means of a specially designed holder.

As shown in Table 4.1, for many years we used Penthrane because it was the agent with the least influence on the IOP. However, Penthrane is no longer produced and in the last 10 years, we have been using Sevorane. We currently use Sevorane (sevoflurane). Sevoflurane is a new-generation fluorinated methyl isopropyl ether with particular physicochemical and pharmacodynamic characteristics, which, after almost 40 years, has displaced Halothane as an inhalant agent in daily anesthetic practice (Fig. 4.1).

Fig. 4.1 Fluoromethyl-2,2,2-trifluoro-1-(trifluoromethyl) ethyl ether

Table 4.1 Anesthetics and intraocular pressure in children

Anesthetics modifying intraocular pressure in children		
Ether	Bronchial secretion	> IOP
	Bronchoconstriction	
	Valsalva test	
Barbiturates	Difficult to measure exact dosage	
	If insufficient	> IOP
	If excessive	Blood pressure reduction	< IOP
		Respiratory depression	< IOP
	Deep anaesthesia		< IOP
	Blood pressure reduction	
	Succinylcholine	Paralysis of respiratory movements	> IOP
		Blood pressure increase	
Halothane (Fluothane)	Blood pressure reduction	< IOP
Anesthetics not modifying intraocular pressure		
Penthrane (Methoxyflurane)		< IOP

First used by Sampaolesi and Carro, 1967, 1969, 1974, 1975 [1–4]

Like all inhalatory agents, it reduces intraocular pressure, relaxing extraocular muscle tone, depressing the CNS, encouraging the outflow of aqueous humor, and diminishing venous and arterial blood pressure. With controlled ventilation and normocapnia, it reduces the IOP in proportion to the depth of anaesthesia. Given that it is well-accepted on inhalation, its rapid induction, the precise control of alveolar concentration, its hemodynamic stability, and the rapid recovery, Sevoflurane is the nearest we currently have to an ideal inhalatory agent for anesthesia in children.

In all cases, when we have given general anesthesia to children, we have used an oximeter, a device for determining oxygen saturation in the blood (Fig. 4.2).

Sevorane (sevoflurane) is applied either on a gauze covering the mouth or on a mask through which the drug is administered drop by drop (Fig. 4.3).

Macroscopic examination is carried out by opening the eyelids as much as possible (Fig. 4.4a). Funduscopy with the ophthalmoscope follows (Fig. 4.4b).

Once general anaesthesia has been induced, the examination continues as follows:

1. Two drops of a local anesthetic (Novesine, Anestalcon, etc.) are instilled in each eye so that they fall directly on the cornea, to produce the best effect (Fig. 4.5a).

2. Fluorescein paper strips are applied on the eyes (these are paper strips with dry fluorescein on the edge, which is dissolved by the tears, manufactured by Haag Streit) (Fig. 4.5b).

Since the head of newborns up to 2 years of age is much smaller than that of adults, a wooden supplement (Fig. 4.6a) covered with disposable paper towels is put on the chin holder of the slit lamp so that the infant's eyes are suitably positioned, at the level of the horizontal black strip of the slit lamp (Fig. 4.6b). Of course, the sleeping child is seated on the lap of the nurse or anesthetist, who holds the child's head (Fig. 4.6b).

An important advantage of Halothane and Sevorane is that they keep the eye looking straight forward, which helps make an accurate examination with applanation tonometry and gonioscopy (Fig. 4.7).

Biomicroscopy of the anterior segment is performed, with special emphasis on the presence of tears in the Descemet membrane (Haab striae) on the cornea, and their location is illustrated in a cir-

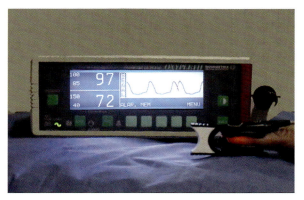

Fig. 4.2 Oximeter

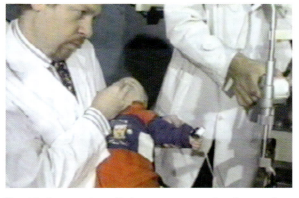

Fig. 4.3 Sevorane is applied on a gauze covering the mouth

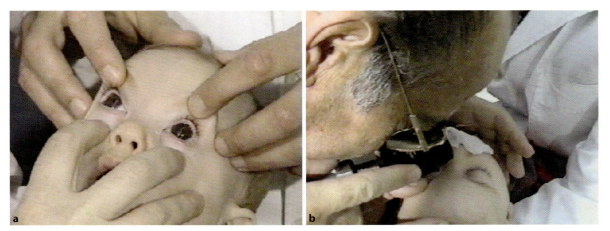

Fig. 4.4 **a** Macroscopic examination of both eyes. **b** Fundoscopy with the ophthalmoscope

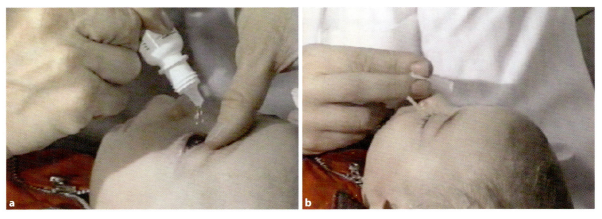

Fig. 4.5 **a** Two drops of local anesthesia in each eye. **b** Fluorescein paper strips are applied to the eyes

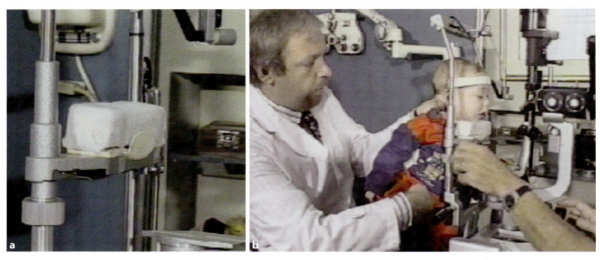

Fig. 4.6 a Wooden supplement so that the the infant's eyes are in a suitable position. **b** Sleeping child is seated on a nurse or anesthetist lap

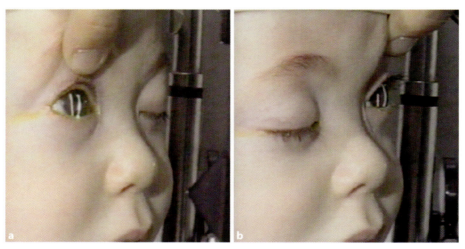

Fig. 4.7a,b Halothane and Sevorane keep the eye looking straight forward

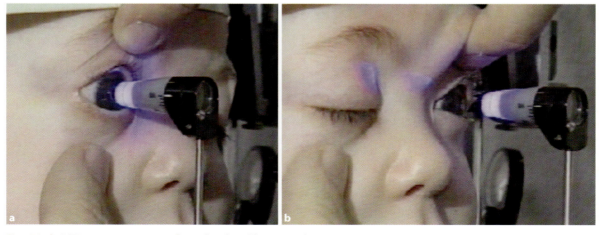

Fig. 4.8a,b IOP measurement is performed with Goldmann applanation tonometer

cle with the pupil drawn in it. Tears in the Descemet membrane located at the level of the pupil produce amblyopia and strabismus. In these cases, perforating corneal grafts have been required. These procedures have a good prognosis if performed properly (see Chap. 18, clinical history no. 238).

3. At this stage in the examination, the pupil should be thoroughly examined to find any pigment ectropion and to check whether there is hypoplasia of the superficial mesenchymal layer of the iris or if it is still under development. Special attention should also be given to the presence of anomalies characteristic of secondary congenital glaucomas at the posterior corneal surface, such as posterior embryotoxon, Rieger syndrome, etc.

4. The presence of cataract, and, finally, the presence of an anterior embryotoxon, which is typical in children with congenital glaucoma, are ruled out. It should be kept in mind that this embryotoxon influences corneal diameter measurements at the vertical axis. Therefore, as is explained later, the corneal diameter should be measured at the horizontal meridian.

5. IOP measurement is performed with Goldmann applanation tonometry (Fig. 4.8). The position of the eye is crucial for this measurement. At present, before this measurement, the IOP is measured with Pascal's tonometry (Fig. 4.9) to avoid the influence of corneal thickness on IOP values.

Gonioscopy is performed with a Goldmann three-mirror lens specially manufactured by Haag Streit for children. Unlike the one designed by Goldmann for adults, there is a 10-mm lens and an 11-mm lens designed for children (Fig. 4.10)

Gonioscopic examination is more accurate with the use of the lens designed by Fankhauser and Roussell, (Fig. 4.11), since this provides a perfectly defined greatly magnified image. In addition, with this lens, a perfect evaluation of the two types of congenital glaucomas is possible (type 1, primary congenital glaucoma, and type 2, refractory congenital glaucoma), as well as the identification of congenital anomalies of the chamber angle in secondary congenital glaucoma.

6. In goniophotography, photographs are taken with the highest illumination of the slit lamp, with a Tungsten 160 ASA film for night lighting. A Nikon camera was adapted to perfectly fit the eyepiece of the slit-lamp by means of a ring specially manufactured by Pfortner Laboratories (Fig. 4.12a,b).

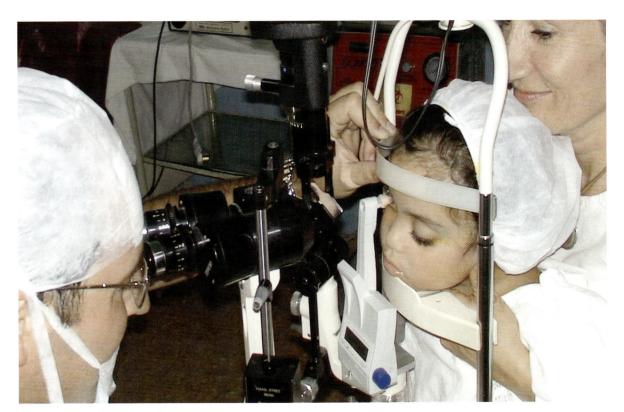

Fig. 4.9 Measured with Pascal's tonometer

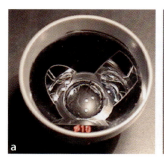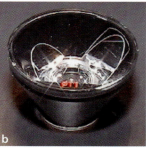

Fig. 4.10a,b Gonioscopy with Goldmann 3-mirror lens of 10 and 11 mm diameter for babies

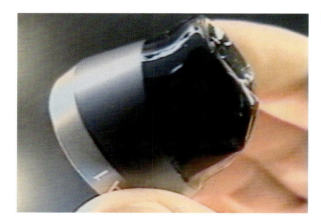

Fig. 4.11 New Gonioscopic lens designed by Roussel and Fankhauser with more resolution

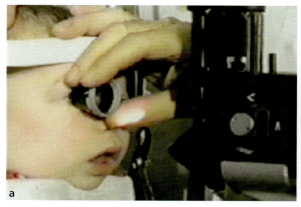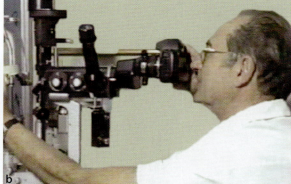

Fig 4.12a,b Gonioscopic examination at the slit lamp

Fig. 4.13 Video. Camera 1 works as video camera. Camera 2 works as digital video recorder

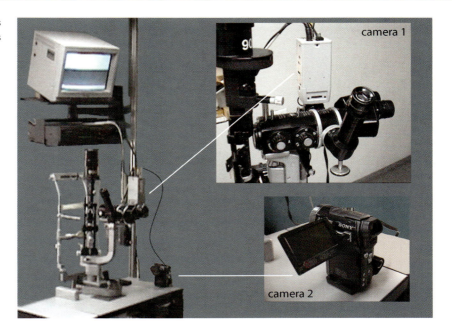

In the last 5 years, we have obtained complete images or slit images by means of movie camera 1, connected to a monitor which is, in turn, connected to camera 2. Camera 1 works as a video camera. Camera 2 works as a digital video recorder (Fig. 4.13).

7. Echometry is used to obtain the axial length. Firstly, the eyelids are separated by means of an Ossoinig shell (Fig. 4.14). A drop of methylcellulose is administered inside the shell to seal off the scleral contact area (Fig. 4.15a), so that the saline solution with which the cylinder is filled does not leak through the contact area between the shell and the eye (Fig. 4.15b). The probe of the echometer can thus be placed in the saline solution with no contact with the cornea (Fig. 4.16a) (noncontact echometry). An echogram is obtained, which not only provides the axial length measure, but also offers more details on the configuration of the anterior chamber, as well as of the lens and corneal thickness. Figure 4.16b shows that the peaks representing the anterior and posterior corneal surfaces are well apart from each other (thereby reflecting the great thickness of the cornea) due to the corneal edema caused by ocular hypertension.

8. The last step involves the measurement of the corneal diameter with a strabismus caliper, at the horizontal meridian (Fig. 4.17a, b).

Once the examination has been completed, as the anesthesia is very superficial, the anesthesiologist squeezes the ear lobe of the infant to wake him up (Fig. 4.18a–c). This is very important, since one of the parents, who has been present in the office during the entire examination, can see how short this examination is and leave with the baby awake. The parents will then be willing to attend the subsequent follow-up visits, during which general anesthesia is used again.

Even though I have been working in a University Hospital for 54 years, during which we have examined more than 4,000 infants under general anesthesia as described, with the method taught to all the residents, at present the examination under general anesthesia is performed in the operating room, with the infant in the supine position and the IOP measured with hand-held applanation tonometry. This failure to apply the method described is all the more surprising since it is taught thoroughly and is extensively used worldwide. These ophthalmologists even fail to use the method they have been taught by Dr. Manzitti. He made the child lie in a supine position, with the chin-holder removed from the slit-lamp, and measured the IOP and performed gonioscopy correctly by placing the slit-lamp at different heights.

9. The chamber angle can be examined with the SL-OCT (Heidelberg Engineering, Heidelberg, Germany) (Fig. 4.19), a very important new device for the study of congenital glaucoma.

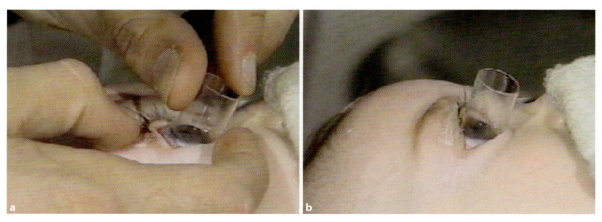

Fig. 4.14a,b Opening of the eyelids by means of an Ossoinig shell

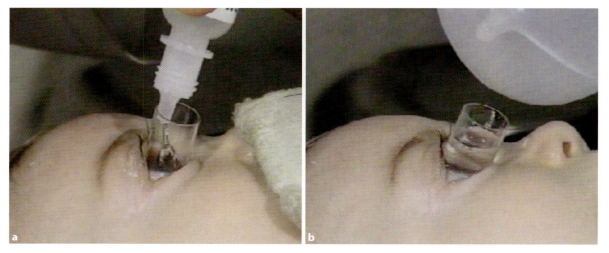

Fig. 4.15 **a** Drop of methylcellulose to seal off the scleral contact-area. **b** The Ossoinig shell is filled with saline solution

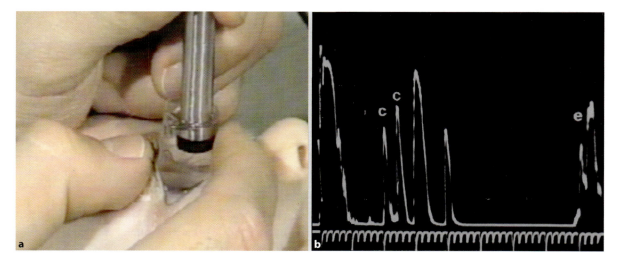

Fig. 4.16 **a** Probe of echometer in Ossoinig shell. **b** Echogram provides axial length, anterior chamber and corneal thickness

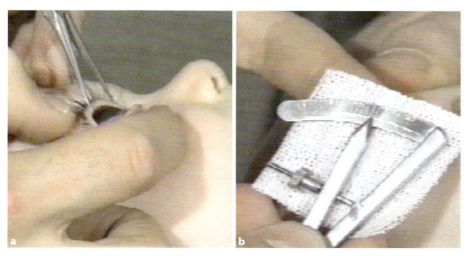

Fig. 4. 17a,b Measurement of corneal diameter

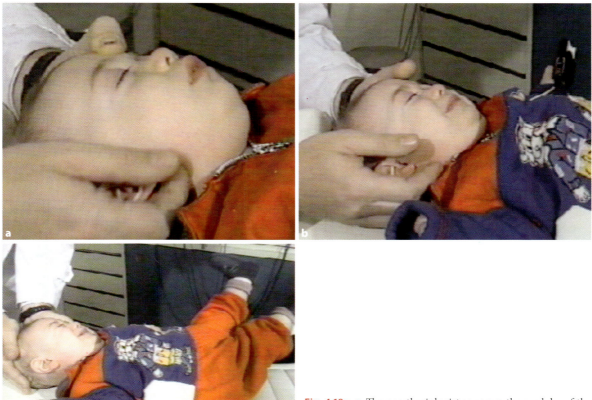

Fig. 4.18a–c The anesthesiologist squeezes the ear lobe of the infant to wake him up

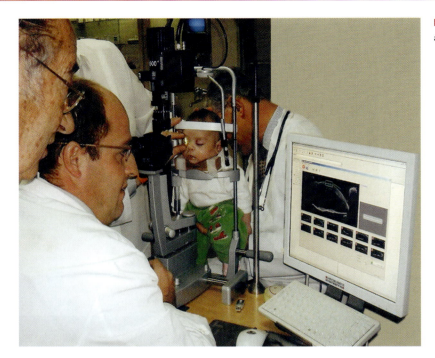

Fig. 4.19 Examination of the chamber angle with SL-OCT. (see Chap. 13)

References

1. Sampaolesi R, Reca R, Carro A (1967) Presión ocular en el niño hasta los 5 años bajo anestesia con Pentrane (Metoxifluorane). Arch Oftal B Aires XLII:180–185
2. Sampaolesi R (1969) La pression oculaire et le sinus camerulaire chez l'enfant normal et dans le glaucome congénital aux dessous de l'âge de 5 ans. Docum Ophthal 26:497–515
3. Sampaolesi R, Reca R, Carro A, Armando E (1975) Estado actual del estudio continuado de la presión ocular de los niños desde el nacimiento hasta los 5 años de edad. Arch Oftal B Aires 50:321–333
4. Sampaolesi R, Reca R, Carro A, Armando A (1976) Normaler Intraokularer Druck bei Kindern bis zu 5 Jahren mit und ohne Allgemeinnarkose. Seine Wichtigkeit fur die Fruhdiagnose des anegborennen Glaukoms. In: Glaukom Symposium Wuerzburg 1974, Enke, Stuttgart, pp 278–289
5. Ferreira AA, Lobo De Morais L (1965) Emprego do Metoxifluorano en anestesia para otorrinolaringologia e oftalmologia. Rev Brasil Anest 1:143–146

Contents

Tonometers Used for Measuring Intraocular Pressure in Children

The examination is generally carried out with the child supported at the slit lamp by the anesthesiologist (see Chap. 4). Goldmann's applanation tonometer is generally used (Fig. 5.1a). Today we also use Pascal's tonometer, which gives us the pressure corrected for corneal thickness (Fig. 5.1b). After operating, only the ocular pressure and the axial length need to be checked. This can be done on a stretcher while the child is under anesthesia in a supine position. In this case, Draeger's hand applanation tonometer is very useful (Fig. 5.1c). We sometimes also use the Goldmann hand applanation tonometer (Fig. 5.1d), which is very precise, but there are very few units manufactured by Haag-Streit. The Perkins tonometer can also be used.

Before discussing this subject, the following should be taken into consideration:
- Intraocular pressure measurement is technically difficult in children up to 5 years of age.
- Statistical reports of normal intraocular pressure in children are scarce worldwide.
- The different types of anesthetics available influence intraocular pressure values (see Chap. 4).

Normal Intraocular Pressure in Children from Birth to 5 Years of Age Under General Anesthesia

In 1967, we established that the normal intraocular pressure in children under general anesthesia with Methoxyflurane (Penthrane) has a mean value (X) below the normal X found in adults [1]: X = 10.56, S = 1.01.

The study involved 48 eyes of 24 healthy children. In 1969, we continued the study with the inclusion of 85 eyes of 48 children, thus extending the statistics, and obtained a mean intraocular pressure for children under general anesthesia of X = 10, S = 2.9. We therefore concluded that intraocular pressure in children is 5 mmHg lower than in adults [2] (Tables 5.1–5.4).

In the study conducted in 1975 [3–5], I extended the statistics to 93 normal children (139 eyes), who had consulted for other disorders not influencing intraocular pressure values. These eyes were divided into six age groups: 63 eyes of children under 1 year; 36 eyes of children within the 1st year; nine eyes of children within the 2nd year; eight eyes of children within the 3rd year, 11 eyes of children within the 4th year, and 12 eyes of children within the 5th year.

The normal intraocular pressure was measured with either the Goldmann-Schmidt, Draeger, or Perkins hand applanation tonometers, with the child in the supine position. In some children, it is sometimes necessary to open the palpebral slit slightly with a lid speculum, which can be easily prepared with a paper clip.

We do not use Halothane. Halothane induces strong blood pressure reductions [6], and therefore a large drop in intraocular pressure.

Normality Criteria

The following normality criteria were taken into account: corneal diameter under 12 mm, normal chamber angle, normal eye fundus, echometry with values within the normal range normal intraocular pressure in normal children until 5 years of age.

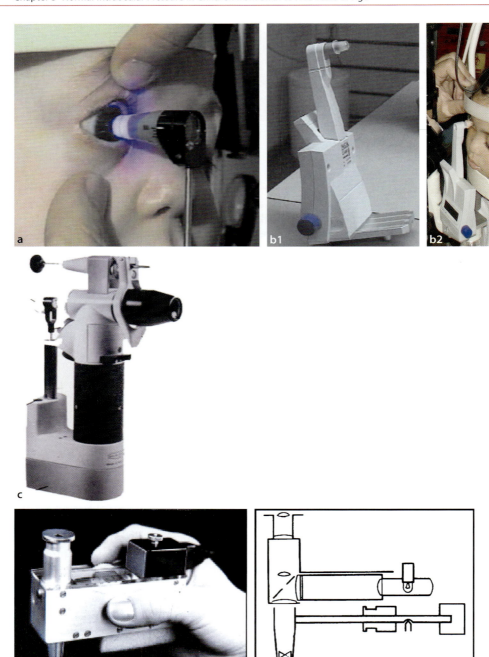

Fig. 5.1a–d Different kinds of tonometers used for measuring IOP in children with congenital glaucoma: **a** Goldmann applanation tonometer at the slit lamp. **b** 1 and 2- Pascal Dynamic contour tonometry at the slit lamp. **c** Draeger hand applanation tonometer. **d** 1 and 2- Goldmann hand applanation tonometer

In Fig. 5.2, the ordinates show intraocular pressure values in millimeters of mercury and the abscissas, the age in years. This chart should be kept hanging on the wall of the operating room so that, when measuring intraocular pressure under general anesthesia, the ophthalmologist can check whether the readings fall within the normal range. For instance, when measuring intraocular pressure in a child aged 6 months, the mean intraocular pressure should be 8 mmHg, the maximum 14 mmHg, and the minimum 4 mmHg. Values above 14 mmHg or below 4 mmHg are strongly suggestive of hypertension or hypotension, respectively (Figs. 5.2, 5.3).

Table 5.1 Intraocular pressure at different ages

Years of age						
	Below 1	1	2	3	4	5
Arithmetic mean (mmHg)	8.9	9.8	10.4	11.5	13.3	12.5
Number of eyes	63	36	9	8	11	12
Mean, standard deviation	2.4	2.7	1.2	1.7	2.6	2.9
Scatter	0.3	0.4	0.4	0.6	0.8	0.8

Table 5.2 Statistical comparison of ages

Types of variation	Addition of squares	Degrees of freedom	Mean of the squares
Between the ages	291.55	5	58.31
Within the ages	805.27	133	6.05
Total	1,096.82	138	

Table 5.3 Statistical test

F 5.33, 95% = 2.29

F 5.133 = 9.63; $p<0.001$

Regression of intraocular pressure in relation to age up to 5 years (Fig. 5.2)

$y = 8.5 + 0.85\ x$

y = intraocular pressure

Regression coefficient = 0.85

x = years of age

Mean deviation s y.x = 2.4

Student t test = 6.83; $p<0.001$

95% confidence interval for normal IOP values until the age of 5 years (mmHg)

Table 5.4 Maximum and minimum intraocular pressures at different ages

Age	Minimum	Maximum
Below 1 year	8.4	9.4
1–2 years	9.4	10.2
2–3 years	10.4	11.1
3–4 years	10.9	12.0
4–5 years	11.6	13.1
5–6 years	12.2	14.2

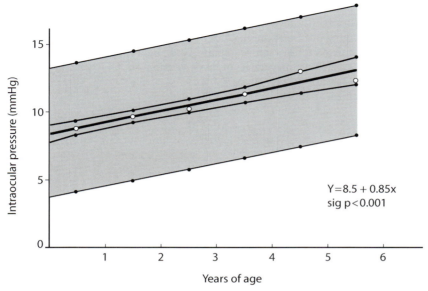

$$Y = 8.5 + 0.85x$$
$$\text{sig } p < 0.001$$

Fig. 5.2 The regression line (*thick line*) shows the annual IOP rise from birth to 5 years of age. On the ordinates, IOP in mmHg. On the abscissas, years of age. This graph is very useful for physicians, who should have it visible whenever they measure IOP under general anesthesia in children. For example, at 6 months of age, the maximum possible IOP is 14 mmHg

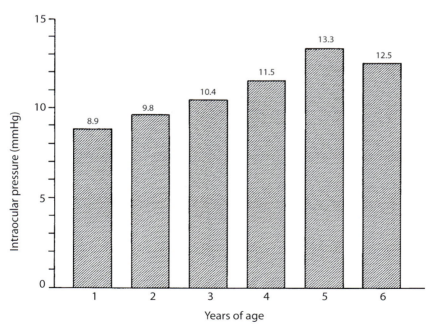

Fig. 5.3 Distribution of IOP values in normal children up to 6 years of age

The thick line, the regression line, in the chart, shows the annual intraocular pressure increase which occurs from birth up to 5 years of age (Fig. 5.2). It is very important for the ophthalmologist to understand this concept clearly: intraocular pressure is a variable that steadily increases throughout life, from birth to old age.

We have calculated the normal intraocular pressure values according to age, up to 5 years. The analysis of variation shows that intraocular pressure varies according to age. This is consistent with the significant intraocular pressure increase showed by the regression line at this stage of growth (from 1 to 5 years of age). The regression coefficient shows that intraocular pressure increases by 1 mmHg per year, starting from 8.5 mmHg (actual increase: 0.85 mmHg per year). The intraocular pressure reading should, therefore, be related to the child's age, in order to set a diagnostic criterion of normal intraocular pressure, which, in children under 2 years of age is 5 mmHg lower than in adults.

Intraocular pressure in children from birth to the 5th year of age shows a slow increase, and Fig. 5.3 shows that intraocular pressure in babies under 1 year of age is 8.9 mmHg. During the 1st year, it is 9.8 mmHg, during the 2nd year, 10.4 mmHg, during the 3rd year, 11.5 mmHg, during the 4th year, 13.3 mmHg, and during the 5th year, 12.5 mmHg. These are the mean values for the different age groups. Intraocular pressure in children is thus seen to be lower than in adults.

Normal Intraocular Pressure in Newborns Between 12 h and 15 Days of Age Under Local Anesthesia and Without General Anesthesia

We have taken many intraocular pressure measurements in newborns without general anesthesia in order to avoid the influence of general anesthetic agents on intraocular pressure. Thus, we have proven that the intraocular pressure values measured in children, which are 5 mmHg lower than in adults, are not caused by the anesthetic agent. The measurement of intraocular pressure in newborns up to 15 days of age can be performed without general anesthesia, using Dr. A. Armando's method, which is a method for calming down and relaxing the baby in such a way that tonometry can be performed [3].

Material

Fifteen normal babies were studied in the maternity ward (six boys and nine girls), ranging in age from 12 h to 15 days.

Method

Using positions that remind the baby of the fetal position, the baby becomes calm and relaxed, and neither sedatives nor general anesthetic agents are required for intraocular pressure measurement.

There are three positions that make it easier to measure intraocular pressure:

1. The baby is placed in fetal position (Fig. 5.4), with the head upward and the body half flexed, the legs flexed and crossed over the belly, and the arms over the chest. In this position, the baby is held in the arms of the physician or the nurse, who must have one hand on the baby's head and one under the buttocks while making flexion movements.

2. Then the baby is placed in a supine position, and, holding the baby's crossed arms with one hand, flexion movements of the crossed and flexed legs are made with the other hand toward the belly (Fig. 5.5a).

3. When the baby is relaxed after these two maneuvers, this condition can be maintained by movements joining and separating the knees, as shown in Fig. 5.5b. Newborns are generally hypotonic, with transient hypertonia of the limbs. This means that newborns tend to have their four limbs flexed. When the baby stops crying and becomes quiet with these maneuvers, two Castroviejo lid speculums are placed, with nylon threads to pull from so that the fingers do not rest on the lids, which may cause the intraocular pressure to rise. This allows a 5- to 7-mm palpebral opening. Local anesthetics and fluorescein are administered and the intraocular pressure is measured with a Draeger hand tonometer (Fig. 5.6a). In our study, we also used a Mackay–Marg tonometer with inscription (Fig. 5.6b).

Without general anesthesia, intraocular pressure in newborns is not significantly different from that of normal children within their 1st year without general anesthesia.

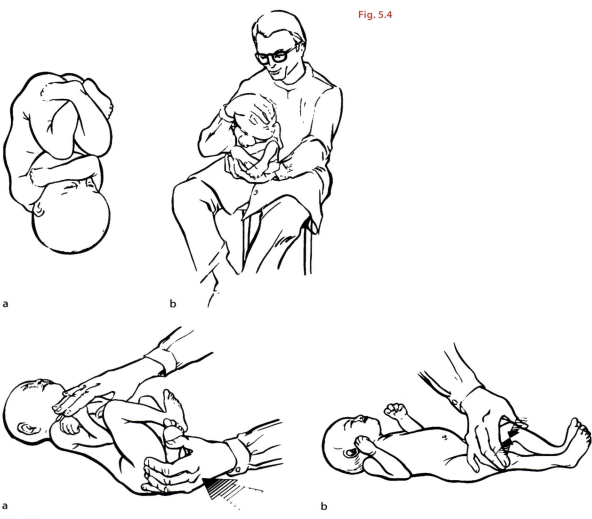

Fig. 5.4

a

b

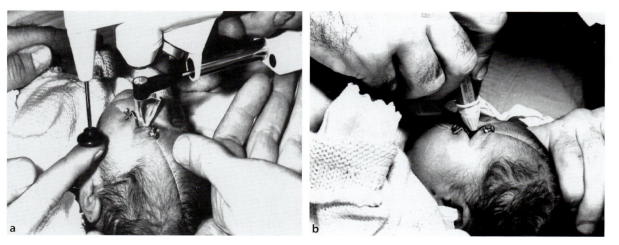

a

b

Fig. 5.5

a

b

Fig. 5.6

Ocular rigidity. Ytterborg's studies accounting for children's intraocular pressure being 5 mmHg lower than in adults

Schiötz´s tonometer should not be used to measure intraocular pressure in children. Although the classical literature already considered that the use of Schiötz´s tonometer in children led to countless mistakes regarding corneal curvature, corneal diameter, etc., the paper giving the reasons why it should not be used in children was written by Ytterborg in 1960 [7]. He explained that:

1. The conversion tables for Schiötz tonometry, like those made by Friedenwald [8], McBain [9, 10], Prijot [11], etc., were based on adults' eyes, with normal corneal diameters, and so they are not applicable to children.
2. The newborn's eye has approximately one-third of the adult's eye volume, the cornea has a more definite curvature, and the ocular walls have a different structure.
3. To prove this, Ytterborg examined 50 eyes enucleated from adults and 16 enucleated from children of different ages. He took tonometric measurements and scleral rigidity measurements with an electromanometer. He found that the scleral rigidity coefficient of children's eyes is much higher than that of adults' eyes. This is shown in Figs. 5.7 and 5.8.

The measurement of clinical ocular rigidity in 109 eyes of children between 5 months and 10 years of age under general anesthesia yielded a rigidity coefficient of 0.024. This means that with Schiötz tonometry there is a risk of diagnosing glaucoma when this is not the case. Ytterborg proved that children's ocular rigidity is double that of adults. In his paper, Ytterborg states, "the lines on the chart represent Friedenwald's normal calibration curves with 5.5, 7.5 and 10-g weights respectively, according to the 1955 tables (Fig. 5.7). The values I found deviate significantly from the ones represented by these curves. For instance, a scale reading of 4 using a 5.5-g weight, corresponds to an intraocular pressure of 20.5 mmHg according to the 1955 conversion tables, but, in fact, corresponds to an intraocular pressure value of 11.5 mmHg. The mean pressure for adults is slightly over 15 mmHg. If the intraocular pressure values are the same for newborns, the scale reading, according to these tables, should normally be slightly lower than 3. This scale reading is a strong indication of glaucoma in adults. The difference is even greater if the comparison is made with Schiötz's pressure curves, whose values are approximately 5 mmHg higher than Friedenwald's."

In 1960, Ytterborg studied the ocular rigidity of newborns, without applanation tonometry. He concluded that children's intraocular pressure, as measured using a Schiötz tonometer, is 5 mmHg lower than the mean for adults. These experimental results were proven later in our clinical papers [1–5].

We highly recommend the papers by Kornblueth et al. [12, 13], Horven [14], Manzitti [15], Manzitti and Damel [16], Degenne et al. [17], Hetherington and Shaffer [18], Grote [19], and Goethals [20] which studied the influence of anesthetic agents on intraocular pressure.

In my opinion, the fundamental work is the study co-authored by Radtke and Cohan [21] because they are the only authors who compared intraocular pressure values of children under general anesthesia and with a new method of their own design in which the child is awake in order to ensure the consistency of these values, thereby ruling out the influence of general anesthesia on intraocular pressure. This paper was the first one to confirm our results in the United States. Their study investigated babies between 19 and 173 h of age, i.e., up to the 7th or 8th day, and they reached the relaxed condition with the baby in its cradle and covered with a blanket to keep it warm. They used a Sauer retractor manufactured by Storz and they pre-

Fig. 5.4a,b For intraocular pressure measurement, the newborn is placed in a position similar to the fetal position

Fig. 5.5 a Then the baby is placed in a supine position, and, holding the baby's crossed arms with one hand, flexion movements of the crossed and flexed legs are made with the other hand toward the belly. **b** When the baby is relaxed after these two maneuvers, this condition can be maintained by movements joining and separating the knees

Fig. 5.6 a Intraocular pressure measurement in a newborn, with Draeger tonometer with local anesthesia and palpebral opening by means of a Castroviejo speculum. **b** Intraocular pressure measurement in a newborn with Mackay–Marg tonometer with local anesthesia

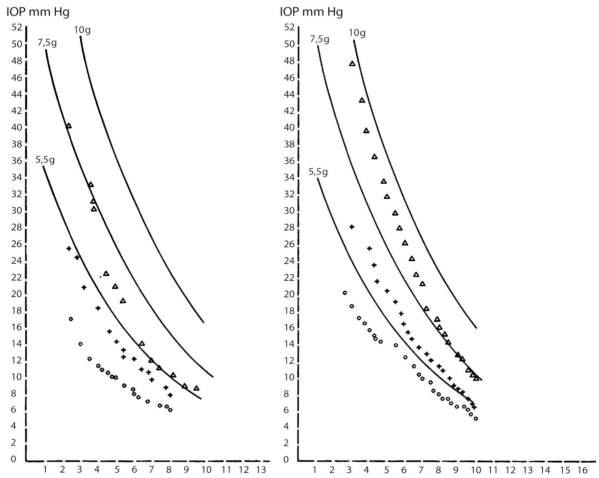

IOP mm Hg

IOP mm Hg

Fig. 5.7 a Tonometric calibration curve in the eye of a newborn. **b.** Tonometric calibration curve in the eye of a child of three and a half months. The *solid lines* correspond to the calibration made by Schiötz in the adult; the *circles*, to the weight of 5.5 g; the *crosses*, to a weight of 7.5 g, and the *triangles* to a weight of 10 g [7]. As can be seen, the ocular rigidity is completely different from that of the adult. This is why it is advisable not to use the Schiötz tonometer in children

vented the Bell phenomenon, according to the blepharostat opening, by waiting for 1 min after placing it. They instilled up to two topical anesthetic eyedrops, to achieve complete relaxation. In some babies, they failed to achieve complete relaxation and repeated their attempt some hours later or on another day.

With this method, they were the first ones in the world after us to present a group of 60 normal newborns with a mean intraocular pressure of 11.4 ± 2.4 mmHg. They presented a table (Table 5.5) listing all the authors who had measured intraocular pressure in children up to the moment of their publication.

This table, as well as Radtke's paper, shows that the first six authors, out of a total of nine, used only the Schiötz indentation tonometer (with the above-mentioned consequent errors), and the other authors, including Radtke, were the first to use applanation tonometry.

The importance of Borrone's paper [22] should also be stressed, in which the intraocular pressure of 50 normal children between 5 and 15 years of age was studied, finding the following values: between 5 and 8 years, 8–11 mmHg; 9–11 years, 12–14 mmHg; and 12–15 years, 15–17 mmHg. If the values of the entire group are taken into account (population mean), an intraocular pressure mean ranging from 11.65 to 12.02 mmHg was obtained.

Table 5.5 Different studies of intraocular pressure in the child with different anesthesia and different tonometers

Author	Anesthesia	Tonometer	Mean IOP (mmHg)	Age	Measurements
Dolcet	Topical	Indentation	(41–56)	24 h	35 children
Brockhurst	Topical	Indentation	26.5 (6.5–33)	Premature	59 children
Giles	Topical	Indentation	25.8 (12–30.4)	1 h	32 years (110 attempts)
Horven	Topical	Indentation	16.3 (10.2–24)	4 h to 10 days	50 children (67 attempts)
Kornblueth et al.	Diethyl ether	Indentation	22.5 (RE), 20.9 (LE), 15.9–29	5–24 h	47 eyes
Westby and Skulbert	Diethyl ether	Indentation	16.9 (8.5–22–4)	1.5–9 years	110 eyes
Gotoh and Kitazawa	Fluothane	Indentation and applanation	14.7 (9–22) 13.4 (7–20)	25 h to 8 days	25 children
Hetherington and Shaffer	Fluothane	Applanation and indentation	12.5 (7–22)	3 months to 5 years	30 eyes
Sampaolesi et al.	Methoxyfluorane	Applanation	10 (7.81–12.19)	A few days to 5 y	135 eyes

Draeger's Home Tonometry

Draeger [23] proposed performing a home tonometry in children operated for congenital glaucoma between 5 and 8 years of age, as well as the measurement made by the ophthalmologist, especially when the children live far from the clinic. This tonometry measurement was taken by members of the patient's family. They learned "under close supervision the correct handling of the applanation tonometer. If marked variations in IOP were found, more frequent checks were made in order to enable early intervention by the doctor. In several cases of congenital glaucoma, it was the parents who carried out the IOP measurement in their school-age children. In one of the cases, this was done by the wife and in another by the step-mother who was the patient's doctor."

Draeger goes on to relate a "particularly striking case: an 8 year-old patient with refractory congenital glaucoma. Extreme oscillations of the IOP were detected early that necessitated a fresh surgical intervention" (Fig. 5.8a,b). Similarly, six more operations were

indicated until finally the IOP was regulated and the progression of the eye disease was stopped.

In the case of children over 8, Dr. Draeger provides them with the Self Tonometer: Ocutome, that he had designed, so that they can check the state of their IOP personally (Fig. 5.9).

Finally, in those operated for congenital glaucoma between 10 and 40 years of age, we have always checked the IOP by means of a daily pressure curve with its own algorithm [5]. We make the curve taking the pressure in bed at 0600 hours with the patient lying in the supine position with a hand applanation tonometer, and then with the patient mobile, with the slit-lamp at 0900, 1200, 1500, 1800, and 2100 hours. The arithmetic mean and the standard deviation (variability) are calculated, which must not pass the limits of 19.1 and 2.1, respectively, the highest normal values (see Vol. 2, Chap. 15). A very interesting example of the IOP value in late congenital glaucomas in a child that I operated in both eyes at the age of 6 years can be found in Chap. 17 (Fig. 17.34–17.37).

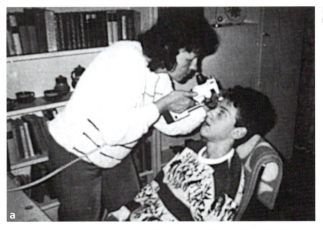
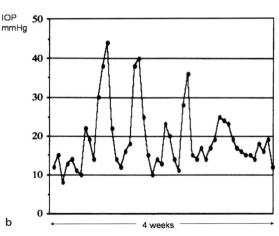

Fig. 5.8 a Home tonometry made by a family member (kindly provided by J. Draeger). **b** Three peaks of pressure of between 30 and 40 mmHg shown by home tonometry (courtesy of J. Draeger)

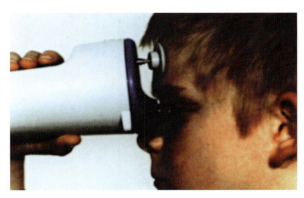

Fig. 5.9 Child operated for congenital glaucoma personally checking his IOP using the Self Tonometer: Ocutome (courtesy of J. Draeger)

References

1. Sampaolesi R, Reca R, Carro A (1967) Presión ocular en el niño hasta los 5 años bajo anestesia con Pentrane (Metoxifluorane). Arch Oftal B Aires XLII:180–185
2. Sampaolesi R (1969) La pression oculaire et le sinus camérulaire chez l'enfant normal et dans le glaucome congénital aux dessous de l'âge de 5 ans. Doc Ophthalmol 26:497–515
3. Sampaolesi R, Reca R, Carro A, Armando E (1975) Estado actual del estudio continuado de la presión ocular de los niños desde el nacimiento hasta los 5 años de edad. Arch Oftal B Aires 50:321–333
4. Sampaolesi R, Reca R, Carro A, Armando A (1974) Normaler Intraokularer Druck bei Kindern bis zu 5 Jahren mit und ohne Allgemeinnarkose. Seine Wichtigkeit für die Fruhdiagnose des angeborenen Glaukoms. In: Glaukom Symposium Wuerzburg 1974, Enke, Stuttgart, pp 278–289
5. Sampaolesi R, Calixto N, de Carvalho CA, Reca R (1968) Diurnal variation of intraocular pressure in healthy, suspected and glaucomatous eyes. First South American Symposium on Glaucoma, Bariloche 1966. Mod Probl Ophthalmol 6:1–23
6. Ferreira AA, Lobo De Morais L (1965) Emprego do Metoxifluorano en anestesia para otorrinolaringologia e oftalmologia. Rev Brasil Anest 1:143–146
7. Ytterborg J (1960) On scleral rigidity. Oslo University Press, Oslo
8. Friedenwald JS (1955) Tonometer calibration: an attempt to remove discrepancies found in the 1954 calibration scale for Schiotz tonometers. Trans Am Acad Ophthalmol Otolaryngol 61:108–122
9. McBain EH (1957) Tonometer calibration: determination of Pt formula by use of strain gauge and recording potentiometer on enucleated normal human eyes. AMA Arch Ophthalmol Chicago 57:520–531
10. McBain EH (1958) Tonometer calibration II. Ocular rigidity. Arch Ophthalmol Chicago 60:1080
11. Prijot E (1958) La rigidité de l'oeil humain. Acta Ophthalmol 36:865
12. Kornblueth W, Aladjemoff L, Magora F, Gabray A (1959) Influence of general anesthesia on intraocular pressure in man. Arch Ophthalmol Chicago 61:84–87
13. Kornblueth W, Abrahanamow V, Aldjemoff L, Magora F, Gomgos (1962) Intraocular pressure in the newborn measurable under general anesthesia. Arch Ophthalmol Chicago 67:750–752
14. Horven I (1961) Tonometry in infants. Acta Ophthalmol 39:911–918

15. Manzitti E (1963) Técnica de examen en el glaucoma infantil. Arch Oftal B Aires 38:345–347

16. Manzitti E, Damel A (1964) Valores de la tonometría aplanática en el lactante normal. Arch Oftal B Aires 39:360–362

17. Degenne S, Benck P, Gerhard JP, Payeur G, Roth A (1967) Les modifications de la Po chez l'enfant sous anesthésie générale. Bull Soc Ophtal France 67:1118–1121

18. Hetherington JJ, Shaffer RN (1968) Tonometry and tonography in congenital glaucoma. Invest Ophthalmol Vis Sci 7:134–137

19. Grote P (1975) Augeninnendruckmessungen bei Kleinkindern ohne Glaukom in Halothanmaskennarkose. Ophthalmologica 171:202

20. Goethals M, Missotten L (1983) Intraocular pressure in children up to five years of age. J Pediatr Ophthalmol Strabismus 20:49

21. Radtke ND, Cohan BE (1974) Intraocular pressure measurement in the newborn. Am J Ophthalmol 78:501

22. Borrone RN (1984) Presión ocular en niños de 5 a 15 años. Arch Oftal B Aires 59:219–234

23. Draeger J (1992) Neue Wege zur Fruhdiagnose und Verlaufkontrolle des Glaukoms, Spektrum Augenheilkd 6:267–272

Contents

Introduction

It is well known that the diagnosis and surgical indications for congenital glaucoma depend on three elements: (1) clinical symptoms, (2) intraocular pressure measurement with applanation tonometry [1, 2], and (3) chamber angle examination.

In 1970, since I was concerned about intraocular pressure readings for children under general anesthesia, because of the deviations produced by different anesthetic agents, and given that Penthrane, one of the only anesthetics that did not modify intraocular pressure, was about to be discontinued, I decided to test a Siemens echograph for measuring the axial length in the eyes of children with congenital glaucoma symptoms, and I found it useful. The first echograms I obtained are shown in Fig. 6.1.

I used Gernet and Hollwich's curves [3] and the first papers of Buschmann and Bluth [4] for normality patterns. Then I bought the first echograph used in Argentina. I went to Spitz, where the company that manufactured the echograph designed by Ossoinig was located, and Dr. Till standardized my echograph.

Since 1966, after the first Glaucoma Symposium was held in Bariloche, the Glaucoma Club has continued working on a multicenter basis (Nassim Calixto in Belo Horizonte, Celso Carvalho in Sao Paulo, and myself in Buenos Aires). I purchased two Draeger hand applanation tonometers and took them to my two Brazilian colleagues, and I persuaded each of them to buy a Kretz echograph so that we would be able to conduct a joint study on intraocular pressure and echometry in the diagnosis and follow-up of congenital glaucoma.

Since 1971, I have been using echometry in congenital glaucoma eyes and I have found that, in cases where intraocular pressure readings were suspect because they did not deviate much from normal values, echometry seemed to be a useful new tool. This encouraged us to conduct a systematic study of ocular echometry in normal children in order to establish the mean values and their deviation according to age. We also studied a group of congenital glaucoma patients who were given echometry in addition to the routine examination under general anesthesia. This allowed us to compare the diagnostic value of echometry with that of tonometry.

The proceedings of the Glaucoma Symposium held in Würzburg in 1973 were published in 1974. This book includes one of my papers on the early diagnosis of congenital glaucoma, and on p. 287 [2], for the first time, the usefulness of echography in the early diagnosis of congenital glaucoma is discussed ("Beispiel

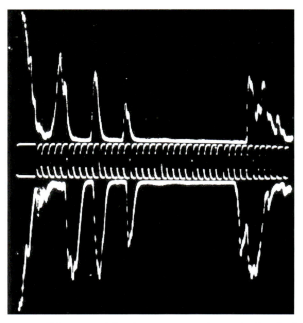

Fig. 6.1 Echogram of the glaucomatous right eye (*top*) and of the normal left eye (*bottom*) arranged as mirror images

für die Nützlichkeit der Echographie": Examples of the usefulness of echography). In this paper, I reported a case in which intraocular pressure values are repeatedly suspect in a child with symptoms of congenital glaucoma and transparent corneas. Figure 6.1, which is a reproduction of Fig. 9 of that paper, is the echogram of this case showing that the eye with symptoms had an axial length of 14.5 mm, whereas its fellow eye measured 12.56 mm.

In 1980, at the 8th SIDUO Meeting, I presented a paper that was published in the book *Documenta Ophthalmologica Proceedings Series 29*, titled "Ocular echometry in the diagnosis of congenital glaucoma" [5].

In 1982, in cooperation with Dr. Caruso, I had the continuation of this paper published in the journal *Archives of Ophthalmology* [6]. In 1982, at the International Glaucoma Society Meeting, I presented a paper that was later published in the book *Glaucoma Update II*, titled: "Ocular echometry and the diagnosis of congenital glaucoma and its evolution" [7]. A. Tarkkanen (Helsinki University Central Hospital, Finland) and G.L. Spaeth (Wills Eye Institute, Philadelphia, PA, USA), respectively, made the following comments on the paper:

I congratulate the author on this excellent paper. Our experience is in agreement with the findings presented. The problem in borderline cases of infantile glaucoma is that the estimates of the intraocular pressure are inaccurate. Applanation tonometry has never been calibrated against infantile corneas in glaucomatous eyes. Our experience of echometry in 20 cases aged from 4 to 48 months shows that the axial lengths in eyes with infantile glaucoma are greater than those of normal controls. Some of the borderline cases show an increase in axial length not attributable to normal growth. After surgery, an early decrease in the axial length down to 0.8 mm has also been noted. The anterior measurements, however, remained unchanged while only the post-equatorial readings showed alterations.

We are impressed with the value of performing ultrasound examinations on children with congenital glaucoma. The test is a very important addition to the other tests that are used in the diagnosis and treatment of children with, or suspected of having, congenital glaucoma. The author is to be congratulated for this important advance.

Reibaldi [8], Tarkkanen et al. [9], Calixto and Cronemberg Sobrinho [10], and Carvalho and Betinjane [11] confirmed the reliability of this method.

During the 12th SIDUO Meeting, Fledelius [12] said that, in the pediatric service he headed in Copenhagen, he had always obtained unreliable false values when measuring intraocular pressure in congenital glaucomas under general anesthesia. He had been very pleased when he read our Nijmegen paper and since then he has been performing only echometries instead of measuring intraocular pressure.

In order to apply echometry to the diagnosis and follow-up of congenital glaucoma, we carried out the following study with normal children with the aim of finding out the values of axial lengths in developing normal eyes and in congenital glaucomas.

Echometry

Material

The first group comprised normal eyes (without ophthalmic symptoms and showing normal applanation tonometry values): 33 eyes of children ranging between 2 and 72 months of age.

The second group was made up of glaucomatous eyes (with characteristic symptoms and pathological intraocular pressure values): 36 eyes in patients ranging from 2 to 24 months of age. This group underwent preoperative as well as immediate postoperative echometry.

The case history plays an important role in the clinical study of a child suspected of having congenital glaucoma. The main factor in this study is the time span between the appearance of symptoms and surgery.

Method

The horizontal corneal diameter was measured. The anterior segment was examined with a biomicroscope, paying particular attention to the chamber angle. The intraocular pressure was measured with applanation tonometry; funduscopy was used to examine the optic nerve, peripheral retina, and macula. The last step involved echometry under cycloplegics.

Echometry Equipment

We used a Kretz 7200 MA echograph (Fig. 6.2a) with a 10-Mhz probe, Ocuscan (SonoMetric Health, Inc., Salt Lake City, UT, USA) (Fig. 6.2b), B Scan S (Quantel Medical, Clermont Ferrand, France) (Fig. 6.2c), or Ocuscan RXP (Alcon Laboratories, Fort Worth, TX, USA) (Fig. 6.2d). We are currently developing a special module for congenital glaucomas for this device. This new module will not only provide information on axial

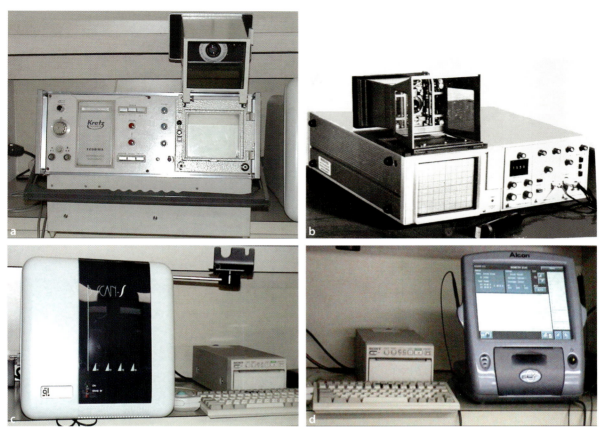

Fig. 6.2 a Kretz echograph. Model 7200 M.A. **b** Ocuscan 400 echograph. (Sonometric). **c** B Scan S (Quantel Medical). **d** Ocuscan RXP (Alcon Laboratories)

length, but will also place this information on the normal eye growth chart in order to determine whether the value is normal or pathological.

An immersion device consisting of a plastic cylinder (Ossoinig Scleral Shell No. 20 manufactured by Hensen Ophthalmic Development Laboratory, Iowa City, IA, USA) (Fig. 6.3a) is fitted to the sclera and four drops of 4,000-centipoise viscosity methylcellulose 2.5% are first instilled in it to seal off the scleral contact area.

The cylinder is then filled with isotonic saline solution. Under general anesthesia (Fig. 6.3b), with the child in the dorsal position, our method enables the eye to be accurately centered, an absolute prerequisite to correct measurement. The probe is then inserted into the cylinder without touching the cornea, up to approximately 0.5 cm from it, thus obtaining echograms at tissue sensitivity and measuring sensitivity.

We take four echograms for each eye.

Figure 6.4 shows a characteristic echogram in which measurements are taken with dividers with the points placed on the base line of the echogram, precisely on the point where each echo arises. Thus the chamber angle, lens, and vitreous body are measured.

Only in cases with corneal edema is the pertinent value taken into consideration, as measured from the two echograms corresponding to the anterior and posterior corneal surfaces; otherwise, a mean value of 0.5 mm is assigned.

With the Ocukretz, the axial length is calculated by the echograph itself, according to the mean sound velocity, and the values appear on the monitor. The peaks representing the cornea, the anterior and posterior surface of the lens, and the posterior ocular wall should be the same height in order to obtain a good measurement. The posterior peak representing the ocular wall should be perfect. It should be perpendicular and start directly at the baseline, with no minor peaks in front of it. The measurement should be performed at measurement sensitivity, i.e., 17 dB.

Since the values are obtained in microseconds, they are converted into millimeters on the basis of the sound velocity in the different transparent media [13]. With

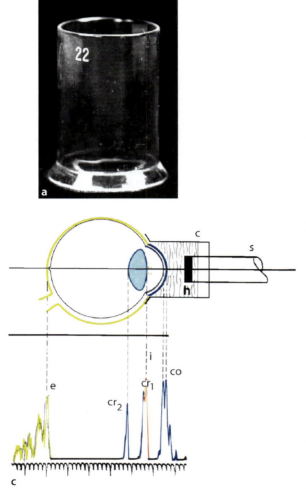

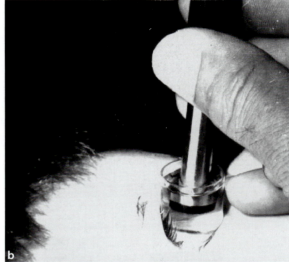

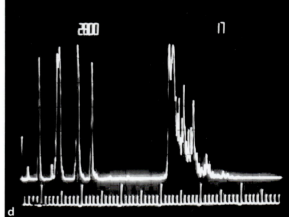

Fig. 6.3 **a** Plastic cylinder for echometry (Ossoinig Shell). **b** To perform echometry, the plastic cylinder is placed on the sclera with some drops of methylcellulose in order to fix it to the sclera. The cylinder is filled with saline solution and when measuring, the proximal edge of the probe should be separated from the corneal vertex by at least 0.5 cm. **c** This sketch correlates the measurement method with the echogram obtained; *s* probe; *c* plastic reservoir; *h* saline solution in the reservoir.

The echogram obtained has been reproduced below; *co* cornea, *i* iris, *cr1* anterior surface of the lens, *cr2* posterior face of the lens, *e* posterior wall of the eyeball, *d* echogram obtained. To obtain good results, it is critical for the peaks representing the anterior and posterior corneal surface, anterior and posterior lens surface, retina, choroid, and sclera, to be at the same level, when the measurement sensitivity is 17 dB

these data, we have built a program for a small Hewlett Packard computer used to calculate the following echometric parameters:

I.   Corneal thickness
II.   Anterior chamber depth
III.   Lens thickness
IV.   Vitreous body length
V.   Axial length

VI. $\dfrac{\text{Anterior chamber}}{\text{Axial length}}$

VII. $\dfrac{\text{Anterior segment (cornea + anterior chamber + lens)}}{\text{Vitreous}}$

VIII. $\dfrac{\text{Cornea + anterior chamber}}{\text{Vitreous}}$

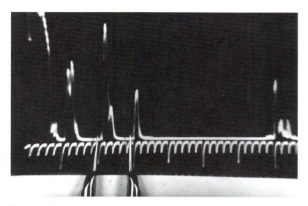

Fig. 6.4 The echogram measures the distances between the posterior corneal surface and the anterior lens surface, between the anterior and posterior lens surface and between the posterior surface of the lens and the retina, in microseconds. Sometimes, in the presence of corneal edema, the distance between anterior and posterior corneal surface is also measured. The use of callipers is very helpful in these measurements

Parameters VI, VII, and VIII are three different indices. It should be taken into account that the axial length is made up by adding I + II + III + IV + the retinal thickness, which is considered a constant, equivalent to 0.35 mm [14].

Statistical Methods Used

The minimum square method was used for the growth curves of normal and pathological eyes according to age. The statistical significance of the echometric differences between groups was calculated by means of the Student t test.

Results

Correlation Between Axial Length and Age in Normal Eyes

A logarithmic growth curve of the population of 36 eyes studied was made according to: $y = a + b (\log x)$, using the following formula:

$$y = 18.7 + 1.245 (\log x)$$

where y is the axial length in mm, and x the age in months.

The correlation coefficient r is 0.9044 ($p < 0.001$) and the significance of the regression coefficient b is $t = 11.82$ ($p < 0.001$). The confidence intervals of the line have also been calculated (for each normal eye studied), as well as the prediction confidence interval for the population of normal children (Table 6.1).

Value of the Prediction Confidence Interval for Normal Eyes in the Differential Diagnosis Between Normal and Glaucomatous Eyes

Figure 6.5 was constructed using the values in Table 6.1. The ordinates show the axial length of the eye in millimeters, and the abscissas, the child's age in months, in logarithmic scale. This is why a straight line, rather than a curve, is obtained.

The dotted band represents the normal range: the values between the mean and standard deviations, upward and downward. The value of this method can be observed in the first statistical analysis presented (Fig. 6.6), where we have included the axial lengths of the 79 eyes with congenital glaucoma. This demonstrates the usefulness of the prediction confidence interval for normal and glaucomatous eyes.

Comparison Between the Echometric Values of the Normal and Congenital Glaucoma Groups

The axial length in normal and in glaucomatous eyes belonging to children up to 2 years of age was presented in the previous section. We will now compare the echometric values of the two groups. First, we will analyze the length or thickness of each of the transparent media independently and then the three indices which can relate these transparent media to each other.

Table 6.2 shows that the measurements of the anterior chamber, vitreous length, and axial length are significantly higher in the population of glaucomatous children. This was previously shown by Gernet and Hollwich [3] and Espildora Couso [15] and explains the influence of elevated IOP on a distensible eye.

The most interesting finding, in our opinion, is the behavior of the lens, which is significantly thinned in the population of glaucomatous eyes. This is an important issue, which contributes to the emmetropization of the glaucomatous eye, whose axial length, if considered in isolation, would justify lower myopia values than those found clinically (the rest of the emmetropization factors are corneal flattening and posterior displacement of the lens via the deep chamber).

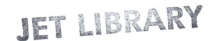

Table 6.1 Correlation between axial length and age in normal eyes

Age in months	Y (mm) Axial length	95% confidence interval Line	Prediction
1	18.7	18.2–19.1	17.3–20.1
2	19.4	19.0–19.7	18.0–20.7
3	19.8	19.4–20.1	18.4–21.1
4	20.0	19.8–20.3	18.7–21.4
5	20.3	20.0–20.5	19.9–21.6
6	20.4	20.2–20.7	19.1–21.8
7	20.5	20.3–20.8	19.3–21.9
8	20.7	20.5–20.9	19.4–22.0
9	20.8	20.6–21.1	19.5–22.2
10	20.9	20.7–21.2	19.6–22.3
11	21.0	20.8–21.3	19.7–22.4
12	21.1	20.9–21.3	19.8–22.4
18	21.5	21.3–21.8	20.2–22.8
24	21.8	21.5–22.1	20.5–23.1
30	22.0	21.7–22.3	20.7–23.3
36	22.2	21.9–22.5	20.8–23.5
42	22.3	22.0–22.7	21.0–23.7
48	22.5	22.1–22.8	21.1–23.8
54	22.6	22.2–22.9	21.2–23.9
60	22.7	22.3–23.1	21.3–24.0
66	22.8	22.5–23.3	21.4–24.1
72	22.9	22.5–23.3	21.5–24.2
78	22.9	22.5–23.3	21.6–24.3
84	23.0	22.6–23.4	21.6–24.4

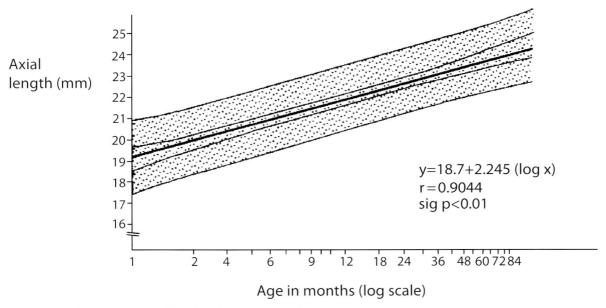

Fig. 6.5 Correlation between axial length and age in 36 normal eyes

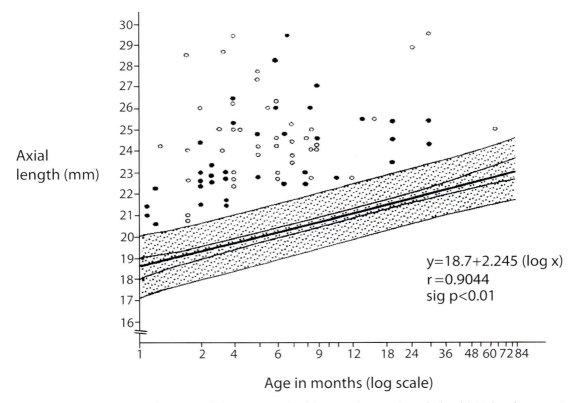

Fig. 6.6 Seventy-nine eyes with congenital glaucoma outside of the normal range, above the band (• Trabeculotomy, ∘ Combined surgery)

Table 6.2 Study of the index correlating the different transparent segments

Echometry	Normal	Glaucomatous	Student t test
Number of eyes	33	22	
Cornea	0.54	0.64 ± 0.24	-3.75^*
Anterior chamber	3.04 ± 0.51	3.57 ± 0.53	5.30^*
Lens	3.85 ± 0.24	3.50 ± 0.25	-4.82^*
Vitreous	13.25 ± 1.18	14.70 ± 0.93	-4.84
Axial length	20.97 ± 1.48	22.75 ± 1.05	

*Significant difference $p < 0.001$

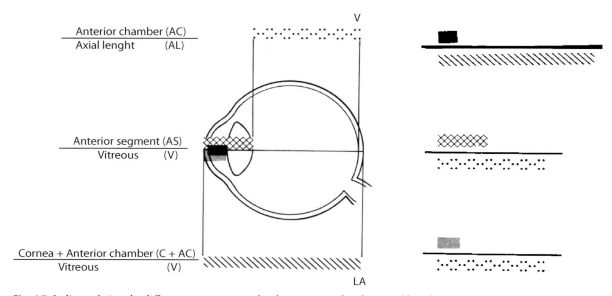

Fig. 6.7 Indices relating the different segments to each other: anterior chamber–axial length, anterior segment–vireous, cornea–anterior chamber–vitreous

Figure 6.7 shows the three indices relating these segments to each other:

VI. $\dfrac{\text{Anterior chamber}}{\text{Axial length}}$

VII. $\dfrac{\text{Anterior segment (cornea + anterior chamber + lens)}}{\text{Vitreous}}$

VIII. $\dfrac{\text{Cornea + anterior chamber}}{\text{Vitreous}}$

The statistical study of these segments demonstrated that for indices VI and VIII, there is no significant difference between normal and glaucomatous eyes. However, the difference is highly significant in index VII. Table 6.2 shows the values of these indices.

Index VI $\dfrac{\text{Anterior chamber}}{\text{Axial length}}$ and

index VIII $\dfrac{\text{Cornea + anterior chamber}}{\text{Vitreous}}$

are significantly different in both populations, because in most cases, eyes exposed to ocular hypertension increase their anteroposterior length harmoniously, i.e., both anterior chamber and vitreous length grow. In contrast, index VII is significantly lower in glaucomatous children, since it includes the lens, whose thickness is lower in eyes with congenital glaucoma.

Echometric Asymmetry in Bilateral Congenital Glaucomas

Of a total of 60 cases studied, 20 were unilateral and 40 bilateral. In the latter, a manifest asymmetry was found in axial length as well as in each of the segments making up the transparent media. This asymmetry might be related to the difference in IOP usually found in the two eyes of the same patient. This finding markedly contrasts with the values obtained both in normal children (33 eyes) and in bilateral megalocorneas (ten eyes) where asymmetry is typical.

The Value of Echometry in the Follow-Up of Pure Congenital Glaucoma

Echometry is a very valuable method for the follow-up of congenital glaucomas after surgery. This was re-

ported for the first time by Buschmann and Bluth [4]. As shown in Fig. 6.8, we have found four different types of progression in pure congenital glaucomas:

a. The axial length stops growing with time, reaching the normal range band and, as the child grows, progressing further within the normal range; then it continues its growth normally. In most cases, this axial length behavior is consistent with IOP regulation up to 4 years of age. The functional results depend on the preoperative axial length. Those cases with axial lengths of 23–24 mm have good functional results, while in those over 25 mm, the results are generally less favorable (Fig. 6.8, solid line).

b. The axial length continues its growth through successive postoperative check-ups, going outside the normal range band. This type is generally associated with ocular hypertension that has not been resolved by surgery. In these cases, if IOP readings are normal, it will have to be measured under general anesthesia on different days at different times, in order to detect IOP peaks. It should be remembered that during the first 24 months of age, the normal IOP values should not exceed 7–14 mmHg (Fig. 6.8, hatched line).

c. In some cases, even though the IOP is regulated, the axial length remains stable for some time, but starts to grow between 2 and 4 years of age, and then becomes stable again. This phenomenon was reported

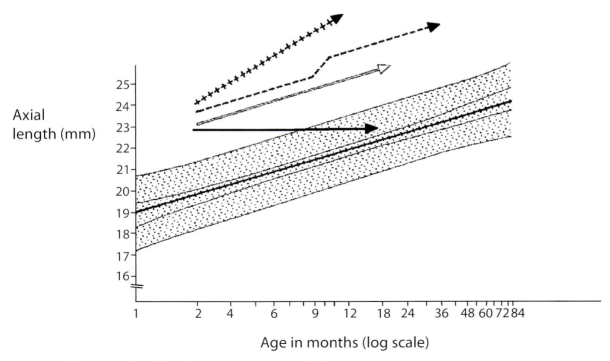

Fig. 6.8 Different types of axial length progression in congenital glaucomas

by M. Massin and B. Pellat (personal communication). The reason for this has not been elucidated, but the IOP in these cases should be monitored more frequently (Fig. 6.8, dashed line).

d. Some cases in which the eye continues to grow parallel to the normal range, while the IOP remains regulated, have a good prognosis (Fig. 6.8, double line).

Figure 6.8 illustrates the four types of progression. When echometry is performed at week 1 or 2 postoperatively, in most cases it yields slightly decreased axial length values compared with those found before surgery, but 2 or 3 months later, they have returned to their previous values. This phenomenon is more evident in myopic eyes with pure congenital glaucoma.

Every time an echometry is performed in the follow-up of a case of congenital glaucoma, an A and B echography of the eye and orbit must always be made, as illustrated by the following case history.

Examples

Case 1

A 4-month old girl, referred to us by another ophthalmologist with a presumed diagnosis of congenital glaucoma. The first measurements of intraocular pressure were:

	Right eye	Left eye
On presentation	15 mmHg	9 mmHg
1 Month later	15 mmHg	6 mmHg
45 Days later	15 mmHg	6 mmHg

The symptoms persisted (marked photophobia), without corneal edema, with normal diameter of both corneas, and with physiological excavation of the optic nerve. The only remarkable point was the pressure difference between the right eye (15 mmHg) and the left eye (9 mmHg). In the normal pressure curve corresponding to the age of this child (4 months), the maximum intraocular pressure should not exceed 12 mmHg. However, it is very difficult to indicate surgery in an eye with an intraocular pressure of 15 mmHg and a clear cornea. We were not sure whether or not to operate.

At 6 months of age, echometry was done. The length of the vitreous in the right eye was 14.55 mm and in the left eye was 12.66 mm. In successive echograms, it continued increasing its axial length. We operated, the growth stopped, and the ocular pressure equaled that of the other eye. This case shows the value of echometry in cases with uncertain diagnosis.

Case 2

A 3-month-old male child presented in October 1978 with symptoms of unilateral childhood congenital glaucoma, with a corneal diameter of 12 in the right eye and 12.5 in the left eye (pathological eye); the intraocular pressure under general anesthesia was 10 mmHg in the right eye and 29 mmHg in the left eye. The cornea of the left eye presented a 0.78-mm edema compared with 0.54 mm in the normal eye. The length of the vitreous and the axial length were significantly greater than in the healthy eye (see table below). We successfully performed a trabeculotomy in the affected eye. Two months later, in December 1978, he came back for a check-up and, as can be seen in the table below, the ocular pressure was 8 mmHg in the right eye and

Date	Corneal diameter	Intraocular pressure	Vitreous	Echometry	
				Axial length	Anterior segment
October 1978	12	10	12.26	20.29	0.63
	12.5	**29**	13.02	21.15	0.60
November 1978	12	8	**13.41**	**21.44**	0.57
	12.5	8	12.64	20.53	0.60
February 1979	**13.5**	**25**	**13.79**	**21.71**	0.56
	12.5	12	12.64	20.29	0.58

Compare the values in black with the Fig. 6.9

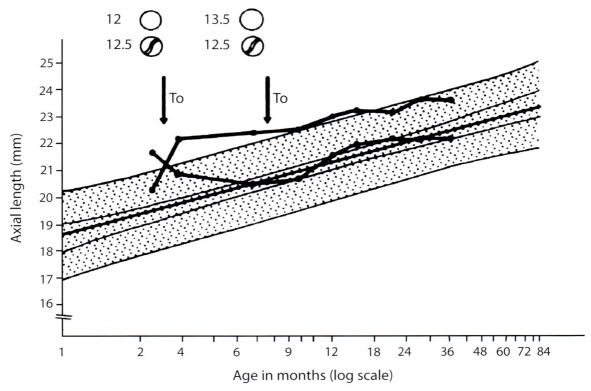

Fig. 6.9 Case 2. *Double arrow*, right eye, *solid arrow* left eye. The *arrows* indicate surgery. *To* trabeculotomy, *small circles* cornea with or without breakage of the endothelium and Descemet membrane. The *numbers near the circles* represent the corneal diameter in millimeters

8 mmHg in the left eye, and the corneal diameter had not changed. However, note the length of the vitreous body and the axial length of the healthy eye that had no symptoms; at that time, they were greater than those of the operated unhealthy eye. We took these data into account but, with no symptoms and no increased ocular pressure, with a normal optic nerve, we did not feel it was right to operate.

Two months later, in February 1979, when the child came for a check-up, everything was found to be perfectly under control in the operated eye, but the ocular pressure in the previously healthy eye (right eye) was 25 mmHg and the length of the vitreous body and the axial length, as well as being greater than those of the operated eye, were also greater than they had been in December. The cornea had also progressed from 12 mm to 13.5 mm. We immediately operated on the eye and, as can be seen in Fig. 6.9 and the measurements table for Case 1, the intraocular pressure dropped to normal values and the rapid, progressive increase in echom-

etry values stopped. In time, when the child reached 1.5 years of age, the dimensions were normal. For the family, the treatment was a complete success, but we know that the second eye, instead of being operated at 7 months, should have been done at 4 months.

Case 3

A male patient came to us at the age of 8 years. In each eye another colleague had done four surgeries for congenital glaucoma. The right eye had normal pressure and the optic nerve was normal, while the left eye presented phthisis bulbi.

One examination per year was done during the follow-up. When he was 12 years old, while doing the echography after the echometry, I found a mucocele invading the orbit after breaking through the orbit's inner wall, extending as far as the ethmoidal and frontal sinus (Fig. 6.10).

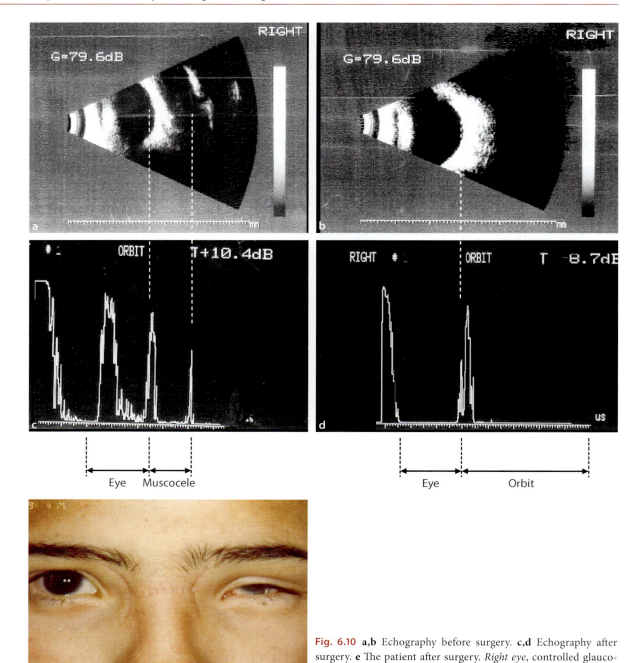

Fig. 6.10 a,b Echography before surgery. **c,d** Echography after surgery. **e** The patient after surgery. *Right eye*, controlled glaucoma. *Left eye*, phthisis bulbi. The patient is now 22 years old, has good vision and good visual field

Conclusions

Axial length enlargement in children with congenital glaucoma is not a recent discovery, since the word "buphthalmos" was coined by Ambroise Paré in 1561 for its resemblance to a bull's eye.

The value of echometry for an accurate comparison of the growth of normal and glaucomatous eyes was stressed by Gernet and Hollwich [3] and the importance of the follow-up of congenital glaucomas was highlighted by Buschmann and Bluth [4]. Based on these studies, we [5, 6] have proposed echometry as a vital method for the diagnosis and follow-up [7] of congenital glaucomas.

The study of axial length in children with congenital glaucoma is a very valuable parameter, and this has been widely confirmed since 1983. It is very useful in the diagnosis of congenital glaucoma cases in which the IOP is slightly above the normal range, or in the diagnosis of glaucoma in the fellow eye of children thought to have unilateral congenital glaucoma. IOP was considered the most important variable in the diagnosis of congenital glaucoma until this new application of echometry was found. The main difference between tonometry in adults and children is that it is impossible to perform diurnal pressure curves in children. The second difference lies in the fact that in some places it is necessary to measure IOP under general anesthesia. The literature around the world indicates that Penthrane cannot be used in some countries, or other types of anesthetic agents are used, though these give inaccurate values since they modify the blood pressure or they influence the central nervous system. In other places, intubation is used. Using the method we have introduced, with Penthrane, the values obtained are highly accurate.

Even if the IOP is measured according to our method, and the reading is accurate, we cannot monitor IOP for 24 h as we can in adults (diurnal pressure curve). The IOP varies greatly over the 24-h period, while the axial length growth in congenital glaucoma reflects only long-term variations (days, months, or years), as a result of IOP rises in distensible eyes. An IOP reading is true only for that particular moment, when it was measured, while axial length values yield information on what has happened in the course of the disease, for a longer period up to the moment of the measurement.

Moreover, IOP readings are influenced by different anesthetic agents, but not echometry. Echometry is therefore the first vital parameter for diagnosis, followed by IOP measurement and other clinical studies.

Echometry is also vital in the follow-up of the disease. In one of our cases, both the family and the ophthalmologist thought surgery had been successful because the child, who had come for consultation with 40 mmHg of IOP, had reduced it to 20 mmHg. Nevertheless, they were wrong, because the normal maximum IOP for a child aged 12 months is 14 mmHg. In cases like this one, since echometry shows that the eye has not stopped growing and that the axial length is growing further outside the normal range, the ophthalmologist will be aware of this and will prescribe medical therapy or reoperation; otherwise the eye will develop irreversible optic nerve, visual field, and macular function damage.

Some cases have very elevated IOP with no axial length growth, but these are late congenital glaucomas in which the IOP started to rise at 5 years of age, when the sclera has already lost its elasticity. Leydhecker [17], Ytterborg [18], and Dannheim [19] called attention to the variations of scleral rigidity in children of different ages.

Many other authors have confirmed our findings and added further data on the value of echometry in the diagnosis and follow-up of congenital glaucoma (B. Schwartz, personal communication; G. Quigley, personal communication).

References

1. Sampaolesi R (1969) La pression oculaire et le sinus camerulaire chez l'enfant normal et dans le glaucome congénital aux dessous de l'âge de 5 ans. Docum Ophthal 26:497–515
2. Sampaolesi R, Reca R, Carro A, Armando A (1976) Normaler Intraokularer Druck bei Kindern bis zu 5 Jahren mit und ohne Allgemeinnarkose. Seine Wichtigkeit für die Frühdiagnose des angeborenen Glaukoms. In: Glaukom Symposium Würzburg 1974, Enke, Stuttgart, pp 278–289
3. Gernet H, Hollwich F (1969) Oculometrie des kindlichen Glaukoms. Ver Zusammenkunft Dtsch Ophthalmol Ges 69:341–348
4. Buschmann W, Bluth K (1974) Ultrasonographic follow-up examination of congenital glaucoma. Graefes Arch Ophthalmol 192:313–319
5. Sampaolesi R (1980) Ocular echometry in the diagnosis of congenital glaucoma. In: Thijssen JM, Verbeek AM (eds) Doc Ophthalmol Proc Series, Vol. 29. Dr. W. Junk, The Hague, pp 177–189
6. Sampaolesi R, Carusso R (1982) Ocular echometry in the diagnosis of congenital glaucoma. Arch Ophthalmol 100:574–577
7. Sampaolesi R (1983) Ocular echometry and the diagnosis of congenital glaucoma and its evolution. In: Krieglstein GK, Leydhecker W (eds) Glaucoma update II. Springer, Berlin Heidelberg New York, pp 175–184
8. Reibaldi A (1982) Biometric ultrasound in the diagnosis and follow-up of congenital glaucoma. Glaucoma editorial. Ann of Ophthalmol pp 707–708
9. Tarkanen A, Uusitalo R, Mianowicz J (1983) Ultrasonographic biometry in congenital glaucoma. Acta Ophthalmol 61:618
10. Calixto N, Cronemberg Sobrinho A (1981) Glaucoma cortisônico. Etudo de 15 casos. Rev Bras Oftalmol 40:19–42
11. Carvalho CA, Betinjane AJ (1983) Variações da biometria ultrasonografica em olhos normais nos primeiros 50 meses de idade. Arq Bras Oftalmol 46:96–99

12. Fledelius HC (1990) Eye size of the premature infant around presumed term. In: Sampaolesi R (ed) Ultrasonography in ophthalmology, 12. Kluwer, Dordrecht, pp 165–172

13. Jansson F, Kock E (1962) Determination of the velocity of ultrasound in the human lens and vitreous. Acta Ophthalmol Kbh 39:899

14. François J, Goes F (1975) Oculometry of progressive myopia. In: François J, Goes F (eds) Ultrasonography in ophthalmology. Bibl Ophthalmol 83:277–282

15. Espildora Couso J, Vicuña R (1979) Alteraciones biométricas en el control tardío del ojo con glaucoma congénito operado. Glaucoma Symposium. The Panamerican Congress of Ophthalmology, Miami, 1979

16. Leydhecker W (1973) Glaukom. In: Ein Handbuch, 2. Springer, Berlin Heidelberg New York, pp 58–75

17. Ytterborg J (1960) On scleral rigidity. Oslo University Press, Oslo

18. Dannheim R (1968) Bericht über die 69. Zusammenkunft der DOG, p 248

Contents

For the ophthalmologist, just as for any medical doctor in any other clinical or surgical speciality, the advances in molecular biology, which include those in genetics, are difficult to understand because of the terminology used and the modern biological concepts involved.

These advances are one of the best examples of so-called translational research (translating basic research into clinical practice and vice-versa), for the practical management of these new concepts deriving from this research [1].

Our goal here is to give an easily understood account of the genetics of glaucoma and the diseases within glaucoma and the new therapies becoming available today.

Different statistics from a variety of countries show that today at least one in 50 newborns suffers from a significant congenital anomaly, one in 100 has a single-gene abnormality, and one in 200 a severe chromosome disorder.

What Is a Chromosome?

Chromosomes are organelles located in the nucleus of normal human cells with a set number of 46 (Fig. 7.1), 44 of which are autosomes and two sexual chromosomes (XX or XY). Chromosomes are structures composed of deoxyribonucleic acid that are arranged in the shape of a paired double helix, one of which comes from the father and the other from the mother.

They can be classified with hematological stains such as Giemsa according to the position of their cen-

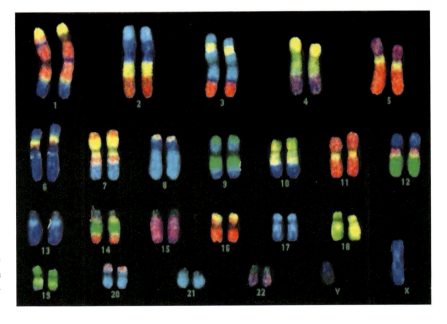

Fig. 7.1 Fluorescent in-situ hybridization (FISH) identification of human chromosomes: chromosome painting

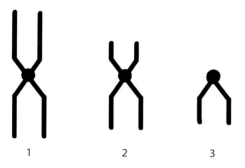

tromeres, a primary construction within them. The centromere is the point where the identical double helixes of deoxyribonucleic acid (DNA) join – this makes it possible for the chromosomes to be classified as (Fig. 7.2):

1. Metacentric;
2. Submetacentric;
3. Acrocentric.

In metacentric chromosomes, the centromeres are in the middle (these are chromosomes 1, 3, 19, and 20).

In the submetacentrics, the centromere divides the chromosomes into a short arm (called p from the French *petit*) and a long one (called q as this is the next letter in the alphabet).

Acrocentric chromosomes are those that have very short arms and also, different from the former, have satellites (deoxyribonucleic acid sequences) joined to the centromere (these are chromosomes 13, 14, 15, 21, 22, and the sexual Y chromosome).

Chromosome abnormalities can thus be classified by modifications in their number and shape. On this basis, with each cell, for example the endothelial cell of the human trabecular meshwork, having 46 chromosomes with different shapes depending on the position of the centromere, and each chromosome being made up of various genes, it is logical to think that at least part of the etiology of a disorder can be detected in these structures.

Chromosome Abnormalities

Chromosome abnormalities are those in which their number, shape, or internal characteristics are altered. The internal characteristics are the number of genes, type of genes, dominant or recessive, change in location, and mutation leading to a change in function. These alterations give rise to serious anomalies in the phenotypical and functional characteristics to which these genes respond.

Chromosome abnormalities are seen in numerical or morphological alterations. Numerical alterations involve an increase or reduction in chromosomes.

The best example of an increase in chromosome quantity is the trisomies: one example is Down syndrome, in which the general anomalies manifest as a mental deficit, cardiac abnormalities, and short stature. Ophthalmological alterations are mongoloid palpebral fissure, cataract, myopia, nodules in the iris, hypoplasia of the peripheral iris, keratoconus, etc.

In other trisomies such as 13, or Patau syndrome, and 18, or Edward syndrome, there are multiple ocular abnormalities, but glaucoma is rarely found.

As mentioned above, the alterations in the number of chromosomes can manifest as a reduction in the normal number. One example of these numerical alterations is monosomy, where instead of two chromosomes there is only one.

Turner syndrome is an example of monosomy, in which the somatic manifestations are short stature, skeletal anomalies, prominent ears, and mental retardation.

In the anterior segment, its ocular manifestations include epicanthus, ptosis, blue sclera, microcornea, eccentric pupil, cataracts, posterior embryotoxon, and fundamentally all have glaucoma as well as nystagmus.

In the posterior segment, the retina will show tortuosity of the retinal blood vessels, pseudopapillitis, optic atrophy, Coats disease, retinitis pigmentosa, macular aplasia, and basically glaucoma, color blindness, and strabismus. As a result of these manifestations, nystagmus may appear.

A second very interesting example is cri-du-chat syndrome, another monosomy, like Coats disease. Its somatic manifestations are severe abnormalities of the intestines, microcephaly and mental retardation, short metacarpal bones, and micrognathia. Ocular manifestations are hypertelorism, epicanthal folds, coloboma of the eyelids, tear reduction, exotropia, cataracts, and tortuous retinal blood vessels, but glaucoma is very rare.

Another very important example of monosomy presenting with glaucoma is Degrouchy syndrome, which

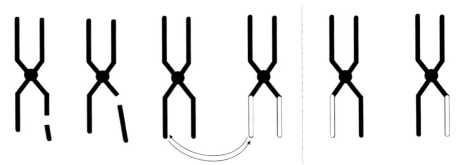

Fig. 7.3 Partial loss of some chromosomes   **Fig. 7.4** Translocation

also presents mental retardation, short stature, and cardiac, visceral and general anomalies.

Alterations in the Shape of Chromosomes

There may also be arm deletion, a partial loss of a segment (Fig. 7.3), or translocation, a misplacement of a chromosome fragment or from one to another (Fig. 7.4). Retinoblastoma, a typical example of this type of alteration, must also be remembered.

Gene Abnormalities

What Is a Gene?

A gene is a region of a chromosome, consisting of units of DNA and containing codes of information for producing a particular protein or enzyme. It can potentially mutate, and some genes exist in several copies of the genome (the set of all the genes expressed in DNA), while others are unique. Genes are located at specific sites of the homologous chromosomes and exist in pairs called alleles [2].

When an individual is homozygotic in relation to a phenotypic character (e.g., hair or eye color), this is because both the genes or alleles are identical. When they are heterozygotic, each gene of the pair or allele is different and specifies different characteristics.

There are dominant genes and recessive ones. If one of the genes of the pair is dominant, the phenotypic expression will be exclusively of the dominant one. Within this group, the dominance of a gene can be absolute or partial. Thus in some examples, such as aniridia, dominance is absolute; this means that the existence of just one altered gene is sufficient for the lack of iris to manifest itself.

In cases where the dominance is not absolute, both the altered genes, maternal and paternal, are needed for the disease to be expressed. This is also known as penetrance. The higher the penetrance, the greater the percentage of descendants affected by the disease.

If both genes are recessive, the phenotypic expression will be the result of that recessive gene. Naturally, if both are dominant, the result in the phenotype will be dominance.

Genes are classified into various types:

- Structural: according to the protein it generates;
- Regulator: when it controls an enzyme activity within the metabolism;
- Topographic: when it determines the location of a protein or enzyme within the cell, for example, that the enzyme be situated in the cell membrane or in an organelle.
- Temporal: when it determines the activity of other genes at different stages of life.

Thus the pathology of a gene or various genes, simultaneously or otherwise, can cause multiple disorders as a result of mutated proteins, poor enzyme control, wrong location, or wrong stage of life.

The most common genetic defect is mutation, i.e., a change in the information for forming a protein or enzyme (Fig. 7.5).

The gene information is codified in messages by DNA sequences.

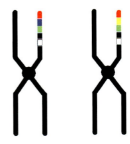

Fig. 7.5 Mutation

The term "gene" is given to a definite, limited portion of a chromosome that can be seen sometimes morphologically, and at others, more often used today, by gel densitometry, or by polymerase chain reaction (PCR), which are molecular biology techniques. These are the ones where etiology is related with a modification of the normal structure of more than one gene.

The next question must be: where are genes located?

Genes constitute very small parts of the chromosomes, and their anomalies consist of abnormalities of one or more genes (polygenic/multifactorial inheritance). In the first case, the alteration is simply a mutation or modification within the structure of a particular gene, which is expressed by a mutated protein, or some form of morphological expression such as the loss of homozygosity, microsatellite alterations (of the gene satellites), etc.

Each Mendelian feature is represented by two variants of the same gene, maternal or paternal, which are called alleles and occupy the same locus or place of two homologous chromosomes. Genes in turn may be autosomal if they belong to an autosome, or sex-linked if they are located in the X or Y chromosome. It should be remembered that the father and the mother each provide one of the pair of genes, and this is why it is important to study the Mendelian features of the genealogical tree. Nowadays, the ability to map the genes of the chromosomes enables genetic defects to be linked with specific structural chromosome defects, establishing a biologically very important bridge between Mendelian genetics and modern cytogenetics, based on more precise techniques such as the study of DNA.

Every genetic message is coded in DNA sequences, with the codon as the basic genetic unit, consisting of a triplet of DNA bases. This sequence is transmitted in a series of amino acids, forming a polypeptide chain, i.e., a protein, the basic principle of modern genetics.

To sum up, we have chromosomes that are made up of pairs of genes, which are in turn made up of DNA. Based on this information (of the DNA), the proteins will come out as normal or as mutated.

In glaucoma, the study of these gene alterations is being fully applied [3], through numerous mappings of loci in different genes, such as the lq23, Chr2, 3q21-q24, 8q23, as well as other genes on Chr7 and Chr10. Thus primary open-angle glaucoma (POAG) could be a variety of diseases at the molecular level (molecular pathology), explaining certain cases of different clinical behavior, based simply on forms that are molecularly different [4–6]. In some cases, chromosomes 2, 14, 17, and 19 may be involved in this pathology, suggesting for example that POAG constitutes a heterogeneous genetic disorder.

An ophthalmologist who wishes to put this research into practice could do the chromosome, gene, and DNA sequence studies using different methods, and the studies can be done on affected tissues removed for therapeutic reasons, such as filtering operations, or on the patient's blood cells. In the not too distant future, gene therapy may be included in the alternative protocols.

To apply the knowledge of genetics in glaucoma, we will classify it as follows:
1. Congenital glaucomas:
   – Primary [7];
   – Primary refractory [8];
   – Associated with ocular alterations: Rieger, Peters, Axenfeld, aniridia, sclerocornea, cornea plana, isolated retinal dysplasia, persistent hyperplastic primary vitreous;
   – Associated with ocular and somatic alterations: neurofibromatosis, Sturge–Weber and Klippel–Trenaunay syndromes, Norrie disease, Warburg syndrome, and retinal dysplasia;
   – Associated with metabolism errors: hyperaminoaciduria, Lowe syndrome – (oculocerebrorenal syndrome), Fanconi syndrome, homocystinuria, Hurler syndrome (mucopolysaccharidosis), ochronosis (alkaptonuria);
   – Associated with mesodermic dystrophies: Marfan syndrome, Marchesani syndrome;
   – Associated with goniodysgeneses [9, 10]: late congenital glaucoma, Busacca metaplasia, pigmentary;
   – Associated with the nevus of Ota and other ocular melanocytosis;
2. Nonhereditary congenital glaucomas:
   – Rubeola;
   – Toxoplasmosis;
3. Secondary pediatric glaucomas:
   – Retinopathy of prematurity.

Therefore, if we examine the above and our practical experience in observation, especially of the angle, we will recognize:
- Glaucomas with an altered phenotype: Barkan's membrane, pathological mesoderm remains, etc.
- Glaucomas with a normal phenotype and normal gonioscopic angle.

In both cases, there is gene alteration (in one or more genes) and consequently the molecule, the filtration-related protein or proteins in question, are altered; knowing their names will help gene therapy [11].

In the international nomenclature, it was arbitrarily decided that the chromosomes affecting open-angle

Table 7.1 Molecular genetics of primary congenital glaucoma: gene references and protein results

Locus name	Gene symbol	Chromosome locus	Protein name
GLC3A	CYP1B1	2p22-p21	Cytochrome P450-1B1
GLC3B	Unknown	1p36.2-p36.1	Unknown
GLC3C	Unknown	14q 24.3	Unknown

From [12]

glaucomas should be identified as GLC1, those of closed-angle as GLC2, and congenital glaucomas as GLC3. Stone [4, 5] for example, described a family with congenital glaucoma in which the alteration was found on chromosome 1, on its long arm, so the name given was GLC3,1q, where GLC3 means congenital glaucoma, the number "1" indicates that the chromosome affected is chromosome 1, and the letter "q" means the long arm.

There are numerous chromosomes already detected in congenital glaucomas, for example:

- GLC3,1q21-q31;
- GLC3,1p36-6p25;
- GLC3,2p21.

In other disorders such as Rieger syndrome, the affected chromosomes have been recognized: 4q25 and d13q14.

In aniridia, there are two types of aniridia: (1) an1 in Chr. 2p and (2) an2 (wagr) 11p 13 – where the "w" means Wilms tumor, the "a" is for aniridia, the "g" for genitourinary disorders, and the "r" for mental retardation.

Ophthalmology is one of the areas where the greatest number of genes have been found to be affected in ophthalmologic diseases. It is calculated that there are currently from 50–100,000 genes, 10% of which may be involved in some ocular disease (between 5 and 10,000). See Table 7.1 for an example.

Genetic Counseling

The mode of inheritance in primary congenital glaucoma there is autosomal recessive, and prenatal testing can determine the risk for this disease. With a *CYP1B1* (GLC31) mutation, an individual has a 25% chance of being affected, a 50% of being asymptomatic, and a 25% chance of being unaffected. However, further studies are necessary for the proper implementation of this risk evaluation method. The detection of phenotype (goniodysgenesis) is very important for the genetic counseling in ophthalmological practice.

References

1. Santillo C, Brinelli M (2003) Eziopatogenesi dei glaucomi infantili. Boll Oculi 82:103–116
2. Musarella MA (1992) Gene mapping of ocular diseases. Surv Ophthalmol 36:285–312
3. Gonzalez EO, Rodriguez MM, Gonzalez Garcia AD y Cruz AL (1999) Avances en la genética de los glaucomas. Rev Cubana Oftalmol 12:77–83
4. Stone E.M, Fingert JH, Alward WLM, Nguyen TD et al (1997) Identification of a gene that causes primary open glaucoma. Science 275:668–670
5. Sheffield VC, Stone EM, Alward WLM, Drack AV, Johnson AT, Streb LM, Nichols BE (1993) Genetic linkage of familial open-angle glaucoma to chromosome 1q21-q31. Nat Genet 4:47–50
6. Aldred MA, Baumber L, Hill A, Schwalbe EC, Goh K, Karwatowski W, Trembath RC (2004) Low prevalence of MYOC mutations in UK primary open-angle glaucoma patients limits the utility of genetic testing. Hum Genet 115:428–431
7. Walton DS, Katsavounidou G (2005) Newborn primary congenital glaucoma: 2005 update. J Pediatr Ophthalmol Strabismus 42:333–341
8. Cohn AC, Kearns LS, Savarirayan R, Ryan J, Craig JE, Mackey DA (2005) Chromosomal abnormalities and glaucoma: a case of congenital glaucoma with trisomy 8q22-qter/monosomy 9p23-pter. Ophthalmic Genet 26:45–53
9. Kniestedt C, Kammann MTT, Stürmer J, Gloor BP (2000) Dysgenetische Kammerwinkelveränderungen bei Patienten mit Glaukom oder Verdacht auf Glaukom aufgetreten vor dem 40. Lebensjahr. Klin Monatsbl Augenheilkd 216:377–387
10. Richards JE, Lichter PR, Boehnke M, Justine LA, Uro, Torrez D, Wong D, Johnson T (1994) Mapping of a gene for autosomal dominant juvenile-onset open-angle glaucoma to chromosome I q". Am J Hum Genet 54:62–70

11. Bergen AA, Leschot NJ, Husman CA, De Smet MD, De Jong PT (2004) From gene to disease: primary open-angle glaucoma and three known genes: MYOC, CYP1B1 and OPTN. Ned Tijdschr Geneeskd 148:1343–1344

12. Bejjani BA, Edward DP (2007) Primary congenital glaucoma. Gene Reviews. http://www.ncbi.nlm.nih.gov/bookshelf/br.fcgi?book=gene&part=glc. Cited 29 July 2008. University of Washington, Seattle

Contents

Embryology of the Chamber Angle

Embryological Development of the Chamber Angle. The Normal and Abnormal Chamber Angle in Newborns up to 1 Year of Age and Its Importance with Respect to Pathology

We will leave aside the discussion of the two most widely accepted theories regarding the mechanism by which the chamber angle is formed: whether it results from atrophy and resorption [1] or from cleavage and separation into layers [2].

The primordium of the chamber angle appears between the 3rd and 5th month of gestation. It is ring-shaped and its periphery is bounded by a triangular area with its base facing it.

In 1906, Seefelder and Wolfrum [3] described the formation of the anterior chamber and chamber angle, which can be summarized as follows:

1. The ciliary processes develop at the end of the 3rd month of gestation.
2. The Schlemm canal appears in the second half of the 4th month.
3. The anterior chamber appears at the end of the 5th month and its development finishes in the middle of the 6th month.

At the end of the 3rd month, a primordium of the anterior chamber can be seen at the periphery, even when there is no mesoderm there.

At the beginning of the 6th month, the lens touches the posterior surface of the cornea only at its posterior pole.

The iridopupillary membrane, the central part of which later gives rise to the pupillary membrane, and its peripheral part to the iris stroma, is located in front of the lens capsule.

"Mesodermal tissue can be found at the chamber angle, between the corneoscleral trabecular meshwork (ciliary muscle tendon) and the ciliary processes and the iris. In the fetal stage, this corneoscleral trabecular meshwork reduces the anterior chamber" [3]. These authors named it the pectinate ligament, as did Hüeck, since it is very similar to this characteristic formation of ungulates (rabbits and horses). Since the Symposium on Congenital Glaucoma held in Venice, we have preferred to call it normal mesodermal tissue.

Figure 8.1 shows the histologic appearance of the primordium of the chamber angle at the 7th, 8th, and 9th months of gestation with corresponding graphics.

The chamber angle develops by enlarging in two directions: toward the periphery and backward. It has a loose and definite mesenchymal tissue (squared in the graphic).

It is triangular in shape, bounded toward the front by the longitudinal part of the ciliary muscle and by the scleral trabecular meshwork, which is its tendon, and to the rear by the future iris root, the bundles of the radiated ciliary muscle (Ivanoff's muscle) and the ciliary processes. The third side is formed by the anterior chamber at that location (Fig. 8.1). As shown in the figure, in the 7th month, both the Schlemm canal and the spur are clearly distinguishable: the black circles represent the circular part of the ciliary muscle, which is starting to develop, and the thick black band, its longitudinal part. The squared areas represent the mesodermal tissue.

It should be noted that the Schlemm canal extends posteriorly to the peripheral limit of the anterior chamber.

By the 8th month (Fig. 8.1b), the anterior chamber has extended toward the periphery, the radial part of the ciliary muscle has developed further (in an antero-posterior direction), the mesodermal tissue has shortened and thickened, and the separation between its layers is greater (large squares).

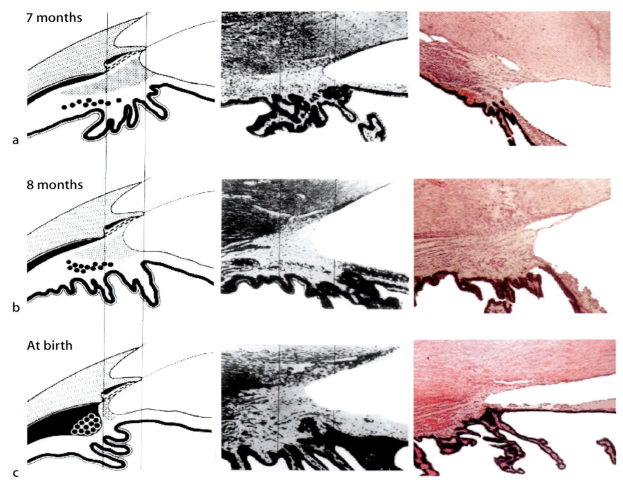

Fig. 8.1a–c Intrauterine development of the chamber angle. **a** Chamber angle at the 7th month; **b** chamber angle at the 8th month. In **a**, the anterior chamber just reaches the Schwalbe line. Behind it, the mesodermal tissue has a very tight mesh (*small squares*); it extends over the whole area from the scleral trabecular meshwork (*dotted line*) to the radiated muscle and the ciliary process. In **b**, the anterior chamber enlarges in a distal direction. The meshes of the mesodermal tissue are looser (*larger squares*). In **c**, at birth, the anterior chamber enlarges even further and the mesodermal tissue is reduced to a thin layer that will later become the Busacca trabecular conjunctival layer, also known as the Rohen iridoscleral membrane. (The histologic sections on the *right*, from [3]). The corresponding graphics are displayed on the *left*. On the *right* (in color) an original specimen confirming the specimen from Seefelder and Wolfrum [3]

At birth, the 9th month (Fig. 8.1c), the limit of the anterior chamber has extended past the spur, and the radial part of the ciliary muscle has become attached to the longitudinal part (the circular part will derive from the radial part, since it develops after birth). The mesodermal tissue has reduced to one layer with bigger inner spaces (the largest squares in the graph), which is the Busacca trabecular conjunctival layer or the Rohen iridoscleral membrane.

Figure 8.2 shows the great similarity between the histologic appearance of the normal chamber angle at the 7th month of gestation and the chamber angle in congenital glaucomas.

Figure 8.3 shows a sequential histology of different histological sections in the chamber angle in the 7th month: a broad anterior chamber showing the abundant mesenchyma tissue and the Barkan membrane (Fig. 8.3a); an image similar to the previous one, with a more closed angle (H-E) (Fig. 8.3b); the Masson trichrome stain shows the position of the ciliary muscle and also marks the Barkan membrane in an even more closed angle (Fig. 8.3c); an image with H-E stain-

Normal chamber angle at 7 months   Congenital glaucoma at birth

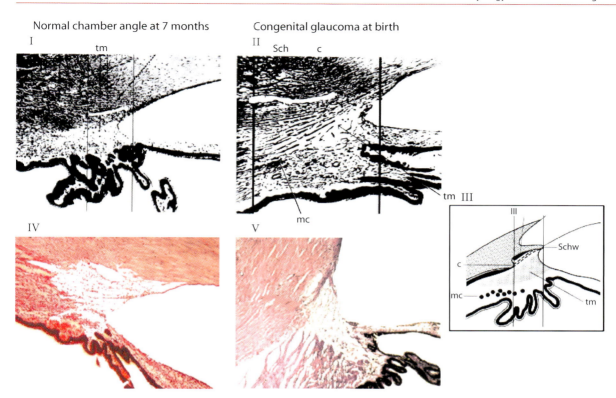

Fig. 8.2 The histology of congenital glaucoma has the same appearance as that of the chamber angle at the seventh month of gestation. *I* Chamber angle of the normal fetus at the seventh month [3]. *II* Chamber angle in congenital glaucoma. *III* Graph representing I and II. *tm* mesodermal tissue, *Sch* Schlemm canal, *mc* radiated ciliary muscle, *c* anterior ciliary vein and collector. *IV* and *V* original specimen from Sampaolesi and Zarate confirming Seefelder and Wolfrum

ing shows an extremely narrow angle with mesodermal remains simulating a high iris insertion (Fig. 8.3d).

Chronodynamics of Normal Anterior Segment Development

After ovulation, the ovum passes into the fallopian tube where it meets the sperm cells, one of which fertilizes it. As a consequence of fertilization, the diploid number of chromosomes is restored, the sex is determined, and the cleavage process starts. This is a succession of mitoses that determine the formation of a number of smaller cells called blastomeres, which thus take on a volume in accordance with the usual human tissue cells (remembering that the fertilized egg is a large cell). Seventy-two hours after ovulation, the egg has reached approximately 16 cells. Then, as liquid penetrates between the cells, which continue dividing, the blastocyst develops, which is a cystic structure in which the peripheral cells become flattened (they will constitute the trophoblast), with a group of them remaining concentrated in one of the poles (inner cell mass) (Fig. 8.4a). The trophoblast will form the caul and the placenta, while the inner cell mass gives rise to the embryo and the amnion.

Implantation occurs in the endometrium at this blastocyst stage where an inner cell mass and a cavity surrounded by the trophoblast is found. The inner cell mass gives rise to the ecto- and endodermic embryo layers. A space appears between the former (ectoderm), which are cells arranged in a flat shape, and amniogenic cells derived from the trophoblast, and this will constitute the amniotic cavity. Thus in a 15-day-old embryo, we have the amniotic cavity, the embryonic ectoderm and endoderm, and the vitelline sac (Fig. 8.4b). The ectoderm and the endoderm constitute the embryonic disc. In the caudal part of the disc, at only 15 days, a cellular thickening of the ectoderm appears, which swells out into the amniotic cavity, called the primitive streak. It becomes spherical and begins to settle between the ectoderm and the primitive endoderm, to form the

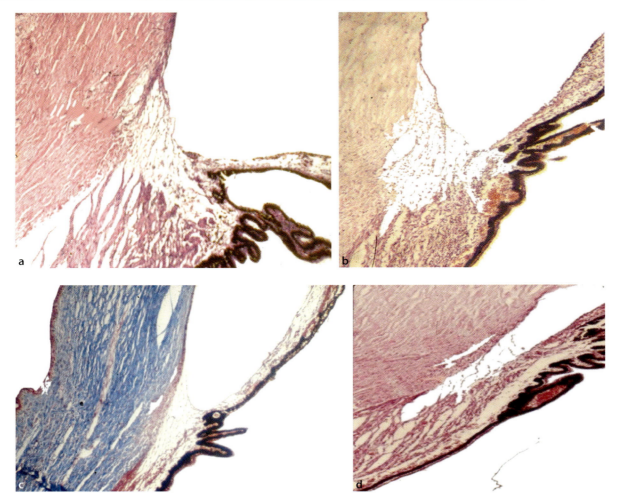

Fig. 8.3a–d Sequential histology of different histological sections in the chamber angle in the 7th month. **a** Broad anterior chamber showing the abundant mesenchymal tissue and the Barkan membrane. **b** Image similar to the previous, with a more closed angle (H-E). **c** The Masson trichrome shows the position of the ciliary muscle and also marks the Barkan membrane in an even more closed angle. **d** Image with H-E staining with an extremely narrow angle with mesodermal remains simulating a high iris insertion

third germinal layer, called the intraembryonic mesoderm, which, as it spreads toward the edges, joins the extraembryonic mesoderm, situated in relation to the trophoblast. The embryonic disc is now trilaminar: ectoderm, mesoderm, and endoderm (Fig. 8.4c).

From the ectoderm are successively formed the plate, the groove, and the neural tube. At the same time, the paraxial mesoderm and the somites are formed, which are segmentations of this tissue starting on day 21 at the anterior level and continuing in a caudal direction until by day 30 there are 44 pairs. The endoderm develops into the embryonic intestine.

The anterior (cranial) part of the neural tube constitutes the prosencephalon, and the primitive optic groove is formed on its sides and then the optic vesicle, which is thus a lateral evagination of the prosencephalon.

On day 26, the optic vesicle approaches the embryonic ectoderm (Fig. 8.5a). On day 27, the crystalline plaque can be distinguished in this ectoderm (Fig. 8.5b). This initial crystalline placode goes on to form a crystalline vesicle, which then separates from the primitive ectoderm on day 33, and corneal differentiation begins [4].

Fig. 8.4a–c Early stages of development (1st month). **a** Drawing of a blastocyst on day 10 of development. **b** Drawing of an embryo on day 15, where the amniotic cavity can be seen (*CA*), ectoderm (*Ect*), endoderm (*End*) and vitelline sac (*SV*). **c** Drawing of the trilaminar embryo disc, where the mesodermal layer has been added (*Mes*)

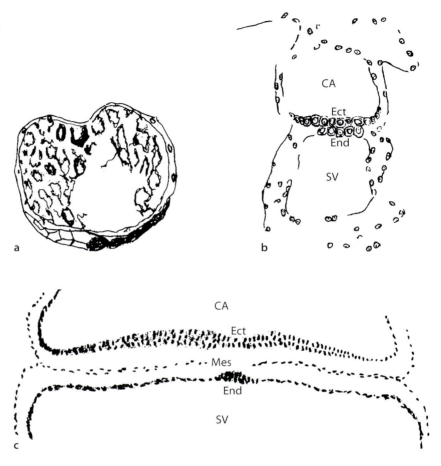

Fig. 8.5a,b Initial development of the interrelation between the ectoderm and the optic vesicle. **a** Optic vesicle as at day 26 of development, approaching the ectoderm of the embryo. **b** The crystalline placode is differentiated

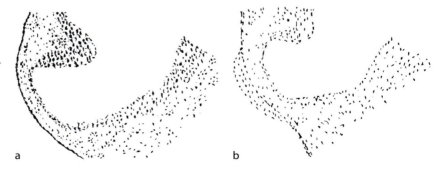

The crystalline placode is a thickening of the superficial ectoderm in the region adjacent to the neural ectoderm (optic vesicle). This thickening happens after the 2nd week and is induced by the optic vesicle, although the nature of the agent that acts to cause this is not precisely known and could be related with the extracellular matrix produced either by the neuroectodermic cells of the optic vesicle, or by those of the crystalline placode.

The thickening that makes up the crystalline placode looks like a stratified epithelium, but it is really a monolayer of cells that become columnar, whose nuclei are found in different sites, i.e., they form a true pseudostratified epithelium. This different position of the nuclei is caused by them migrating from the basal layer to the apical sector before mitosis. Later the crystalline placode begins a central depression, starting to form the crystalline vesicle, accompanying the invagination of the optic cup, which thus forms its double layer (Fig. 8.6).

The lens vesicle separates from the (corneal) ectoderm in the 4th week. In this way, the cells making up the lens vesicle have their basal part in the outer side, which explains why the basal lamina they secrete, con-

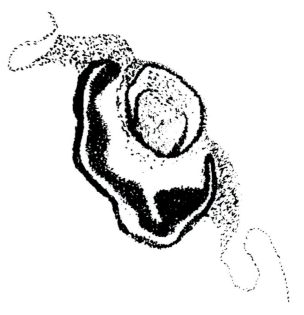

Fig. 8.6 Invagination of the lens. Invagination of the optic cup coinciding with the penetration and initial differentiation of the crystalline vesicle

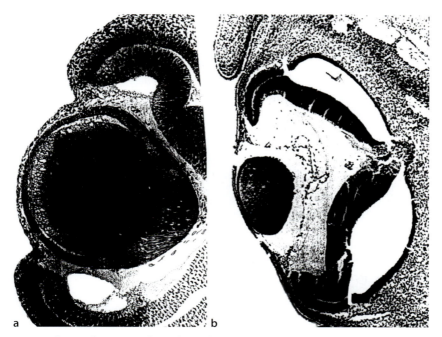

Fig. 8.7a,b Development in the 2nd month. **a** Close-up showing the large size of the crystalline vesicle with its real central space and the tunica vasculosa lentis. **b** Note the double row of the cornea in formation

Fig. 8.8a,b Structures in formation between 2nd and 3rd months of development. **a** 2.5-month embryo where fused eyelids (*PF*), developing cornea (*C*), anterior chamber (*CA*), iris membrane (*Ir*), crystalline vesicle (*VC*), primary vitreous (*k*), internal layer of the developing retina (*IR*), real space (*ER*) between this layer and the pigmentary epithelium (*EP*) can be seen. **b** The same structures in greater detail

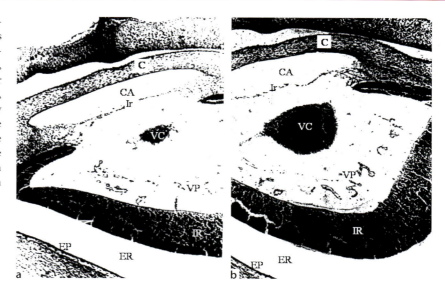

stituting the lenticular capsule, is located in an external position. This happens around the 6th week, appearing at the same time as the vessels of the tunica vasculosa lentis (Fig. 8.7a), which arise from the hyaloid circulation and are located in the posterior part of the crystalline, and out of which come the vessels surrounding the equator and going to the pupillary membrane, constituting the anterior vascular capsule [5, 6].

At this stage (day 34–36), we can see the cornea in formation (two layers) and the recently separated crystalline vesicle, in which a central space can be distinguished between the anterior epithelium and the fibers being formed from the equator. To the sides and behind, the optic layer can be seen with its two layers; note that the outer layer corresponds to the pigmentary epithelium that has grains of melanin (Fig. 8.7b).

It should be remembered that by day 33–34 (around the 1st month) we have a cornea in formation, a crystalline vesicle separated from the ectoderm, and an optic layer (lateral projection of the prosencephalon) with a double cell layer: the outer one, the pigmentary epithelium, and the inner layer, the remaining layers of the retina. This real space dividing the two layers will later become virtual. However, in pathological states (retinal detachment), this space explains why the pigmentary epithelium generally remains attached to the choroids.

Then the different corneal layers are differentiated and the iris begins to develop, initially as a thin layer of

the pupillary membrane. At the same time, on the ectodermic side, the fundi of the sacs are already formed and both eyelids fused (Fig. 8.8a).

This stage, from day 60 onward, already shows us a formed anterior chamber with abundant endothelized mesenchyme; this can be seen in the image of a histological section of an ocular globe in its 3rd month of development, where we can recognize the cornea with all its layers, an anterior chamber with abundant mesenchyma tissue in the fetal chamber angle, the iris in the initial stages of formation, the lens surrounded by the tunica vasculosa lentis, vascularized primary vitreous, and in the posterior part, the internal layer of the developing retina separated by a real space from the external layer corresponding to the pigmentary epithelium (Fig. 8.8b).

Embryological development continues with some important details, summarized in Table 8.1, which mentions specifically the appearance of the Schlemm canal in the 4th month, the characterization of the fibrillocellular trabeculae in the 5th month coinciding with the functional start of the circulation of aqueous seen in the vacuoles present in the canal [7].

The 6th month is marked by the start of the formation of the aqueous humor and the posterior displacement of the ciliary muscle.

Is very interesting to consult the thesis of Dr. Francisco Contreras, titled *Development and anomalies of the chamber angle* [11].

Table 8.1 Chronodynamics of normal anterior segment development (gestation days and months)

1st months	
Day 15	Bilaminar embryo (ectoderm and endoderm)
Day 17	Trilaminar embryo (ectoderm, mesoderm and endoderm)
Day 20	Neural groove
Day 24	Optic pits in neural groove
Day 26	Optic vesicles
Day 27	Crystalline placode
Day 28	Crystalline vesicle joined to ectoderm
Day 34	Crystalline vesicle separated from ectoderm
Day 40	Paraxial mesenchyme appears around lens
Day 50	Incipient anterior chamber
2nd Month	Crystalline vesicle separated from ectoderm
	Abundant endothelized angle mesoderm
Day 60	Anterior chamber with abundant endothelized mesenchyme
3rd month	Iris and ciliary body formation starts ciliary processes development of ciliary muscle
	Abundant endothelized angle mesoderm
4th month	Ciliary processes: ciliary channels (nulle)
	Schlemm's canal.
	Uveal trabecular and corneoscleral differentiated (cellular)
	Abundant endothelized angle mesoderm
5th month	Schlemm's canal (endothelial vacuolization)
	Mesodermal resorption begins
	The core of the trabeculae starts to form (cellular-fibrillary)
6th month	Formation of aqueous humor
	Mesodermal resorption continues
	Posterior displacement of ciliary muscle starts
	It is in the 8th month when the fenestration of the endothelial membrane covering the anterior chamber (the Barkan membrane) begins and the posterior displacement of the ciliary muscle, accelerating in the 9th and 10th month, then completing the formation of the angle recess. All of this is summarized in Fig. 8.9, stressing the great similarity between the angle in the 8th month of development and that of congenital glaucoma, as mentioned in the first part of this chapter (Fig. 8.2)
7th month	Fenestration of the pretrabecular endothelial (Barkan) membrane
	Posterior displacement of ciliary muscle
8th and 9th months	Disappearance of endothelial membrane, displacement of ciliary muscle, and resorption of mesoderm are completed
4th and 5th years	Formation of chamber angle recess completed

From [8–10]

Fig. 8.9 Chronodynamics of normal anterior segment development

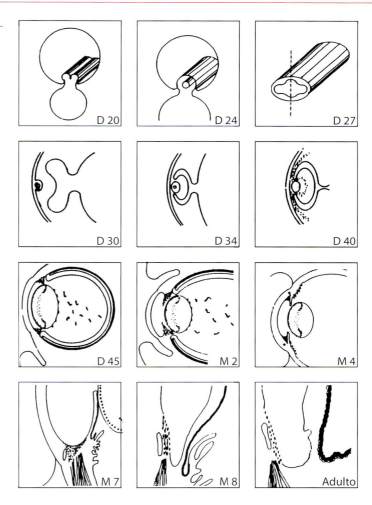

References

1. Mann I (1964) Development of the human eye. Grune & Stratton, New York
2. Burian HM, Braley AE, Allen L (1956) A new concept of the development of the angle of the anterior chamber of the human eye. Arch Ophthalmol 55:439–442
3. Seefelder R, Wolfrum (1906) Zur Entwicklung der Vorderen Kammer und des Kammerwinkels beim Menschen nebts Bemerkungen uber ihre Entstehung bei Tieren. Grafes Arch Ophthl 63:430–451
4. Ehlers N, Matthiessen ME, Andersen H (1968) The prenatal growth of the human eye. Acta Ophthalmol 46:329–349
5. Barber AN (1955) Embryology of the human eye. Mosby, St Louis
6. Wilmer HA, Scammon RE (1950) Growth of the components of the human eyeball. Arch Ophthalmol 43:599–619
7. Kupfer C, Ross K (1971) The development of outflow facility in human eyes. Invest Ophthalmol 10:513–517
8. Ozanics V, Jakobiec FA (1982) Prenatal development of the eye and its adnexa. In: Jakobiec FA (ed) Ocular anatomy embryology and teratology. Harper Row, Philadelphia, pp 11–96
9. Noden DM (1982) Perocular mesenchyme: neural crest and mesodermal interactions. In: Jakobiec FA (ed) Ocular anatomy embryology and teratology. Harper Row, Philadelphia, pp 97–119
10. Tripathi RC, Tripathi BJ (1982) Functional anatomy of the anterior chamber angle. In: Jakobiec FA (ed) Ocular anatomy embryology and teratology. Harper Row, Philadelphia, pp 197–248
11. Contreras Campos F (1972) Development and anomalies of the chamber angle in the eyes, Universidad Nacional Mayor de San Marcos, Lima, Peru

Contents

Anatomy of the Chamber Angle

The chamber angle is the outermost part of the anterior chamber, where the anterior or scleral wall converges with the posterior wall of the iris in a curved segment made up of the inner surface of the ciliary body.

Despite its simple definition, the anatomy and histology of this area reveal its great complexity. Figure 9.1, schematic representations made by Benninghoff and reproduced and quoted for the first time by Rohen and Unger in 1959 [1], show the variety of systems converging in the area of the chamber angle.

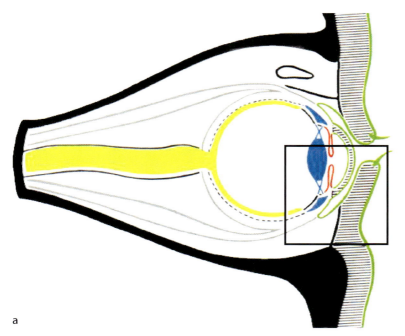
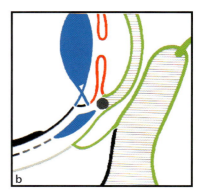

a

b

Fig. 9.1 a Benninghoff's schematic representation of the five ocular functional systems. The main system (*yellow*): the retina and optic nerve 1; accommodation system 2 (*light blue*); crystalline lens, zonule, ciliary body with muscle and elastic choroid: diaphragm-iris system 3 (*red*); transparency and protection system 4 (*green and striped area*): eyelids, lacrimal system, conjunctiva and cornea; motility system 5 (*gray*): sclera and extrinsic muscles. **b** Magnification of the area within the rectangle in **a**. The *black dot* marks the place where all five systems described in **a** come together: the chamber angle. This is why this zone is so complicated

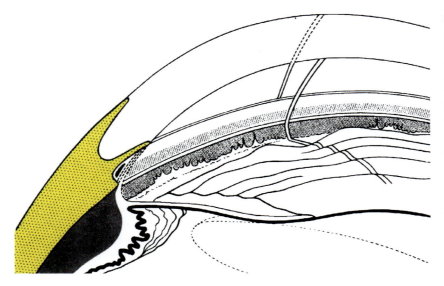

Fig. 9.2 Anatomy of the chamber angle. The sclera (*yellow*) extends into three prongs in its anterior end. Two are longer – the anterior chamber: the limbus – and the middle chamber – the scleral septum – and the posterior chamber is smaller: the spur. These three prongs form two channels: the anterior chamber lodges the optical element – the cornea – and the posterior chamber houses the filtration element – the Schlemm canal and the trabecular meshwork

These systems are:

1. Main system: retina-optic nerve;
2. Accommodation apparatus (lens, zonule, ciliary body with ciliary muscle and choroid);
3. Diaphragm-iris;
4. Motility apparatus (sclera and extrinsic muscles);
5. Eyelids, lacrimal system, conjunctiva, and cornea.

The complexity of the chamber angle is evident in these schematic representations (Fig. 9.1a,b), since there are tissues of different origins and five systems with different functions involved. This complex anatomy has a correspondingly complicated physiology.

The eyeball has a spherical shape and lodges the optical apparatus for transmission, consisting of three parts: the transparency system (4), the accommodation system (2), and the diaphragm system (3). This apparatus produces inverted images that are smaller in size than in the outer world.

The images are formed on a layer of nerve cells embryologically derived from the brain tissue in an anterior prolongation, and which are differentiated into photoreceptors: the retina-optic nerve system (1), which is the receptive sensory part of the optical system.

The role of physiological ocular pressure is to keep the dimensions of this optical system constant, a vital prerequisite for adequate image formation.

The explanation will be simplified as much as possible without sacrificing accuracy.

In its anterior edge, the sclera (yellow in Fig. 9.2) has three finger-like prongs, two of which are longer – the limbus and scleral septum – and the third, which is shorter – the spur.

Two channels are formed between these three prongs: an anterior angle that lodges the optical element – the cornea (Fig. 9.3) – and a posterior one, the scleral channel, lodging the filtration system (Fig. 9.4) – the Schlemm canal and the trabecular meshwork.

The scleral septum and spur form the posterior channel of the anterior end of the sclera. This is the filtration channel, which lodges the Schlemm canal and the trabecular meshwork (blue and green, respectively).

The ciliary muscle (red, Fig. 9.5) is located between the sclera and the iris.

The root of the iris is always inserted in the internal face of the ciliary body, in the middle in emmetropic eyes, in the anterior part in hyperopic eyes, and in the posterior part in myopic eyes. The iris can be seen in brown with the posterior layer of the iris with the pigmentary epithelium in light brown, and in dark brown, the superficial mesenchymal layer of the iris with the circular folds. The root of the iris is formed only by the deep layer (Fig. 9.5).

The intermediate wall of the chamber angle is formed by the anterior part of the inner surface of the ciliary muscle (red) and the inner wall of the chamber angle is formed by the iris and its root.

Fig. 9.3 Anatomy of the chamber angle. The cornea (*light blue*) is lodged in the anterior optical channel formed between the limbus and scleral septum

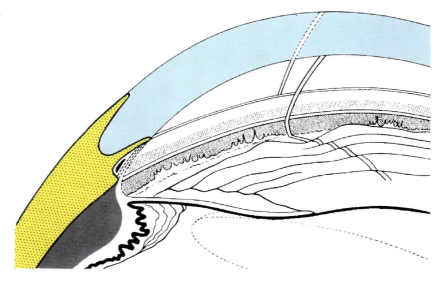

Fig. 9.4 Anatomy of the chamber angle. The scleral septum and spur form the posterior channel of the anterior end of the sclera. This is the filtration channel which lodges Schlemm´s canal and the trabecular meshwork (*blue and green respectively*)

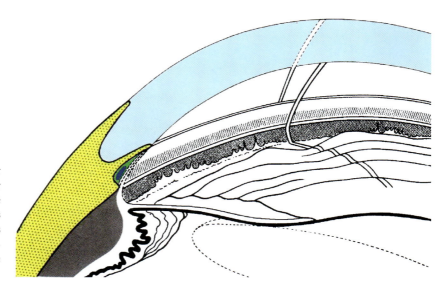

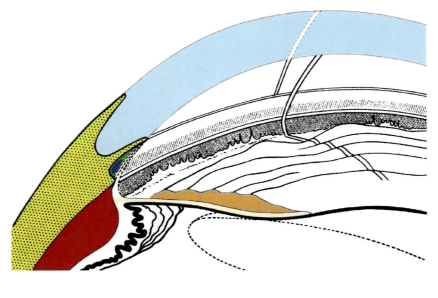

Fig. 9.5 Anatomy of the chamber angle. The intemediate wall if the chamber angle is formed by the anterior part of the inner surface of the ciliary muscle (*red*) and the inner wall of the chamber angle, by the iris and its root

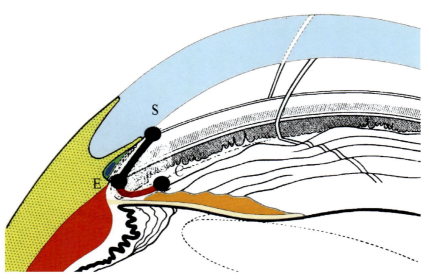

Fig. 9.6 Anatomic division of the chamber angle. The area in *blue* between the Schwalbe line (*S*) and the spur (*E*) is the scleral part, and the uveal part (*red*) is located between the spur *E* and the line of the last fold of the iris (*C*). The former is rigid and fixed and the latter, which is soft and variable

Boundaries

The anterior boundary is a circular white line which is more or less visible depending on each individual case, and the line known as the Schwalbe line (the Schwalbe ring; S, Fig. 9.6). The posterior, or iris, limit is located over the line of the last roll of the iris (C, Fig. 9.6), which is the highest part of the outermost circular fold of the iris.

Constituents

The chamber angle has the following components: the anterior edge of the sclerotic coat, the inner surface of the ciliary body, and the iris root (Fig. 9.7).

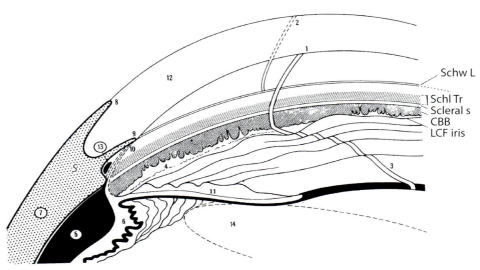

Fig. 9.7 Schematic representation of the chamber angle. The image on the *left* is a section of the chamber angle, combined with the gonioscopic image on the *right*. The following elements can be seen in the section: *7* sclera, *5* ciliary muscle, *6* ciliary body, *8* anterior prong of the sclera:limbus, *9* scleral septum, *10* Schwalbe line, *11* iris, *12* cornea, *13* Schlemm canal, *14* crystalline lens. The gonioscopic image shows the following elements: *S* spur, *Tr* trabecular meshwork, *Tr. Schl* trabecular meshwork lining the Schlemm canal, *L. Schw* Schwalbe line, *BCC* ciliary body band, *UPC* iris, last circular fold of the iris, *4* iris processes. In addition, the optical section shows the following elements: *1* posterior corneal profile line, *2* anterior corneal profile line, which is no longer visible at the level of the Schwalbe line, *3* iris profile line, *10* trabecular meshwork above the Schlemm canal. There are three dotted lines in the figure: the anterior one bends forward until it joins the anterior iris line; this is the uveal trabecular meshwork. Below it, the second dotted line represents the tendon where the ciliary muscle is inserted. The third one represents the trabecular meshwork fibers that run from the septum to the spur

Anatomic Components of the Chamber Angle

The chamber angle is divided into the following anatomic elements (Fig. 9.6): the scleral area (black line in the figure) running from the Schwalbe line (S) to the spur (E), a uveal area (red line) running from the spur to the line of the last roll of the iris (C). The former is fixed and the latter is variable.

Scleral Area

The scleral area of the chamber angle extends from Schwalbe's ring to the spur line. This is the fixed part of the chamber angle.

The scleral channel, which contains the Schlemm canal and the trabecular meshwork (Fig. 9.5, the former in blue and the latter in green), is located between the limits mentioned above.

Schwalbe Line

The Schwalbe line is a narrow band of an apparent thickness of 1 mm, located at the dividing line between the wall of the chamber angle and the Descemet membrane. In some pathological conditions, some parts are thickened or sometimes it extends into the anterior chamber.

Most authors believe it to be the anterior end of the trabecular meshwork. Busacca, based on its gonioscopic appearance, considered it to be the distal end of the scleral prong viewed between the corneal tissue and the scleral trabecular meshwork. He named it scleral septum.

Some authors describe the Schwalbe line as a protrusion into the anterior chamber, but this is not the case and there is no evidence for this in histologic sections. The appearance of an uneven surface stems from the contrast produced when there is an opaque tissue (scleral septum) between two transparent tissues (cornea and scleral trabecular meshwork).

Scleral Channel

In the inner surface of the sclerotic, in the area in which it passes into the corneal tissue, there is a posteriorly concave channel known as the scleral channel. This channel has two walls: an external (or anterior) wall formed by the scleral septum: a prong prolonging the sclera forward like a finger, and an inner (or posterior) wall formed by another smaller scleral protrusion, known as the scleral spur.

Scleral Spur

This is a protrusion of the scleral tissue viewed between the tendon of the ciliary muscle and the Schlemm canal. It is the point of insertion of the longitudinal part of the ciliary muscle and the trabecular meshwork fibers.

Its development varies depending on the individual, and it may be strong and thick, or long and thin. It is made up of a set of scleral fibers that are circular in shape, the same as those forming the scleral septum, and reaching posteriorly as far as the pars plana (orbiculus ciliaris) of the ciliary body (formation of the spur).

The same happens as with the Schwalbe line: it looks as if it goes into the anterior chamber, because it is an opaque tissue adjacent to a transparent one. When there is pigment present on the trabecular meshwork, it is clear that the spur is behind it.

Schlemm Canal

This is located in the scleral channel and its walls are formed by endothelial cells. In its external wall, it lies directly on the scleral fascicles and is in contact with the intrascleral veins. The inner wall is bounded by the juxtacanalicular tissue. The external wall is smooth and the inner wall is irregular.

Scleral Trabecular Meshwork

The scleral trabecular meshwork (Fig. 9.8) is a triangular system made up of small lamellae known as trabeculae. It has the shape of an isosceles triangle with its upper vertex seen under the Descemet membrane at the level of the Schwalbe line. Its three sides have three surfaces:

1. The inner surface (Fig. 9.8, AC) is adjacent to the anterior chamber at this site and opens into it through several small spaces between the trabeculae (intertrabecular spaces).

2. The outer surface (Fig. 9.8, SS and SchC) is in direct contact with the scleral septum (SS) at its anterior part and is part of the inner wall of the Schlemm canal (SchC) at its posterior part.

3. The base or posterior surface (Fig. 9.8, SSp) is adjacent to the spur, and depending on its developmental stage, there may be more or fewer trabecular fibers inserted into it.

There are three types of trabecular fibers (Fig. 9.9):

1. Fibers inserted into the spur (light blue);
2. Fibers coming from the longitudinal ciliary muscle (ciliary muscle tendon) (red);
3. Fibers extending over the ciliary trabecular meshwork (brown).

The fibers (light blue) extending from one sclera to the other, from the spur to the scleral septum near its end at the Schwalbe line, form an arched bundle surrounding the Schlemm canal and separated from it by the porous tissue. In red, trabecular meshwork fibers represent the tendon where the ciliary muscle is inserted. They bridge the spur and insert themselves into the Schwalbe line and are the tendinous continuation of muscular bundles of the ciliary muscle. In brown, one can see the fibers originating at different levels between the Schwalbe line and the spur and also ending at different levels from the insertion of the iris root to the last rolls of the iris. These form the ciliary trabecular meshwork and are actually normal mesodermal remnants, also known as mesoderm of the chamber angle or iris processes.

The innermost fiber layer of the trabecular meshwork (Fig. 9.9, light blue) is made up of conjunctival fibers that will form the Busacca conjunctivo-trabecular layer, which will be described in the next section on the uvea. These fibers extend over the interfascicular conjunctival tissue that separates the muscle fascicles from the ciliary muscle.

Trabeculae are made up of a central core of fibers surrounded by a homogeneous substance. This, in turn, is surrounded by a thick transparent layer known as vitreous membrane. Finally, all these constituents are covered with endothelial cells with their nuclei, continued in the cells of the Schlemm canal to the outside and leaving an open space toward the anterior chamber to the inside.

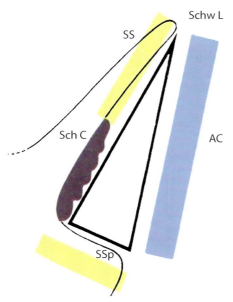

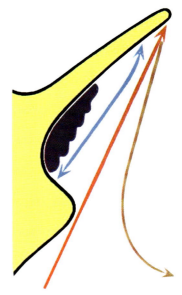

Fig. 9.8 Scleral trabecular meshwork. In the drawing, the scleral trabecular meshwork is represented as a black isosceles triangle. The inner surface (*AC*) is the boundary of the anterior chamber at that site, opening up to it through numerous small spaces and coming into contact with the aqueous humor. The outer wall of the triangle is in contact with the scleral septum (*SS*) in the half proximal to the center of the cornea, while in the distal part it forms the inner surface of the Schlemm canal (*SchC*) through porous tissue. The base or posterior surface is bounded by the scleral spur (*SSp*). *Schw L* marks the Schwalbe line

Fig. 9.9 Trabecular fibers. The fibers (*light blue*) extending from one sclera to the other, from the spur to the scleral septum near its end at the Schwalbe line, form an arched bundle surrounding the Schlemm canal and separated from it by the porous tissue. In red, trabecular meshwork fibers represent the tendon where the ciliary muscle is inserted. They bridge the spur and insert themselves into the Schwalbe line and are the tendinous continuation of muscular bundles of the ciliary muscle. In brown, one can see the fibers originating at different levels between the Schwalbe line and the spur and also ending at different levels from the insertion of the iris root to the last rolls of the iris. These form the ciliary trabecular meshwork and are actually normal mesodermal remnants, also known as mesoderm of the chamber angle or iris processes.

Uveal Area

The uveal area is defined as the variable part of the chamber angle. Its length depends on:
1. The thickness of the ciliary muscle (greater in hyperopic eyes and smaller in myopic ones);
2. The apparent insertion of the iris root.

Boundaries

The uveal area extends from the spur line to the line of the last rolls of the iris.

Constituents

The uveal area has a ciliary part and an iris part.

Ciliary Body

The ciliary body (circular portion of the muscle) is part of the chamber angle at this site between the spur and the insertion of the iris root. The inner surface of the muscle mass forms this segment of the chamber angle. In gonioscopic terminology, it is known as the ciliary body band (CBB).

At the side adjacent to the anterior chamber, it is covered by a conjunctival tissue layer that contains the ciliary trabecular meshwork in its thickness. This is the Busacca trabecular conjunctival layer (or the Rohen iridoscleral membrane). This layer is posteriorly adjacent to the tissue of the iris root and to the ciliary body and has extensions between the fascicles of the ciliary muscle at a deeper level. The peripheral end of the pupillary dilating muscle ends here. This layer is the tissue that separates the anterior chamber from the ciliary muscle (Fig. 9.10).

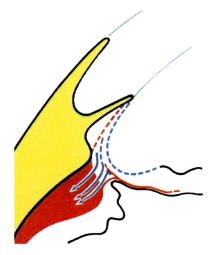

Fig. 9.10 Fibers coming from the trabecular meshwork (*light blue*), which form a layer over the anterior surface of the ciliary muscle known as the Busacca conjunctival trabecular layer. The conjunctival fibers of this layer (*arrows*) are adjacent to the interfascicular conjunctival tissue of the ciliary muscle. These fibers are clearly seen in iridocyclitis cases as they become edematous

Iris Zone

This is usually known as the iris root. It is a ring-shaped narrow band of the periphery of the iris implanted in the ciliary body (Fig. 9.6E, C). Its anterior surface forms part of the anterior chamber. Its posterior surface is in front of the heads of the ciliary processes, from which it is separated by a recess (recessus minimus of the posterior chamber).

The iris channel is the depression of the anterior chamber of the iris at the level of its root, produced by the disappearance in this zone of the superficial mesodermal layer. The limit is marked on the pupil side by the line of the last rolls of the iris, and on the ciliary body side by the insertion of the iris tissue into the trabeculoconjunctival layer (ciliary body band). This line of the last roll of the iris shows interindividual variation and varies in different zones of an individual's chamber angle. In some individuals, the iris channel is so developed that there is a true recess of the chamber angle and this hampers gonioscopic examination.

The iris root is sometimes very short and almost absent. The insertion of the iris in the ciliary body rarely forms a neat line. The superficial mesodermal layer rises to partly cover the trabeculoconjunctival layer, becoming hook-shaped. This band of iris tissue covering part of the anterior surface of the ciliary muscle is known as the Busacca baseline layer of the iris processes.

The anterior edge of this layer is not definite and fine prongs of iris tissue expand from it and branch over the ciliary and scleral walls of the trabecular meshwork; these are the Busacca iris processes, remnants originating in the period of the chamber angle formation. They are Gomori-negative when stained and are normal mesodermal remnants.

Figure 9.11a shows a cross section of an angle of an human eye. Figure 9.11b shows a histological section of an normal chamber angle and in 9.11c the corresponding schema for locating the anatomical formation.

This section shows the iris root formed solely by its deep mesenchymal layer, the recess of the chamber angle, and the fibers of the ciliary muscle, which are adjacent to those of the trabecular meshwork (its tendon) and which have the shape of a perfect isosceles triangle. The external wall of the trabecular meshwork is bounded directly by the Schlemm canal from which it is separated by a denser tissue (juxtacanalicular tissue). One of its external collectors can be seen originating in the Schlemm canal.

Figure 9.12 is an original preparation that I made when I studied the surface electron microscopy of the chamber angle. The specimen was collected from a normal eye enucleated from a 45-year-old man who had died in an accident.

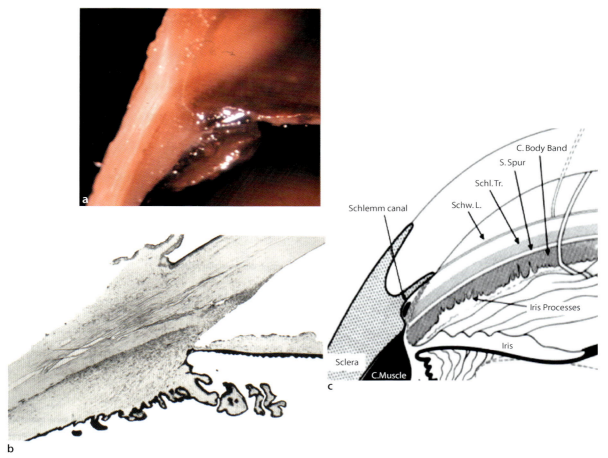

Fig. 9.11 **a** shows a cross section of an human eye. **b** histological section of an normal chamber angle, **c** the corresponding schema for locating the anatomical formation

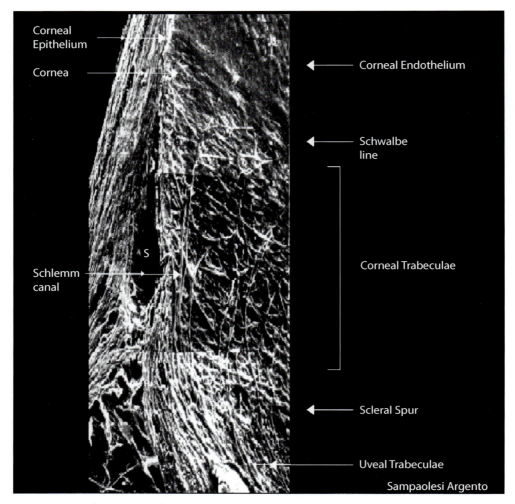

Fig. 9.12 Original preparation that I made when I studied the surface electron microscopy of the chamber angle

Summary

The chamber angle is an area of the anterior chamber that should be studied in depth, since the aqueous humor outflow pathways start here (conventional and nonconventional, or posterior pathways).

Its macroscopic structure can be studied by means of an anatomic dissection, but a correlation of this dissection with the gonioscopic image of an optical section (possible with magnification between 9 and 40) is more useful. In addition to this knowledge, histology enables the study of the structures that are visible gonioscopically, as well as those that are not, showing the complex architecture of this region where the five ocular functional systems and the three embryologic layers are involved.

The gonioscopic image should be correlated with the macroscopic anatomy and histology, both in normality and pathology. Only in this way will the semiology be truly useful.

The chamber angle has a fixed external wall and a mobile inner wall, which come together in a curve (the sinus or camerular gulf) at the spur. Knowledge of the ciliary muscle is very useful to clarify the concepts on the morphologic variations of the chamber angle under pathologic conditions and under the effect of drugs.

Reference

1. Rohen JW, Unger HH (1959) Zur Morphologie und Pathologie der Kammerbucht des Auges. Abhandlungen der Mainzer Akademie der Wissenschaften und Literatur Franz Steiner, Wiesbaden, pp 1–206

Examination of the Chamber Angle

Contents

Chemical composition of Methocel Dispersa
Methylcellulose 2%
Phenylmercuric borate 0.0002%
Sodium chloride
Distilled water

Gonioscopic Contact Lenses

To examine the chamber angle, we use one-, two-, or three-mirror Goldmann lenses (most commonly, the three-mirror lens), as well as the lens designed by Roussel and Fankhauser. The Goldmann lenses can be used with or without a scleral rim [1].

Sterilization of Gonioscopic Contact Lenses

Sterilization of the cone of gonioscopic contact lenses is recommended after using them, with sodium hypochlorite for 3 min on a Petri dish with a hole in its cap, so that only the edge that is in contact with the cornea can be sterilized with the solution. Then it is washed with water.

In this way, both HIV and adenoviruses are inactivated. The American Centers for Disease Control and Prevention (CDC) has reported that transmission of HIV through tears occurs at a rate of 0.04%. Other methods for inactivation are a fresh hydrogen peroxide solution, and ultraviolet light. The Draeger tonometer is sold with a sterilization device using ultraviolet light.

Placing the Lens

1. Anesthesia: one drop of Novesine 0.4% instilled deep in the lower conjunctival sac.
2. Preparation of the gonioscope: one drop of Methocel Dispersa (Dr. E. Baeschlin AG, Winterthur, Switzerland): Methylcellulose (Alcon Laboratories, Fort Worth, TX, USA) in its concave surface.

The liquid used for placement of the gonioscope is highly important. It should allow for a long examination, with neither corneal hazing nor discomfort to the patient.

Methylcellulose 2% has a viscosity of 4,000 centipoises (a poise is a unit in the CGS system of dynamic viscosity: dyne per second per square centimeter). If methylcellulose is not available at this concentration, a gel can be used that is composed of carbomer 980 (polyacrylic acid) 200 mg, benzalkonium chloride 10 mg, sorbitol 400 mg, sodium hydroxide to adjust pH c.s., purified water c.s.p. 100 g.

The use of unsuitable liquids for gonioscopy is the reason why many ophthalmologists consider gonioscopy to be a complicated examination, since the corneal haze produced by many liquids prevents them from viewing the delicate structures of the chamber angle clearly.

3. The patient rests his chin and forehead on the slit-lamp.
4. He is instructed to look up without moving his forehead from the slit-lamp support (Fig. 10.1a).
5. For the right eye, the gonioscope is placed with the left hand and the slit-lamp is moved toward the right. Conversely, for the left eye, the lens is placed with the right hand and the slit lamp is moved to the left.
6. With the free hand, and particularly with the fifth finger, the lower eyelid is pressed in order to rest the lower margin of the gonioscope in the deep lower conjunctival sac (Fig. 10.1b).
7. The gonioscope rests completely on the eye while the patient is directed to look to the front (Fig. 10.1c).
8. The patient is asked to look to the front and the lens is placed on the eye.

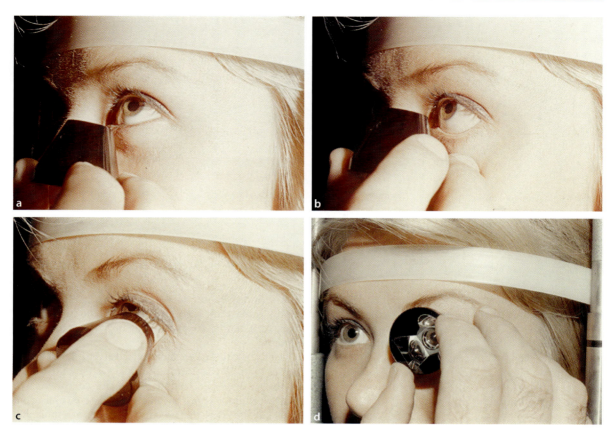

Fig. 10.1a–d Placement of the three-mirror contact lens. **a** The lens is held with the thumb and index finger. **b** With the ring finger or pinky, the lower eyelid is pressed and the patient is directed to look up. **c** Once a good palpebral opening has been achieved, the lens is placed in contact with the eye with the eyelashes outside. **d** The patient is asked to look to the front and the lens is placed on the eye

Examination with the Slit-Lamp or Biomicroscope

The chamber angle should always be examined with a biomicroscope that allows for an optic cut and with a suitable contact lens.

However, in some departments where the Köppe lens is still used, the ophthalmologist performs the examination with a hand-held microscope while holding a small lamp, which is moved around the supine patient. This provides only a rough estimate of the chamber angle structures, with no details.

The examination starts with a broad slit and then proceeds with a narrow one. The examination with a fine slit enables a good optical cut of the visible structures of the chamber angle.

To obtain a good optical cut with a fine slit, one must be familiar with the necessary maneuvers, which vary according to whether one wishes to observe the chamber angle at the vertical meridian at 6 or 12 o'clock or at the horizontal meridian at 3 or 9 o'clock (Fig. 10.2).

The elements that change their position depending on the structures to be observed are the direction in which the patient is looking, the anterior surface of the contact lens, and the direction of the light bundle of the slit-lamp.

If the purpose is to observe the chamber angle at 6 or 12 o'clock, the patient should look laterally, as shown in Fig. 10.2, so that the light bundle of the slit falls normally (perpendicularly) on the anterior surface of the gonioscope (90° angle). The image thus obtained will be clear and useful for diagnosis.

In practice, if the slit lamp's arm is on the right side of the observer, the patient should be asked to look slightly to his left, i.e., to the side where the light source is located.

For an observation of the chamber angle in the horizontal plane at 3 or 9 o'clock with a fine slit, the following steps should be followed (Fig. 10.3):

- Place the slit in a horizontal position.
- Bend the illumination arm forward.
- Dip the anterior plane of the gonioscope, while the patient is asked to look slightly downward (Fig. 10.3b).

This examination can only be done with a Haag-Streit 900 slit-lamp, the first one to enable the slit plane to be inclined horizontally. Mr. Littman (Carl Zeiss, Meditec AG, Jena, Germany) designed a prism at our request so that the Zeiss slit-lamp could be inclined without bending the arm.

Figure 10.3 illustrates the reason for this maneuver, based on the geometric optical principles of light reflection on the mirrors.

The patient can be asked to fix the fellow eye on the small fixation lamp, instead of looking away, since some patients do this abruptly, causing air to come between the contact lens and the eye.

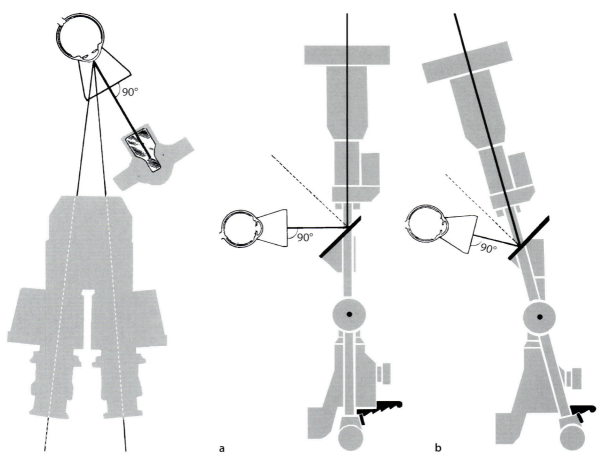

Fig. 10.2 Observation of the chamber angle with a fine slit. Optical cut at 6 and 12 o'clock. The patient should be instructed to look to the side where the illumination arm of the lamp is located so that the light bundle of the slit falls normally on the anterior surface of the gonioscope: a 90° angle

a   b

Fig. 10.3a,b Observation of the chamber angle with a fine slit. Optical section at 3 and 9 o'clock. The following steps should be followed for this observation. First, place the slit in a horizontal direction, as in **a**. Then, as shown in **b**, bend the light arm to the front; the patient is then asked to look down so that the anterior surface of the gonioscope forms a 90° angle with the luminous axis. As shown in **b**, when the light arm is bent, the angle of incidence of the mirror is lower than when the arm is in the vertical position. Since the angle of incidence to the mirror is lower than normal and the reflection angle is the same as that of incidence, the reflected ray that illuminates the gonioscope is deviated upward. This is why the patient should look down

Summary

Goldmann's three- and one-mirror lenses are probably the most useful ones for this examination. In addition, it is vital to use a good contact liquid (Methocel Dispersa). Knowledge of the application technique, and especially of the optical pathway of the slit-lamp and gonioscopic lens rays, is also important. The entire circumference of the chamber angle can thereby be observed in an optical section. From a practical point of view, to obtain good optical sections, the light bundle should fall perpendicular to the contact lens. When the areas at 6 and 12 o'clock are examined, the patient should look toward the light source, whereas when the chamber angle is examined at 3 and 9 o'clock, the slit, which has been previously shifted horizontally, should be inclined, and the patient should look slightly down so that the light rays fall perpendicular to the lens, which is moved in this direction by the ophthalmologist.

To examine the chamber angle in children, there are two new models of Goldmann lenses available, manufactured by Haag Streit, one with a 10-mm diameter and the other an 11-mm diameter. The Roussell Fankhauser goniolens with its high resolution is very useful.

Reference

1. Sampaolesi R (1994) Glaucoma. 2nd edn. Panamericana, Buenos Aires, Argentina

Contents

Lenses for Gonioscopy

Figure 11.1a (upper and lower parts) illustrates the one-mirror Goldmann lens and the two-mirror Goldmann lens, respectively; Figure 11.1b, upper and lower parts, illustrate the three-mirror-Goldmann lens; and Figure 11.1c, upper and lower parts, the Goldmann lens with three 10- and 11-mm-diameter mirrors, respectively, for studying the chamber angle in children.

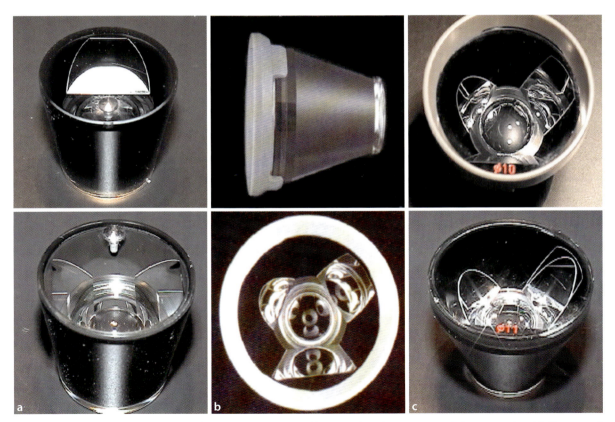

Fig. 11.1 a (*upper part*) Goldmann goniolens with one mirror, **a** (*lower part*) with two mirrors, **b** (*upper part*) and **b** (*lower part*) with three mirrors, **c** (*upper part*) and **c** (*lower part*) three mirrors, 10 and 11 mm in diameter, for studying the chamber angle in children

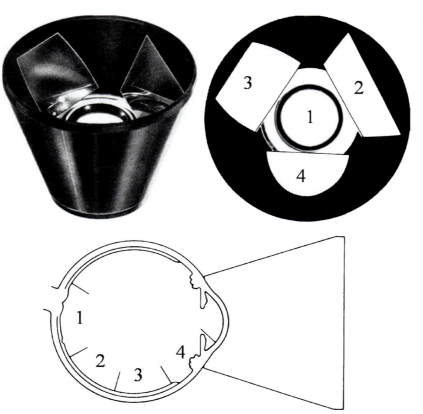

Fig. 11.2 Goldmann goniolens with three mirrors

Looking through the center of the three-mirror Goldmann lens, the posterior pole can be seen from the papilla to the macula. With mirrors two and three, the retina can be seen in the periphery. With mirror four, the chamber angle can be seen (Fig. 11.2).

In order to obtain a comprehensive image, the examination should start with a biomicroscope with a × 10 magnification. The medical practitioner, if still untrained in the observation of the chamber angle, should take the following landmarks into account:

1. The corneoscleral wall (light) can be distinguished easily from the iris wall (dark) by their different colors.
2. In the corneoscleral wall, the Schwalbe line should be found. This landmark will help assess the visibility, or amplitude, of the chamber angle. With a broad slit, it is sometimes very easy to find, since it is clearly visible in the following cases:
   - A nacreous Schwalbe line;
   - The Schwalbe line with pigment deposited on the upper end of the trabecular meshwork;
   - A prominent Schwalbe line at the anterior chamber (pathological), etc.

Usually there are no landmarks in the external wall to make it evident. In these cases, illumination with a fine slit, using the technique already described (see Chap. 10), is required so that the image obtained is clear. At this time, the image resembles Fig. 11.3.

Since the cornea is inserted in a wedge shape (like a watch glass) into the sclera (c) where the anterior channel is located, both lines tend to converge (Fig. 11.3, I).

However, though both lines come together, as shown in Fig. 11.3, I, the consequent image is that shown in Fig.11.3, II, since the anterior profile line (b) is only visible up to the Schwalbe line, because from here downward, the scleral septum (dotted line, c), which is an opaque tissue, obscures it (Fig. 11.3, II). In brief, the position of the Schwalbe line derives from the discontinuation of the anterior profile line (b). This detail is what the ophthalmologist should look for (Fig. 11.3, III). In other words, there are two profile lines above the Schwalbe line (a and b) but only one below it. This is a valuable and meaningful landmark for finding the Schwalbe line in the corneoscleral wall.

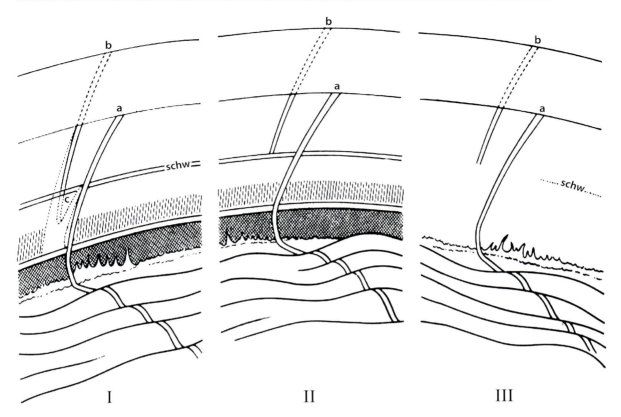

Fig. 11.3 Optical section with a narrow slit in the biomicroscopic examination of the chamber angle. *a* Posterior corneoscleral profile line which runs through the whole chamber angle up to the iris wall. *b* anterior corneoscleral profile line. *c* Optical channel in which the cornea is lodged between two scleral prongs: the limbal prong and the septum. *Schw* Schwalbe line, *Sp* scleral spur

I. The limbal prolongation of the sclera and the scleral septum, which form the optical channel where the cornea (*c*) is lodged, is represented by a dotted line. The posterior corneoscleral profile line is completely visible (*a*). The anterior corneoscleral profile line (*b*) is completely visible up to the Schwalbe line. The small dots continue the invisible part of this line.

II. Image seen through the microscope. The outline representing the sclera in I have been removed. This site where the anterior corneoscleral line becomes invisible represents the Schwalbe line location.

III. When there is neither blood nor pigment in the Schlemm canal, the spur is barely visible, and the ciliary body band is obscured. The point at which the anterior corneoscleral line is discontinued (*b*) shows the position at which the Schwalbe line is placed, located at *schw* in the image. This observation is vital since it is indicative of the fact that the filtrating trabecular meshwork is located between this line and the iris root with no obstacles hindering aqueous humor inflow. *a* Posterior corneoscleral profile line (posterior corneal surface); *b* anterior corneoscleral profile line (anterior corneal surface)

Sometimes, the image observed may be very different from the one shown and be forked-shaped (two points), it is the corneal wedge (Fig. 11.4c), i.e., in the Schwalbe line there are three lines that come together, as shown in Fig. 11.4. This depends on the gonioscope used (Goldmann three- or one-mirror, Worst, etc.) and particularly on the angle formed by the optical observation axis (microscope) with the illumination axis (slit). If the angle is large the image will be like the one illustrated in Fig. 11.4a, whereas if it is smaller, it resembles Fig. 11.4b, and if it is too small, it will be fork-shaped, as in Fig. 11.4c. This is an easily under-

standable optical phenomenon of perspective and parallax. This fork shape is also more visible when the one-mirror Goldmann lens is used (Fig. 11.5), since in this case the direction of the illumination axis is parallel to the posterior corneal surface.

When the anterior chamber is very shallow, the anterior position of the iris and pupil enables the equator of the crystalline lens, the ciliary processes, and the posterior zonular fibers (Fig. 11.6) to be seen with the three-mirror contact lens. It can also be seen in the deep chamber when the pupil is well dilated.

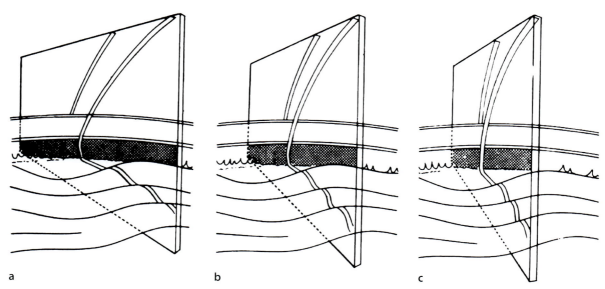

a   b   c

Fig. 11.4a–c Determination of the position of the Schwalbe line. The point of interruption of the anterior corneoscleral profile line, which signals the location of the Schwalbe line may be located either far away from the posterior corneoscleral profile line as in **a**, proximal to it as in **b**, or almost touching it as in **c**. This depends on the angle formed by the observation axis (biomicroscope) and the illumination axis (illumination arm). In **a**, they are widely separated, in **c**, they are very close; **b** represents an intermediate position between **a** and **c**

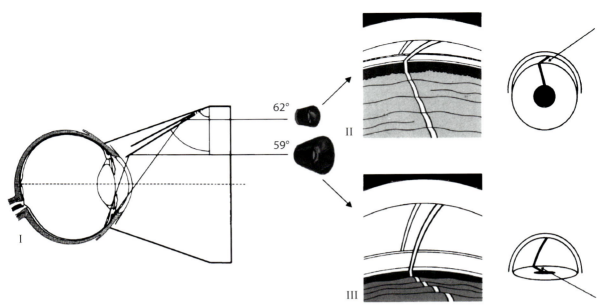

Fig. 11.5 *I* direction of the rays in a gonioscope depending on whether a 62° one-mirror or a three-mirror round rim gonioscope with an inclination of 59° is used. These degrees are measured by the angle formed by the mirror with the anterior surface of the lens. When the one-mirror lens is used, the light bundle follows the posterior corneal surface and permits observation of the chamber angle fundus, as shown by *II*, i.e., the profile of the corneoscleral wall of the chamber angle and the front of the ciliary-iris part are seen. In contrast, when the round mirror of the three-mirror lens is used, the light bundle follows the anterior surface of the iris and then, as shown in *III*, the front of the corneoscleral surface of the chamber angle and the anterior end of the ciliary body band are seen. The iris surface is seen in profile and it obscures the recess of the chamber angle and the posterior part of the ciliary body band. This is the reason why using the 62° one-mirror lens, or a recently manufactured two-mirror lens, also with 62° in each mirror, is recommended. However, the three-mirror lens may be used in children up to 3 years of age since the recess of the chamber angle is absent at this age

Fig. 11.6 The chamber angle highly narrowed by the shifting of the iris-lens diaphragm to the front. The posterior corneoscleral profile line is not attached to the anterior one because the chamber angle is blocked. The anterior position of the iris-lens diaphragm provides a view of the posterior surface of the crystalline lens, the posterior zonular fibers, the Petit canal and, sometimes, the head of the ciliary processes

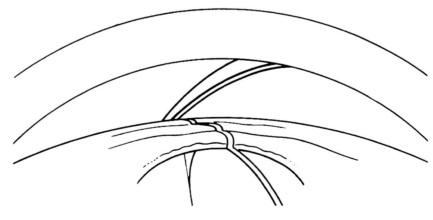

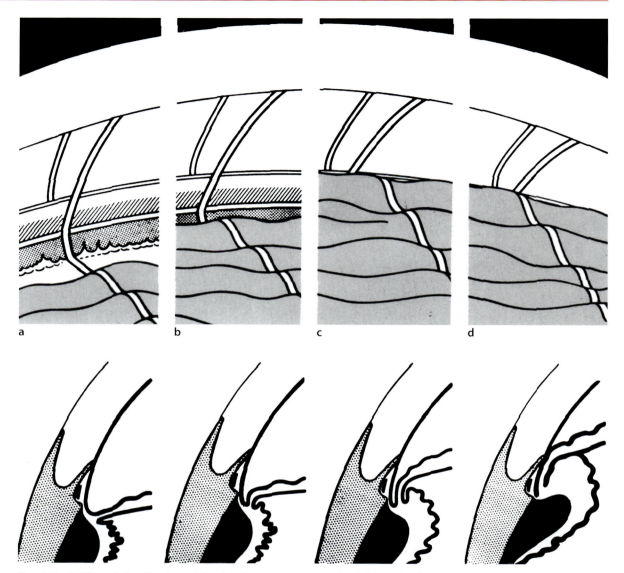

Fig. 11.7a–d *Clinical classification of the chamber angle according to gonioscopic visibility*. Gonioscopic visibility of the chamber angle. **a** Open chamber angle with broad entry; the ciliary body band is complete and the iris root can be seen. **b** Chamber angle with narrow entry; the ciliary body band is visible only in its anterior part. **c** Very narrow chamber angle; the trabecular meshwork is barely visible at its anterior end, at the level of the Schwalbe line. **d** The entry of the chamber angle is blocked, since not only is the trabecular meshwork not seen, but also the posterior corneal profile line is continued directly into the iris profile line with an absence of the parallax image represented by the illustration. At the bottom are the sagittal sections of the chamber angle corresponding to the four gonioscopic images at the top

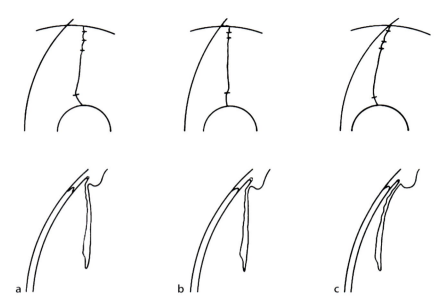

Fig. 11.8a–c *Influence of the shape of the chamber angle and of the depth of the anterior chamber on the visibility of the chamber angle*. At the *top*, the illustrations represent the composition of the anterior chamber, and at the *bottom* of the drawing represents a section of the chamber angle that shows the composition of the chamber angle in each case. **a** Trapezoidal chamber angle and open chamber angle, which is very easy to examine, even when the iris root is long. **b** Planoconvex anterior chamber. There is a direct relationship between the amplitude of the chamber angle and the length of the iris root. **c** Concave-convex anterior chamber; the circular last folds of the iris reduce the amplitude and make the chamber angle difficult to see (reproduced from [2])

The Shape of the Chamber Angle

There is a difference between chamber angle amplitude and its visibility. The amplitude (from the anatomical point of view) depends on the length of the ciliary band. This in turn depends on the iris root insertion into it. The closer to the spur the iris is inserted, the smaller the chamber angle is anatomically.

The gonioscopic visibility (Fig. 11.7) of the chamber angle depends on the position of the inner iris wall relative to the fixed external scleral wall. The entry may be open, and it may be broad, narrow, or very narrow depending on the case. The entry of the chamber angle is broad if the ciliary body band is visible in at least half of the circumference (Fig. 11.7a). It is narrow if the ciliary body band is not visible (Fig. 11.7b) or is only visible at its anterior end. It is very narrow if the scleral trabecular meshwork is visible only in its anterior end or is not visible (Fig. 11.7c). The entry of the chamber angle is blocked when both walls are attached up to the Schwalbe line or even over it (Fig. 11.7d). In short, amplitude is an anatomical concept, while visibility is mostly physiological.

Amplitude and visibility are sometimes dependent on each other: if the iris root is short the chamber angle is easily visible, even when it is anatomically reduced, with a very small ciliary band.

They are sometimes independent: if the iris root is long the chamber angle can only be seen at the site where the last rolls of the iris are short. If there is a place where the last rolls of the iris are tall, the chamber angle cannot be seen, even when it is anatomically broad.

Understanding these concepts becomes even more difficult when the anterior chamber depth is taken into consideration. The anterior chamber may be deep or shallow and this influences visibility.

The illustrations in Fig. 11.8 (modified from [2]) show the relationship between the chamber angle and the depth and shape of the anterior chamber. The depth of the chamber angle depends on the distance between the Schwalbe line and the farthest point in the ciliary profile line. The extension of the iris root is measured between the line of the last roll of the iris and the root insertion.

Chamber angle amplitude has two anatomic variations. Broad chamber angles correspond to a broad ciliary body band and a short iris root. Narrow chamber angles have a narrow ciliary body band and a long iris root.

The New Gonioscopic Lens of Roussel and Fankhauser

In 1983, Fankhauser and Roussel [3] built a new contact lens, CGA1, with a mirror manufactured by Haag-Streit Meridian, for irradiating pathological structures in the chamber angle with high power lasers (Figs. 11.9 and 11.10). Fankhauser explained to the mathematician Roussel the five problems of the three-mirror Goldmann contact lens and Roussel resolved the geometric problem presented by the optical aspects.

Since this lens has a spherical anterior surface, the movements made to focus precisely on the structures to photocoagulate have very little influence on the diameter of the beam and the focus and thus keep it constant. At the same time, the image is independent of any manipulation of the lens. This is why this lens is essential, for example, in laser microphotocoagulation in the trabecular meshwork after nonpenetrating deep sclerectomy (NPDS).

With its extraordinary quality, this lens enables very fine details to be recognized, and the resulting photographs and videos have a quality that is rarely seen. Its convex anterior surface is what gives great amplification and resolution to the image, and it is possible to recognize new structures in the chamber angle that could not previously be seen.

The lasers used for microsurgery today are much more powerful. Argon and krypton have a power of 3 W, while neodymium and others have a power of radiation of the order of 108 W, which can generate mechanical effects used for cutting or perforating the irradiated tissues. It is fundamental to have wide-angle beams, since otherwise the tissues behind or in front of those being treated would be damaged.

Today, even though it was designed for application with these new lasers, the great amplification and resolution it provides means that it is also used in all the diagnostic gonioscopies and for goniophotography.

Optical Properties

Its convex anterior surface enables the convergence of the rays without introducing aberrations, all the while providing high optical resolution. The mirror of this lens has an inclination of 58°, a magnification of 1.5, and its thickness is 17 mm. It reduces the focus of the laser on the structures by a factor of 1.5 in comparison with the Goldmann lens.

It has an antireflective layer. There are two types: CGA7 and CGA8, with a radius of curvature of 7.4 mm and 8.2 mm, respectively.

Figure 11.11 (C) provides a virtual image of the angle corresponding to the center of curvature of the lens. L is the ray of light and R the reflection of the image.

In Fig. 11.12, the vertical axis represents the larger dimension of the laser focus with aberration occurring almost at the level of the vertex of the anterior chamber angle (ordinate). The abscissa represents the angular position of the contact lens on the cornea. For example, if the position of the lens on the cornea has a 4° tilt, the size of the laser focus is around 20 μm, while with the Goldmann lens it would be more than 60 μm. If it were 8°, with the Fankhauser lens it would be 25 μm, while with the Goldmann lens it would be 130 μm.

The aberration of the CGA lens is lower than that of the Goldmann lens when tilting the lens and increasing the rotation angle.

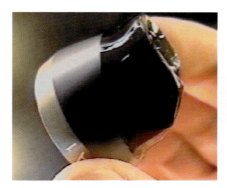 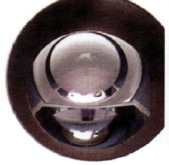 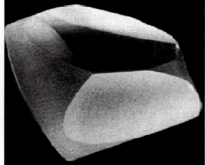

Fig. 11.9 Fankhauser and Roussel gonioscopic lens, lateral view

Fig. 11.10 Front view and spatial configuration of the Fankhauser and Roussel gonioscopic lens

Fig. 11.11 Fankhauser and Roussel gonioscopic lens. L is the ray of the light and R the reflection of the image

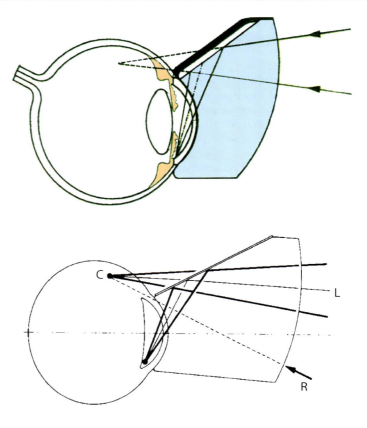

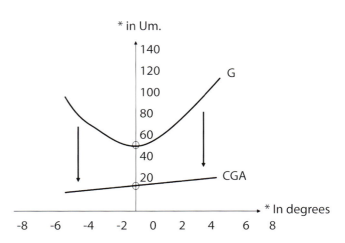

Fig. 11.12 Aberration occurring in the Goldmann lens G and the Fankhauser and Roussel lens CGA

Goniophotographs Taken with the Roussel and Fankhauser Lens

The goniophotographs in Fig. 11.13 enable the normal elements of the angle as well as the angle in open-, narrow-, and blocked-angle glaucoma to be individualized, and the normal angle from cases of goniodysgenesis can be differentiated. To make these goniophotographs, the Roussel and Fankhauser lens described above was used.

Figure 11.13 is a goniophotograph made with a narrow slit and the maximum of light, to obtain the image

in the fork that enables the Schwalbe line to be perfectly located. Figure 11.13a illustrates the corresponding sketch, Fig. 11.13b, the goniophotograph.

Figure 11.14 shows different goniophotographs of the image in fork. In the last goniophotograph, it can be seen that the pigment at the level of the Schwalbe line has two lines, since this is an exfoliative syndrome that presents, above the Schwalbe line, the characteristic waves in the pigment in the posterior face of the cornea.

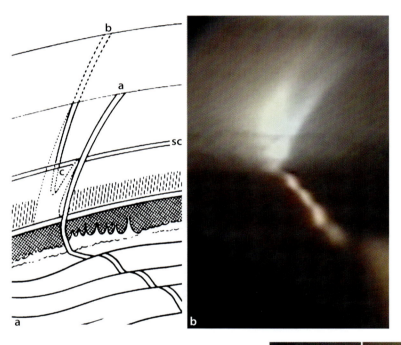

Fig. 11.13a,b Goniophotograph made with a narrow slit and maximum of light to obtain the image in fork which enables the Schwalbe line to be perfectly located. **a** The corresponding sketch. **b** The goniophotograph (*a*, line of anterior profile). The two extensions coming from the sclera are the corneoscleral limbus and the scleral septum. As neither of these is transparent, the fork-shaped image is formed

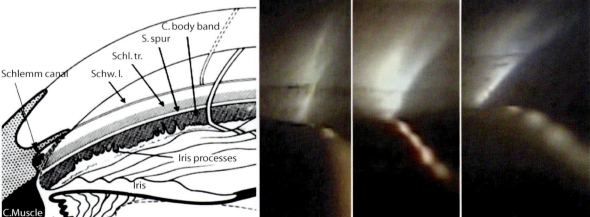

Fig. 11.14 Different drawings and goniophotographs of the fork image

Iris Process

Figure 11.15b shows an iris process, which is a normal mesodermal remnant that is very commonly seen in normal eyes. Figure 11.15b is an illustration of the corresponding histology, and in Fig. 11.15a, the explanatory diagram.

The corneoscleral trabecular network is formed of fibers that run from sclera to sclera (1), by fibers that come from the ciliary muscle, pass by the spur, and reach the Schwalbe line, and then form the ciliary muscle tendon. Fiber 3 represents the iris process.

In Fig. 11.16 illustrates the iris processes that do not normally pass the spur, with the corresponding diagram.

It is important to distinguish these iris processes, normal mesodermal remnants, common in open angles, from goniodysgenesis, as illustrated in Fig. 11.17a, iris processes, and Fig. 11.17b, goniodysgenesis. In cases of goniodysgenesis, there is pathologic mesodermal tissue and similar tree-like extensions that cover the entire trabecular network and reach the Schwalbe line (see goniographs in Fig. 11.17b in Fig. 11.17c).

When the gonioscope is moved backward, suction is produced, and in general, the Schlemm canal fills with blood. Other times it fills with blood spontaneously (Fig. 11.18).

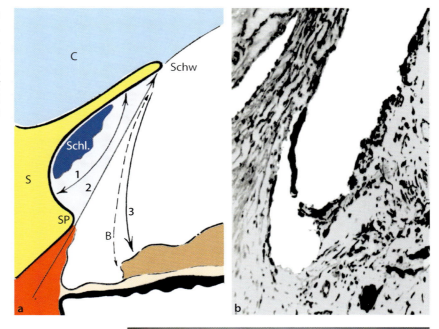

Fig. 11.15 Iris process. **a** Diagram; **b** histology, iris process (*C* cornea, *Schl* Schlemm canal, *S* scleral septum ending in the Schwalbe line, *SP* scleral spur), *1* cornea, corneal trabecular meshwork, *2* tendon of the ciliary muscle between scleral spur and the Schwalbe line, *1–3* uveal

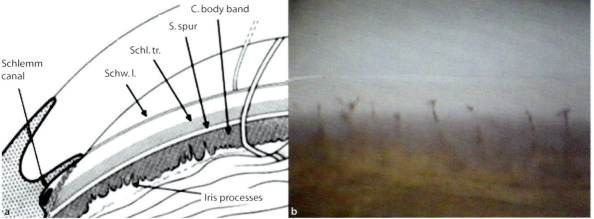

Fig. 11.16a,b The iris processes seen do not normally pass the spur; the corresponding diagram

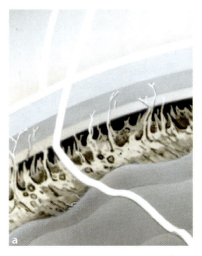 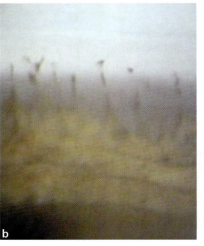 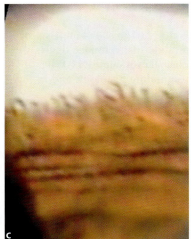

Iris processes
Normal mesodermal remmants

Goniodysgenesis
Pathological mesodermal
remmants

Fig. 11.17a–c Goniodysgenesis

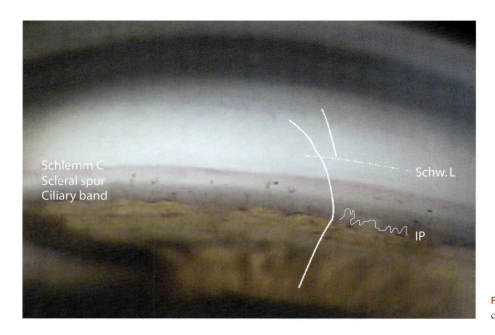

Fig. 11.18 The Schlemm
canal with blood

Narrow Angle Glaucoma

Figure 11.19 shows a narrow angle glaucoma: the flat chamber (Fig. 11.19a), goniophotograph (Fig. 11.19b), corresponding diagram (Fig. 11.19c), and the histological section (Fig. 11.19d).

Figure 11.20 belongs to Goldmann [4] and shows how in a blocked angle, the posterior profile line of the cornea and the anterior profile line of the iris continue directly one from the other (Fig. 11.20a). However, when the angle is narrow and not blocked (Fig. 11.20b), the posterior profile line of the cornea does not continue the anterior profile line of the iris, which is displaced to one side by the parallax.

Figure 11.21a is a steel sheet with three curved, parallel perforations that permit an angle to be drawn easily, an idea from Busacca. Figure 11.21b shows a sketch of the three lines described, traced by the plate, and how they are used to draw an angle. It is a good idea for the ophthalmologist to make these drawings on the patients' clinical histories as well as photographs.

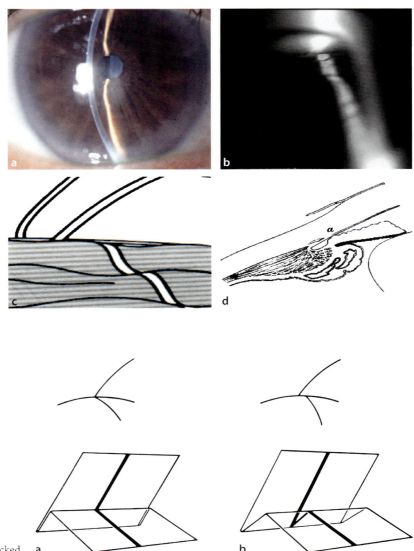

Fig. 11.19 Narrow angle glaucoma. a Flat chamber; b goniophotograph; c diagram; d the histological section

Fig. 11.20 a Blocked and b unblocked

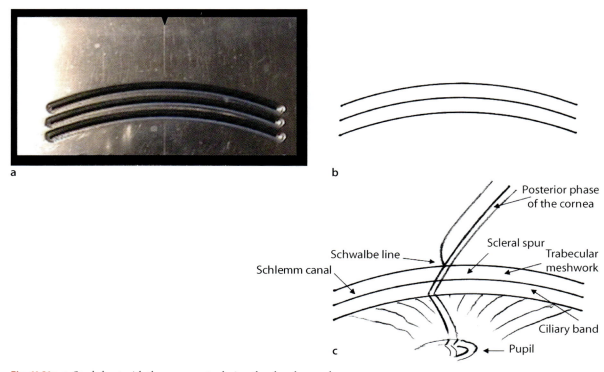

a

b

Posterior phase
of the cornea

Scleral spur

Trabecular
meshwork

Schwalbe line

Schlemm canal

Ciliary band

Pupil

c

Fig. 11.21a–c Steel sheet with three curves to design the chamber angle

Summary

The gonioscopic image depends on the mirror used. The three-mirror lens (the curved mirror of this lens) can be used in children, since they do not have a recess in their chamber angle. This lens enables the observation mainly of the external wall of the chamber angle from the front. In adults, particularly if the chamber angle is narrow, the one-mirror lens should be used. With this lens, the fundus of the chamber angle and the iris wall can be seen from the front.

The different elements, mainly of the external wall, can be studied with the optical section. However, identification of the Schwalbe line is vital, even in the absence of other elements, such as pigment, which may be of assistance. This requires looking for the hook- or Y-shaped (either in an upright or inverted position) image, depending on whether the upper or lower chamber angle is observed (12 or 6 o' clock). The upper arms of the "Y" stand for the anterior and posterior corneal surface above the Schwalbe line, while its single lower line represents the profile line of the trabecular meshwork.

References

1. Rohen JW, Unger HH (1959) Zur Morphologie und Phatologie der Kammerbucht des Auges. Abhandlungen der Mainzer Akademie der Wissenschaften und Literatur Franz Steiner, Wiesbaden, pp 1–206
2. Busacca A (1964) Biomicroscopie et histopathologie de l'oeil, Vol. 2. Schweizer Druck und Verlagshaus. Zurich, p 119
3. Roussel P, Fankhauser F (1983) Contact glass for use with high power lasers – geometrical and optical aspects. Solutions for the angle of the anterior chamber. Int Ophthalmol 6:183–190
4. Goldmann H (1954) Das Glaukom. In: AmslerM, Brückner A, Franceschetti A, Goldmann H, Streiff EB (eds) Lehrbuch der Augenheilkunde. Karger, Basel, p 398

Contents

The Normal Chamber Angle

The description of the chamber angle in children, as well as the graphics presented are based on the study of 76 gonioscopies performed in normal children of the following ages: three children under 1 month, 13 between 1 and 6 months, seven who were 1 year old, three 2 years, three 3 years, two 4 years, four 5 years, three 6 years, one 8 years, and one 10 years.

The chamber angle in children continues its development from birth to 2 years of age, when the gonioscopic appearance stabilizes. Nevertheless, there is still no chamber angle recess at this age, since this will appear at 4 or 5 years of age. Many normal chamber angles that have not completed their evolution have normal mesodermal remnants.

The Chamber Angle in Premature Children

The gonioscopic image of the eye of a premature child born at the 7th or 8th month of gestation is the same as the histological image shown by the sections of the normal chamber angle development taken from Seefelder and Wolfrum [1]. The gonioscopic image corresponding to this histology shows a flat anterior chamber, the bottom of which is covered with a gray band corresponding to the mesodermal remnants (see Chap. 8). Worst [2] has described this gonioscopy remarkably well.

The Normal Chamber Angle in Newborns

In newborns, and within the 1st year of age, the chamber angle has different appearances in accordance with the development of the mesodermal remnants.

When the Mesodermal Remnants Have Reabsorbed

At this stage, the chamber angle shows at the external wall: the Schwalbe line, the scleral trabecular meshwork of a slightly darker gray color, where sometimes the Schlemm canal, the spur, in white, and the ciliary body, in an even darker gray color, can be seen by transparency. The base and root of the iris which can be seen at the internal wall (Fig. 12.1, I).

It is very important to know how to identify the appearance of the internal wall of the chamber angle in its periphery. If, as usually occurs, the superficial mesodermal layer of the iris is poorly developed, is unpigmented, and there are no opaque mesodermal remnants, the pigmentary layer of the iris at the periphery, dark gray in color, almost black, can be seen by transparency (Fig. 12.1, I, *e*) through triangular holes. Let us analyze this appearance in depth. Behind the dark gray ciliary body band, another lighter band can be seen (Fig. 12.1, I, *b*), the latter one is made up of iris tissue of a pinkish orange color. This tissue is located immediately above the iris's major arterial circle, which is visible in some sites. The iris-radiated vessels emerge from this arterial circle. These vessels are surrounded by mesenchymal tissue (Fig. 12.1, I, *c*) (vascular pilars), which are the same color as the orange band described above. These vascular pillars form the sides of the black triangles.

The avascular iris cords, slightly lighter in color, are distinguished inside the triangular black areas (Fig. 12.1, I, *d*). This appearance of the internal wall of the chamber angle, at the areas corresponding to the base and root of the iris, is described in a figure exactly like ours by Eisler [3] and Kupfer [4]. The ciliary body band has a different development depending on age:

the older the child, the wider the band. The width of the ciliary body band depends on the development of the radial and circular portions of the ciliary muscle. It is also related to refraction.

When There Are Transparent Mesodermal Remnants

The appearance described above changes: between the external and internal walls, the chamber angle is filled with mesodermal remnants, which give the chamber angle a more circular shape. The mesodermal remnants are sometimes covered with a gray band with a cellophane appearance (Barkan membrane). Worst [2] made a superb demonstration of this gonioscopy with contact lenses specially designed for this purpose. They are sometimes transparent and slightly pigmented. When it is in the reabsorption process, the Barkan membrane has holes. If all these elements filling the chamber angle are wholly transparent, the iris tissue extending until it ends above the ciliary body band can be seen beneath them and, at the base and root of the iris, the black triangular holes can also be seen. Barkan [5] and Lister [6] presented figures showing this clearly (Fig. 12.1, II, III).

When the Mesodermal Remnants Are Opaque or Pigmented

When the mesodermal remnants are opaque or pigmented, they hide the structures of the chamber angle, which are located below it. The mesodermal remnants extend from the segment between the root and base of the iris and up to the external wall, though sometimes they reach the Schlemm canal or overlap it in tree-like terminations, which may be in direct contact with the scleral wall. Busacca agreed that the iris processes correspond to the mesodermal remnants (Fig. 12.1, IV): "A smooth, bright arch-shaped surface extends from the spur to the iris base and it becomes the chamber angle. This area of the chamber angle may have different appearances and this structure variety depends on the presence, the absence or the number of iris processes, which are the remnants of the pectinate ligament in animals, which is present in the ontogenic development of man" [7].

The dark triangular areas, corresponding to the base and root of the iris, are only visible at this part when both the mesodermal tissue and the Barkan membrane are transparent; but when these formations are opaque, they can only be seen at the level of the Barkan membrane insertion. When the mesodermal remnants are

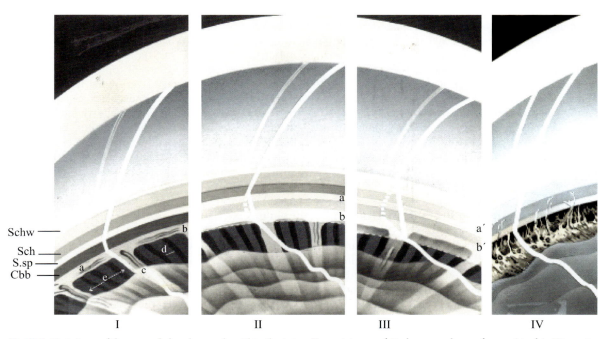

Fig. 12.1 Variations of the normal chamber angle within the 1st year of age. *Schw* Schwalbe line, *Sch* Schlemm canal, *Ssp* scleral spur, *Cbb* ciliary body band, *Ir* iris root, *a*, *b* iris major arterial circle, *c* vascular pillars, *d* avascular pillars, *e* iris epithelial pigmentary layer. *I* chamber angle without Barkan membrane, *II* persistence of Barkan membrane from *a´* to *b´*, *III* persistence of Barkan membrane from *a´* to *b´* (Barkan membrane disappears during the development of the angle), *IV* iris processes

resorbed or missing, the maximum peripheral location these dark zones can reach is the iris root; they can never extend beyond the ciliary body since this is anatomically impossible.

In the chamber angle in normal children, the ciliary body band is generally present and this should always be kept in mind.

It is important to distinguish the base from the root of the iris [7]; the base corresponds to the termination level of the last circular fold of the iris (whose most elevated part is the Busacca iris crest line). Either the mesodermal remnants, when present, or the Barkan membrane, or both, end there. The iris root extends from the base to the ciliary body band. It is covered by mesodermal remnants and it develops after the tearing and resorption of the Barkan membrane and the mesodermal remnants. The entire length of the root is in part made up of the radial fibers of the ciliary muscle (Ivanoff muscle).

The fine slit and the profile lines of gonioscopic images are usually not used in gonioscopies on newborns. This accounts for the common mistake of believing that the vertex of the future chamber angle is located where the corneoscleral profile line joins with the mesodermal profile line, or at the attachment site of the iris profile line with the mesodermal profile line. None of these union points (corneomesodermal and mesodermal-iris) are the vertices of the future chamber angle. The mesodermal profile line is tangent to the corneoscleral and iris profile lines. The actual intersection point of the margins of the future chamber angle is the connection between the extension of the corneoscleral profile line and the iris profile line.

Since the optical section is rarely applied to the study of the chamber angle, its topography is generally

misinterpreted. It should be stressed that the chamber angle in a normal child has its fully developed gonioscopic elements: the Schwalbe line, the clearly visible ciliary body band, and, sometimes, mesodermal remnants undergoing a resorption process or slightly persistent. It should be remembered that in the root of the iris is the peripheral arterial circle of the iris (Fig. 12.2). The excellent description made by Busacca and Carvalho [7] of the mesodermal remnants and the systems making them up, is highly recommended. According to these authors, the mesodermal remnants are developed by three systems.

The reticular system is inside the mesodermal triangle (1, Fig. 12.3). This triangle is bounded to the front by an external longitudinal system of fibers (2, Fig. 12.3) making up the tendon of the Brücke muscle and extending from the Schwalbe line to the longitudinal muscle. Toward the back, it is bounded by the internal longitudinal system (3, Fig. 12.3). This system gives rise to the iris root, especially to the avascular part (radiated cords); it extends from the iris base up to the radiated fibers of the ciliary muscle (Ivanoff muscle) and it is the source of the future iris root. The triangle's side, bounded by the anterior chamber, is made up of the Barkan membrane, known in gonioscopy as the mesodermal band. Remnants of the external longitudinal system will give rise to trabecular formations attached to the external wall of the chamber angle, which are later lined with the Henle layer and with pigment. Remnants of the reticular system will give rise to fibers extending from the iris base or from different points at the iris root, like a bridge on the chamber angle, and up to different heights of the external wall (spur, trabecular meshwork at the level of the Schlemm canal, Schwalbe's line, etc.)

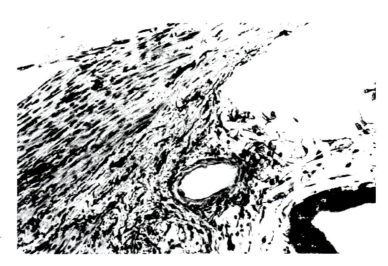

Fig. 12.2 Position of the arterial circle at the level of the chamber angle (original preparation)

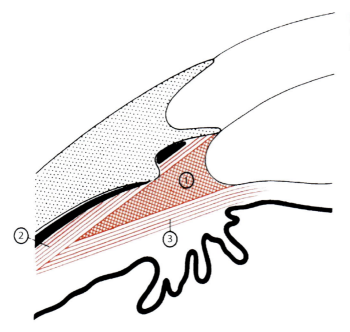

Fig. 12.3 Mesodermal remnants in the fetus (*red*): *1* reticular system, *2* external longitudinal system, *3* internal longitudinal system

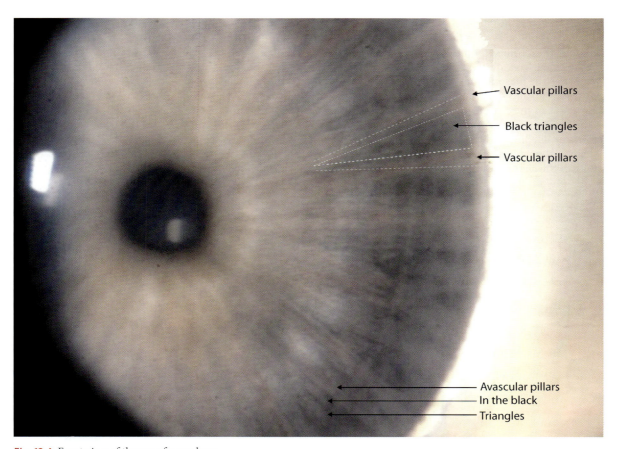

Fig. 12.4 Front view of the eye of a newborn

It is very important to know the direct and gonioscopic appearance of the iris of a normal child. Jerndal et al. [8] state that "the gonioscopic appearance of Barkan's membrane and other goniodysgenetic signs have been a veritable apple of discord, and a number of authors have overlooked or denied the obvious angle maldevelopment in infantile congenital glaucomas."

Figure 12.4 shows a front view of the eye of a newborn. The superficial mesodermal layer of the iris, the clear tissue that follows the pupil, has not developed to the periphery. Therefore, black triangles appear in the peripheral half of the iris, which correspond to its pigmentary layer. The radial sides of these black triangles are the so-called vascular pillars of the iris, which contain very fine red vessels. In the black triangles there are clearer, thin pillars, parallel to the vessels, corresponding to the avascular pillars of the iris.

Figure 12.5 shows normal chamber angles of newborn children. As Jerndal said, many writers do not

know this normal morphology: "Scheie (1968), wrote: I, on the other hand, place almost no diagnostic value on the gonioscopic appearance of the angle of the anterior chamber in infantile glaucoma. Although I do routine gonioscopy, in my opinion, the findings are so nebulous that I cannot distinguish between the angle in a normal eye and one with infantile glaucoma, unless the eyeball is enlarged or some other anomaly known to be associated with glaucoma is present, such as aniridia or Axenfeld's syndrome."

Some authors (Fig. 12.6) present drawings like these and say that they correspond to a chamber angle of congenital glaucoma, whereas it actually corresponds to a normal chamber angle in a normal child.

Figure 12.7 shows four goniophotographs of normal children, with the drawing of a normal chamber angle in a child in the upper right hand corner.

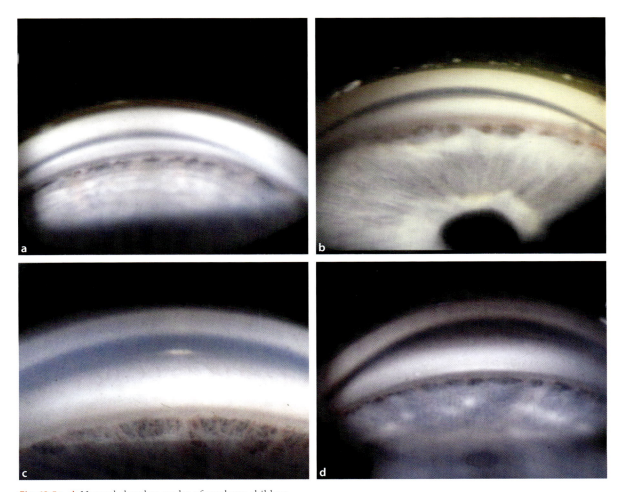

Fig. 12.5a–d Normal chamber angles of newborn children

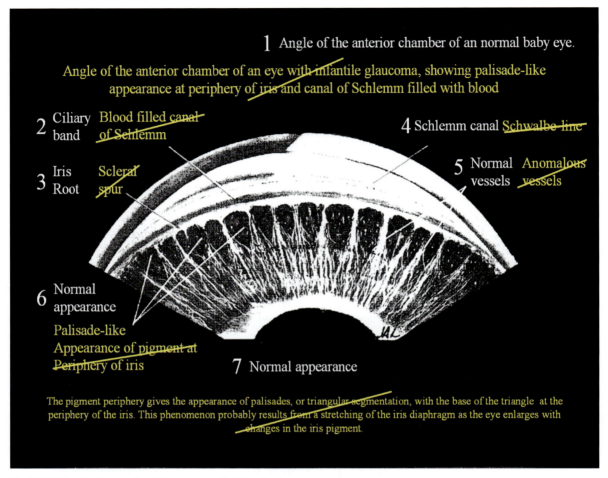

1 Angle of the anterior chamber of an normal baby eye.

Angle of the anterior chamber of an eye with infantile glaucoma, showing palisade-like appearance at periphery of iris and canal of Schlemm filled with blood

2 Ciliary band   Blood filled canal of Schlemm

4 Schlemm canal Schwalbe line

3 Iris Root   Scleral spur

5 Normal vessels Anomalous vessels

6 Normal appearance

Palisade-like Appearance of pigment at Periphery of iris

7 Normal appearance

The pigment periphery gives the appearance of palisades, or triangular segmentation, with the base of the triangle at the periphery of the iris. This phenomenon probably results from a stretching of the iris diaphragm as the eye enlarges with changes in the iris pigment.

Fig 12.6 *Yellow* indicates what is incorrect and *white* what is correct

All the authors who have produced gonioscopy atlases made a drawing of the chamber angle in the child, as we have just shown, calling it a pathological image of the angle in congenital glaucoma, when it is really a normal chamber angle image in a normal child. This Fig. 12.8 is from a very good book: *Color Atlas of Gonioscopy*, by Wallace L.M. Alward [9] (Fig. 12.8).

Goldmann [10] had drawn the anomaly that presents in type II refractory congenital glaucoma, a perfect drawing by his own hand, in which these vessels and black triangles, in an apparent high insertion of the iris, are at the level of the Schwalbe line and do not permit any of the elements of the angle to be seen (Fig. 12.9).

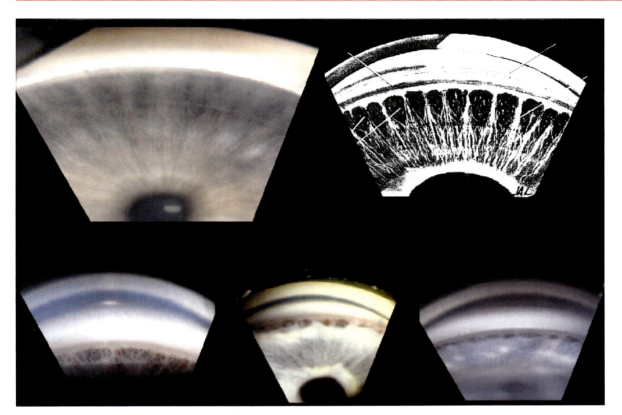

Fig. 12.7 Four goniophotographs of normal children

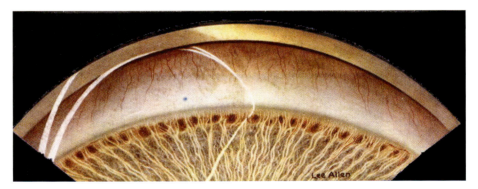

Fig 12.8 From the *Color Atlas of Gonioscopy* by Alward

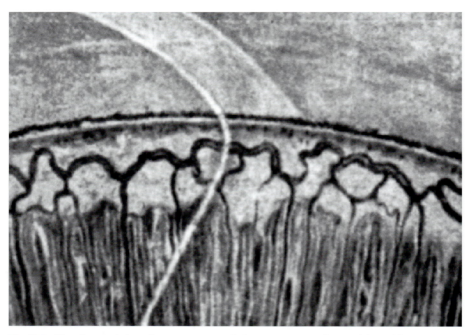

Fig. 12.9 Chamber angle in refractory congenital glaucoma type II, designed by Goldmann in 1948

Contact Lenses for Chamber Angle Examination in Children

For the examination of the chamber angle in newborns and infants up to 2 years of age, there are lenses specially designed by Haag Streit. Their diameter, at the surface that comes into contact with the eye is different from the diameter used for adults, i.e., they have a smaller diameter. There are two alternative lenses for children: one is 10-mm and the other 11-mm. However, recently, Rousell and Fankhauser developed a new contact lens for gonioscopy with greater resolution.

References

1. Seefelder R, Wolfrum C (1906) Zur Entwickliung der vorderen Kammer und des Kammerwinkels beim Menschen nebts Bemerkungen über ihre Entstehung bei Tieren. Arch Ophthalmol 63:430–451
2. Worst JGF (1966) The pathogenesis of congenital glaucoma. Royal Vangorcum Publishers, Assen Netherlands
3. Eisler P (1930) Die Anatomie des menschlicken Auges. In: Shiek F, Brückner A (eds) Shieck und Brückner's Kurzes Handbuch der Ophthal I. Springer, Berlin
4. Kupfer C (1963) Gonioscopy in infants and children. In: Apt L (ed) Leonard's diagnostic procedures in pediatric ophthalmology. Little Brown, London, pp 11–23
5. Barkan O (1936) The structure and functions of the angle of the anterior chamber and Schlemm's canal. Arch Ophthal Chicago 15:101–110
6. Lister A (1960) Some aspects of congenital glaucoma. Trans Ophthal Soc UK 79:163–179
7. Busacca A, Carvalho C (1968) Osservazioni gonioscopiche sul glaucoma congenito. Atti del L Congresso della Societá Oftalmologica Italiana. Arte della Stampa, Roma, pp 64–68
8. Jerndal T, Hansson HA, d Hill A (1978) Goniodysgenesis. A new perspective on glaucoma. Scriptor, Copenhagen
9. Alward WLM (1994) Color Atlas of Gonioscopy (Illustrated by Lee Allen). Wolfe Medical, London
10. Goldmann H (1948) La gonioscopie. Jules François. Rapport sur les informations gonioscopiques, particulerement dans l'étude et le traitement du glaucome. Presenté à la Société Belge de Ophtalmologie. Librairie R. Fonteyn, Louvain, Belgium, p 73

Pathological Chamber Angle in Congenital Glaucoma and Its Implications in Indications for Surgery

Contents

Pathological Chamber Angle in Congenital Glaucomas

The two types of pathological chamber angle in children are type I and type II. Type I (Fig. 13.1) has thin pathological mesodermal remnants that cover the ciliary band of the chamber angles and sometimes slender extensions reach the Schwalbe line. Type II (Fig. 13.1) chamber angles are identified by the presence of thick pathological mesodermal remnants with apparent high iris insertion with black triangles and pillars. In both types, it is impossible to distinguish the ciliary body band.

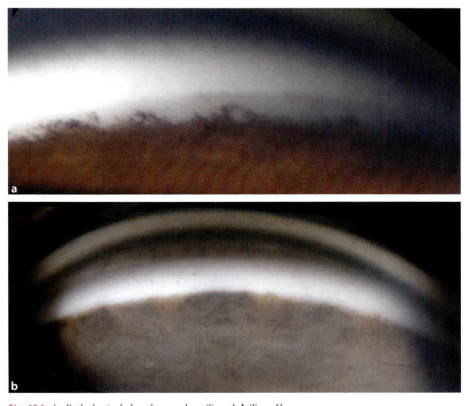

Fig. 13.1a,b Pathological chamber angle. **a** Type I. **b** Type II

Figure 13.2a illustrates type I (Fig. 13.2b type II), with white lines delineating the various elements. Depending on the chamber angle, either trabeculotomy or combined surgery (trabeculotomy + trabeculectomy) is performed.

Figure 13.3 provides a summary of the two types. Figure 13.3a–c corresponds to type I congenital glaucoma: Fig. 13.3b, the goniophotograph, Fig. 13.3a, a schematic drawing of this goniophotograph, Fig. 13.3c, the pathologic anatomy of this condition. Figure 13.3d–f illustrates the diagram and pathologic anatomy of re-

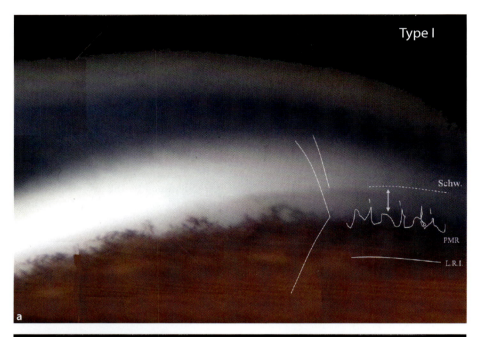

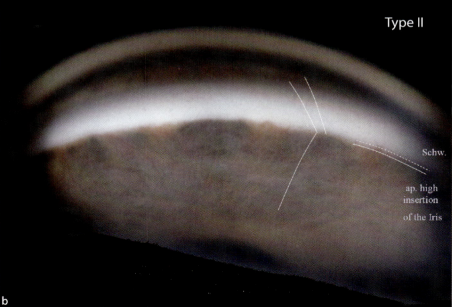

Fig. 13.2 a *Schw* Schwalbe line, *PMR* pathological mesodermal remnants, *LRI* last roll of the iris. **b** *Schw* Schwalbe line, *ap* apparent high insertion of the iris

fractory, type II congenital glaucoma. This gonioscopic differentiation in congenital glaucoma is necessary and knowledge of this will make for success or failure in surgery.

In our early experience, when we did only trabeculotomy, 30% of the children returned for consultation between 1 and 3 years later, the operation having failed, with an increase in IOP and greater axial length of the eye. Looking at the angle, we realized that all of them belonged to type II (apparently high insertion of the iris). This is why it is crucial for the surgical indication to diagnose type I and type II based on the angle, since in type I trabeculotomy should be indicated and in type II a combined operation (trabeculotomy + trabeculectomy in the same session of surgery; see Chap. 16). I proposed this surgery for the first time in 1988 [1, 2].

Ten years later it was proposed by Mandal [3, 4] and in 2000 and 2001 by Meyer et al. and Kiefer et al. [5, 6]. Table 13.1 summarizes this, indicating the principal characteristics, to which are added the axial length and the corneal diameter.

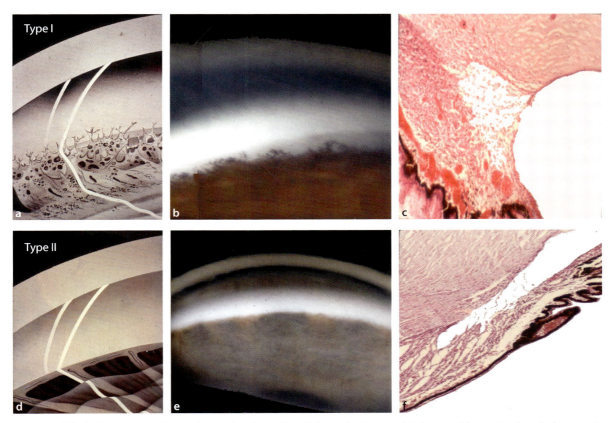

Fig. 13.3a–f *Left*, drawing, chamber angle type I and type II; *middle*, goniophotographic image; *right*, anatomic pathology specimen

Table 13.1 Chamber angle and axial length in the indication of surgery for congenital glaucoma

Type I	Type II
Pathological mesodermal remnants	Apparent high insertion of iris
Axial length: up to 23 mm	Axial length: >23 mm
Corneal diameter: up to 13 mm	Corneal diameter: >13 mm
Trabeculotomy	Combined surgery: trabeculotomy + trabeculectomy
	From Sampaolesi 1988

The Use of SL-OCT in Diagnosis and Follow-Up of Congenital Glaucomas

The recent appearance in the market of a new technology applied to the anterior segment has opened the way to the coherent light tomography. The SL-OCT (slit lamp optical coherence tomography) is coherent light tomography adapted to a conventional slit lamp, produced by Heidelberg Engineering. The Visante is another version of this instrument manufactured by Zeiss, which we have not used.

One of the advantages of the SL-OCT over the Visante is that it is adapted to a slit lamp and is not an additional instrument. The ophthalmologist, used to using the lamp, knows that the slit indicates the section that is seen over the monitor to the right. The lightbeam is located over the structure to be studied, and the ocular section can be seen at that point. In addition, in contrast to the Visante, the SL-OCT makes it possible to perform the Budenz maneuver of indentation gonioscopy, which is fundamental for deciding whether the blockages are functional or organic. Figure 13.4 shows the SL-OCT and Fig. 13.5 the authors studying a child with congenital glaucoma under sedation with Sevorane and monitoring with the same instrument.

Since the SL-OCT can be used in nontransparent media, it is very useful for observing the chamber angle, even in cases where there is a significant corneal edema. Figure 13.6 shows a 2-month-old girl who consulted for pure type II congenital glaucoma (apparent high insertion of the iris) with ocular pressure at 38 mmHg and corneal edema. The gonioscopy can be seen in the genioscopy, with poor resolution due to the edema, while the SL-OCT shows the apparent high insertion of the iris, with peripheral atrophy of the iris, in the same eye at the same time.

The SL-OCT gives a clear idea of the pathogenesis of congenital glaucoma both in the pure congenital glaucomas and in secondary glaucomas or those associated with ocular malformations. Figure 13.7 illustrates type I congenital glaucoma (from pathological mesodermal remnants) with excellent clarity in the tomograph. Pure type II congenital glaucoma (from apparent high insertion of the iris) can be seen in Fig. 13.8, clearly showing the difference between the two phenotypes.

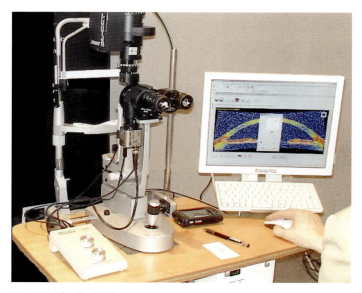

Fig. 13.4 The SL-OCT

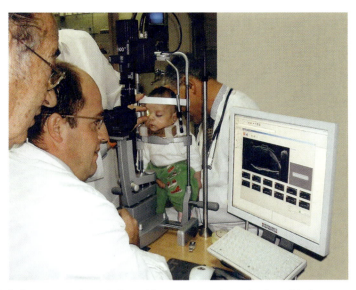

Fig. 13.5 The authors studying a child with congenital glaucoma under sedation with sevorane and monitoring with the same instrument

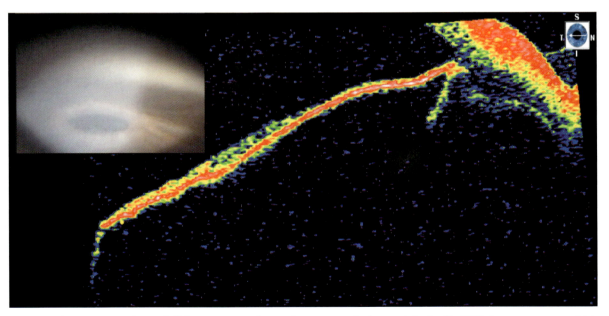

Fig. 13.6 The gonioscopy (*upper left*) has a poor resolution due to corneal edema, while the SL-OCT shows an apparent high insertion of the iris

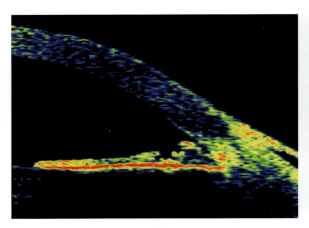

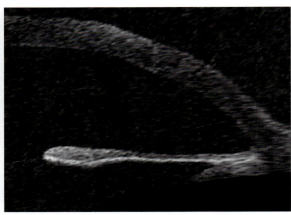

Fig. 13.7 Type I congenital glaucoma

Fig. 13.8 Pure type II congenital glaucoma

Corneal alterations can also be seen with high definition, even though they are microscopic or when there is significant opacity in the media. In the case of Haab striae, when a cross-section is made, the limit of the Descemet membrane can be seen at both sides of the striae, which is visible tomographically as an intracorneal slit or canal (Fig. 13.9).

On the other hand, when the media are not clear, as for example in the leukomas that can accompany congenital aniridia, there are cases in which in anterior segment biomicroscopy, the leukoma prevents a view of the anterior chamber, as shown in the example. Nonetheless, the SL-OCT not only shows its structures, but also the tube of the Ahmed valve that the patient has implanted, with no contact with either the cornea or the crystalline lens (Fig. 13.10).

The same case of secondary congenital glaucoma or associated with aniridia and leukoma can be seen in Fig. 13.11, after performing a penetrating keratoplasty. The biomicroscopy shows how the leukoma has been removed with the transplant and the SL-OCT shows the donor button sutured to the receptor bed, with the tube in the anterior chamber that has no contact with the donor button.

In aniridia, it is also possible to see the detention of the Descemet membrane where the central leukoma begins (Fig. 13.12) and the colobomatous lens, or pear-shaped lens, which is incorrectly mentioned in several texts as superior lens subluxation (Fig. 13.13).

In the angles of normal newborns, there is peripheral thinning of the iris, because at the time of birth the mesodermal layer of the iris is not fully developed. This can be seen in Fig. 13.14. Figure 13.15 shows a different picture, corresponding to a case of peripheral atrophy of the iris in pure type II congenital glaucoma.

In Peters syndrome, congenital glaucoma secondary to or associated with ocular malformations, it is possible in its forme fruste to see the dyscoria, with the pupil drawn toward 12 o'clock behind a partial leukoma, in the biomicroscopy of the anterior segment (Fig. 13.16). The SL-OCT shows the asymmetry in the iris and the posterior ulcer of the cornea described in this syndrome (Fig. 13.17).

In cases in which Peters syndrome is not fruste, a much larger central leukoma is commonly seen (Fig. 13.18) as well as synechiae or adherences between the pupil edge of the iris and the rear face of the cornea, as in Fig. 13.19.

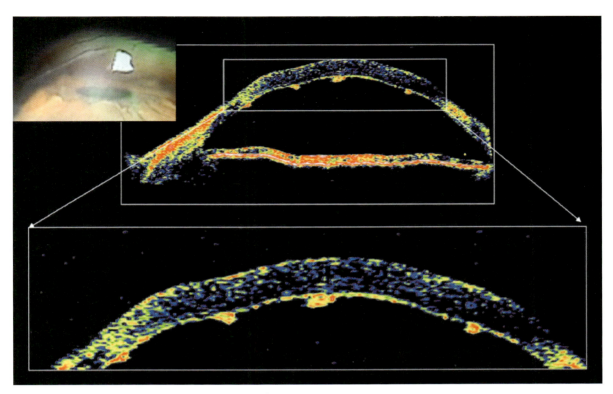

Fig. 13.9 Gonioscopy of Haab striae in Descemet membrane

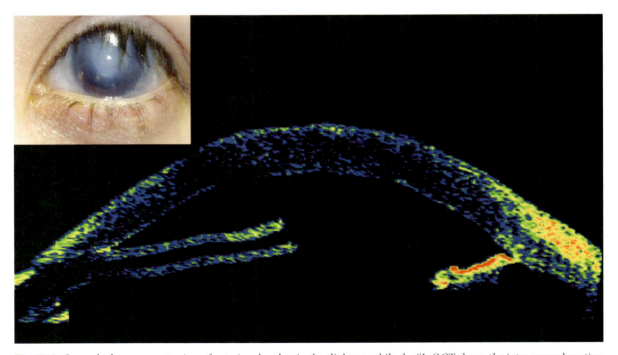

Fig. 13.10 Corneal edema prevents view of anterior chamber in the slit lamp, while the SL-OCT shows the intracameral portion of the tube

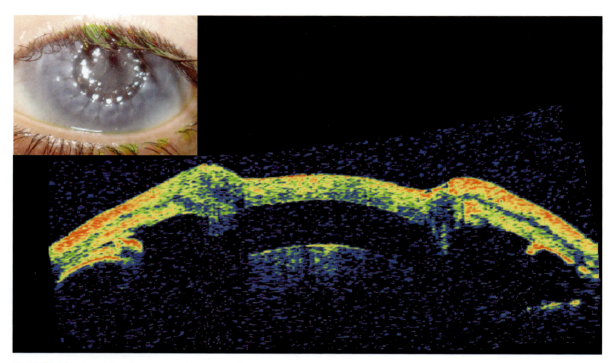

Fig. 13.11 The same eye after penetrating keratoplasty

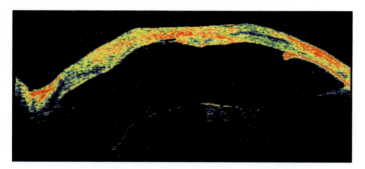

Fig. 13.12 Pear-shaped lens on the left side can be seen, which is often incorrectly mentioned as superior lens subluxation

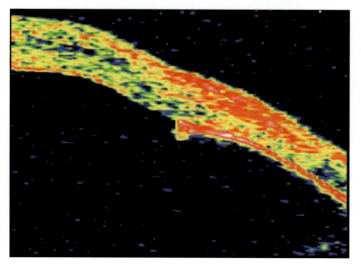

Fig. 13.13 Detention of the Descemet membrane in the peripheral cornea

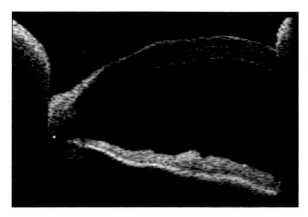

Fig. 13.14 Peripheral thinning of the iris, because at the time of birth the mesodermal layer of the iris is not fully developed

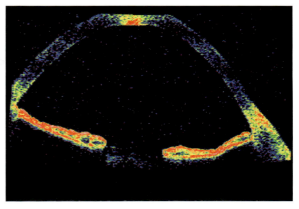

Fig. 13.15 Peripheral atrophy of the iris in pure type II congenital glaucoma

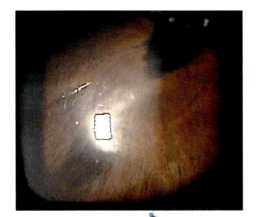

Fig. 13.16 Fruste Peters Syndrome, with central leucoma and dyscoria

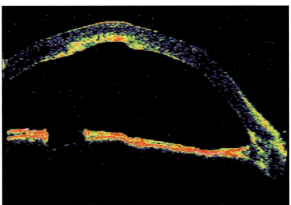

Fig. 13.17 Posterior ulcer of the cornea as described in Peters Syndrome

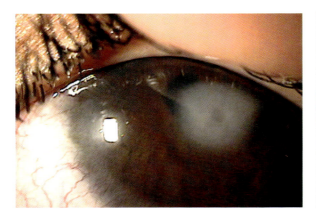

Fig. 13.18 Large leukoma is commonly seen in not fruste Peters Syndrome

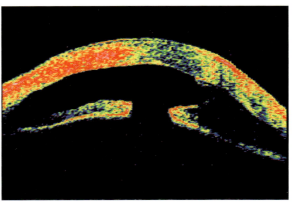

Fig. 13.19 Synechiae or adherences between the pupil edge of the iris and the rear face of the cornea

In late congenital glaucomas, pigmentary glaucomas are found that are characterized by having a trapezoidal anterior chamber and positive peripheral transillumination of the iris. In Fig. 13.20, the anterior chamber can be seen with this aspect, while in Fig. 13.20 the lack of substance in the peripheral iris can be observed, which probably originates the positive peripheral transillumination in these glaucomas.

Among the postsurgical complications are hypothalamia or athalamia, generally seen when atropine was not used during surgery or when there is a positive Seidel phenomenon from poor conjunctival closing. It is important to check both aspects in the surgery with these children, since each reintervention requires general anesthetic.

A case of athalamia can be seen in Fig. 13.21, where the iris was in contact on both sides with the rear face of the cornea, and there is only aqueous humor between the lens and the corneal endothelium. Figure 13.22 shows hypothalamia with hyphema, and the iris can be observed starting to separate from the rear face of the cornea. On the right edge (lower in the eye), a hyphema has accumulated, leaving the visual axis free (blood in red and yellow).

Another frequent complication is when the tube of the Ahmed valve slips out of the anterior chamber. This usually happens when the tube is not left in long enough so that it does not slip out either with the accelerated growth of the ocular globe in decompensated congenital glaucoma or with the normal growth that occurs in the ocular globe of a child. Figure 13.23 shows that the Ahmed tube escapes from the anterior chamber toward the intrascleral portion.

To sum up, this new technology, because it has the qualities of a rapid examination method, high resolution, no need for clear media, and above all, it does not come in contact with the eye, is a very useful tool for evaluating congenital glaucomas in their diagnosis, follow-up, and postsurgical assessment. We believe that it is also superior to ultrasonic ultrabiomicroscopy (UBM) applications, especially in the pediatric glaucoma population.

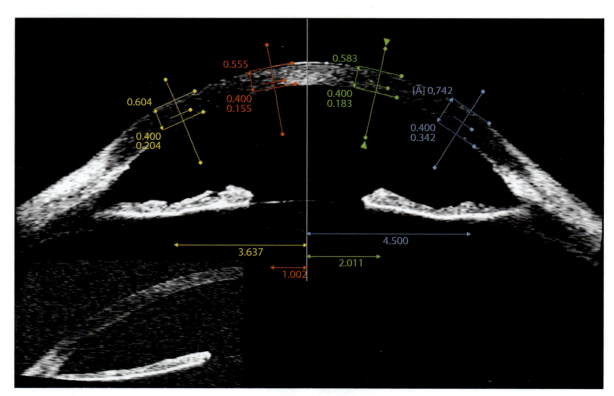

Fig. 13.20 Anterior segment with SL-OCT, pachimetry and peripheral thinning of the iris tissue

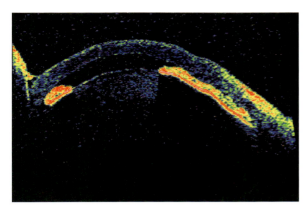

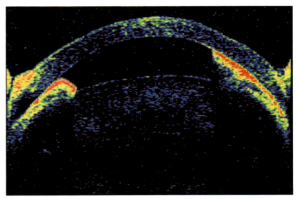

Fig. 13.21 A case of athalamia where the iris was in contact on both sides with the rear face of the cornea

Fig. 13.22 Hipothalamia and hyphema, the iris starts to separate from the cornea on the right side

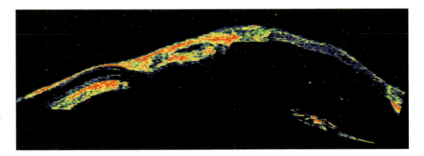

Fig. 13.23 Ahmed tube escapes from the anterior chamber towards the intrascleral portion

References

1. Sampaolesi R (1991) Glaucoma, 2nd edn. Editorial Medica Panamericana, Buenos Aires, Argentina
2. Sampaolesi R (1988) Congenital glaucoma. Long-term results after surgery. Fortschr Ophthalmol 85:626–631
3. Mandal AK (1996) Surgical results of combined trabeculotomy-trabeculectomy for developmental glaucoma. Primary combined trabeculotomy and trabeculectomy in a single session. Ophthalmology 105:974–983
4. Mandal AK (2003) Outcome of surgery on infants younger than 1 month with congenital glaucoma. Ophthalmology 110:1909–1915
5. Meyer G, Schwenn O, Grehn F (2000) Trabekulotomie beim Kongenitalem Glaukom. Ein Vergleich zur Goniotomie. Ophthalmologe 97:623–628
6. Kiefer G, Schwenn O, Grehn F (2001) Correlation of postoperative axial length growth and intraocular pressure in congenital glaucoma. A retrospective study in trabeculotomy and goniotomy. Graefes Arch Clin Exp Ophthalmol 239:893–899
7. Kozlov VI, Bagrov SN, Anisimova SY et al (1990) Nonpenetrating deep sclerotomy with collagen. IRTC Eye microsurgery. RSFSR Ministry of Public Health, Moscow 4:62–66

Clinical History for Congenital Glaucoma

14

This clinical history form is a way of recording all the studies for congenital glaucoma. The tools used for obtaining the data are described in Chap. 4, which discusses examining newborns under general anesthesia.

CONGENITAL GLAUCOMA

Name _____ Surname _____   Glaucoma n° _____

Age _____ Years _____ Months _____ Gender _____   General record n° _____

Address _____

Phone   _____

Referred by   _____

Date _____

OD   OS

DIAGNOSIS

Heredity

General history

Ocular history: Date of onset of symptoms _____

Axial length   _____   _____

**Normal axial length
for this age**   _____   _____

IOP   _____   _____

**Normal IOP
for this age**   _____   _____

**Corneal diameter
Cycloplegia**   _____   _____

Anterior segment

Gonioscopy
  Type 1
  Type 2

Optic Nerve
Peripheral fundoscopy

SURGERY

Date _____

_____
_____
_____
_____
_____
_____

POSTOPERATIVE EXAMINATION

_____
_____
_____

POSTOPERATIVE GONIOSCOPY

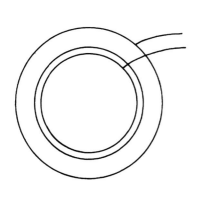
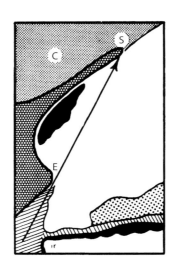
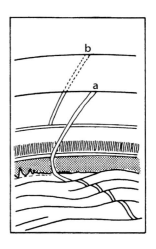

Evolution

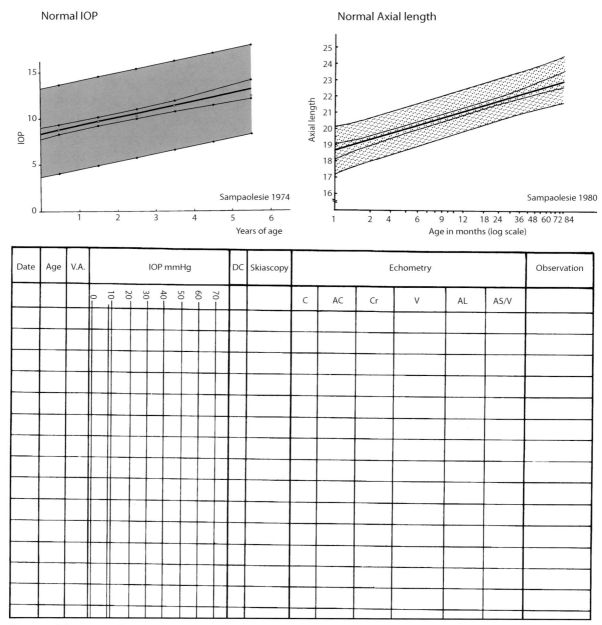

C cornea, **AC** Anterior Chamber, **L** Lens, **V** Vitreous, **AL** Axial Length, **AS/V** Anterior Segment/Vitreous **DC** Corneal Diameter

After 6 years of age

Date	Age	V.A.	IOP mmHg		Myopia	V.A.	A. Length	Visual Field MD	Visual Field CLV	HRT: Phase
			0 10 20 30 40 50 60 70					0 10 20 30	0 5 10 20 30 50	

Date

Summary

Contents

In congenital glaucoma, when pathological mesodermal remnants remain, obstructing the filtration area of the chamber angle, this tissue needs to be surgically removed. Taylor [1, 2] was the first to publish Carlos De Vincentiis's surgical technique for the treatment of glaucoma [3, 4]. Designed in Naples and known as the incision of the angle formed by the iris and the cornea, or internal sclerotomy, this technique had the same requirements as goniotomy, since it was performed with a small sickle-shaped knife (the De Vincentiis knife, specially manufactured to prevent aqueous humor from overflowing), ocular fixation was good, and the incision was nontraumatic and superficial to prevent damage to other structures of the chamber angle. He used the technique for all sorts of glaucomas and it was the first blind goniotomy, though it is actually an *ab interno* trabeculotomy. It was then abandoned for 30 years, perhaps because it was reported only in a local Italian journal and because its author died soon thereafter. In 1900, Scalinci [5] presented 13 cases of congenital glaucoma successfully operated using this technique.

De Vincentiis's technique was perfected by Barkan in 1936 [6], who added visualization of the chamber angle through a lens during the surgical procedure; this newly applied surgical procedure was called goniotomy.

Goniotomy

There are several interesting points to be mentioned concerning goniotomy. Barkan [7] (Fig. 15.1) described the results of this technique in a sample of 51 children (76 eyes with congenital glaucoma). The procedure, performed in the early stage of congenital glaucoma, was successful in 66 cases and failed in ten. There was optic nerve atrophy only in those cases failing to achieve IOP regulation. The procedure was not performed with a microscope, but with a ×5 loupe. The patients were followed up for 10 years.

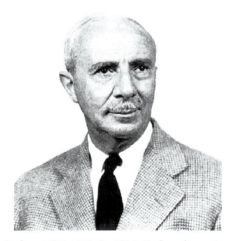

Fig. 15.1 Otto Barkan 1887–1958. In 1936, Barkan dramatically changed the poor prognosis of infantile glaucoma with goniotomy

The author stresses the importance of early diagnosis and prompt operation. He states:

It is essential to operate early, before prolonged distention of the eyeball has caused obliteration of Schlemm's canal. Other important reasons for early diagnosis and prompt operation are: (a) restoration of vision by clearing the cornea ...; (b) prevention of the amblyopia resulting from prolonged obstruction of vision by cloudiness of the cornea; (c) prevention of the development of permanent scarring from corneal cloudiness; (d) prevention of injury to the optic nerve caused by prolonged pressure.

The extensive literature authored by Barkan is very interesting [8–12].

Worst [13] provided a detailed description of this technique as well as of the goniotomy lens he designed himself.

In addition, Broughton and Parks [14] used goniotomy as the initial surgical procedure in 34 patients (50 eyes) with congenital glaucoma. They had an overall success rate of 88% with one or more goniotomies after a follow-up period of 15 years. For these authors, refractive error proved to be a valuable indicator of the success of surgery or of disease progression.

Haas [15] edited the proceedings of a symposium on congenital glaucoma where the outcome of the treatment of 329 eyes of 202 patients with the infantile form of congenital glaucoma was discussed. Patients had undergone between one and five goniotomies, with successful IOP regulation in 77% of cases. Barkan, Shaffer and Haas, among others, contributed material to the discussion. As stated by the author: "early diagnosis with early surgery of the angle will make possible a greatly improved visual prognosis" [15].

Morgan et al. [16] reviewed 37 consecutive patients who had undergone at least one goniotomy or filtering surgery, with a success rate of 78%.

Clothier et al. [17] reported the factors that are relevant to the development of amblyopia in congenital glaucoma, such as: (a) persistent corneal edema, (b) anisometropia, and (c) strabismus. In cases with 7 D or more of anisometropia, the amblyopia was profound. All these factors should be identified early, and they stress the importance of preferential visual tests.

Lister [18] studied a sample of 181 eyes treated with goniotomy as the initial operation. The author stresses the differences in prognosis compared to those reported by Anderson in 1939 [19], for whom the prognosis was very poor, since most patients went blind, while in Lister's sample the IOP was controlled in slightly more than 80% of cases, even considering the most severe cases.

Shaffer [20] also stressed the differences in prognosis from the times of Anderson and the great change observed since the introduction of goniotomy by Barkan, 30 years earlier. He stated that Barkan had actually adapted the De Vicentiis operation (thought to have been reported in 1898). With goniotomy, approximately 85% of cases operated under the age of 1 year achieved IOP normalization. He recommended patching the better eye to counteract amblyopia.

Complications

In a series of 401 goniotomies, Litinsky et al. [21] reported cardiopulmonary arrest in 1.8% of cases as well as apnea, iridodialyses, hyphemas, and anterior synechiae.

Reporting a series of 290 eyes treated at Moorfields Eye Hospital between 1960 and 1979, Cooling et al. [22] observed retinal detachment in 13 eyes.

Surgical Indications

To identify pathological mesodermal remnants and the two main types of chamber angles – vital for deciding which surgical technique to use – the relation between the anatomy, histology, and gonioscopy of normal eyes and those with congenital glaucoma in newborns must be familiar (Chaps. 13, 14).

Surgery is mandatory in all types of congenital glaucoma. In centers such as Shaffer, Hetherington, and Hoskins's center in San Francisco, specializing in this pathology, which may be the most severe of all glaucomas, any infant with symptoms of congenital glaucoma is examined under general anesthesia directly in the operating room, and if necessary, with the parents' previous consent, can be operated immediately after the examination, since a delay of days, weeks, or months may turn a small eye into an enlarged one, and, even if surgery succeeds in regulating IOP, the macular and optic nerve alterations lead to impaired visual acuity.

For the first time, I examined a case in which IOP was regulated spontaneously because the tears in the Descemet membrane and the endothelium continued up to the trabecular meshwork. This child has been followed up for 25 years and at present he has normal IOP, visual acuity, and visual field. The tears extended over the trabecular meshwork, thus causing an automatic goniotomy. Dr. Manzitti and Dr. Damel (personal communication) have studied two cases of the spontaneous regulation of IOP.

Lockie et al. [23] studied 61 cases of primary congenital glaucoma in which they detected six cases of spontaneous cures. All the cases had large corneas and tears in the Descemet membrane.

There are two techniques to be used in children's eyes in the first 6 months of life:

- With angle type I and ocular axial length values 23 mm or less, with no tears in the endothelium and the Descemet membrane or enlarged corneal diameter (see Fig. 13.2, Chap. 13), trabeculotomy is the best technique.
- With angle type II (refractory congenital glaucomas) and an axial length over 23 mm, enlarged corneal diameter, tears in the endothelium and the Descemet membrane, combined surgery (trabeculotomy + trabeculectomy) is better, because trabeculotomy alone fails to regulate IOP.

Though we have abandoned the practice of goniotomy, the next section provides details since many ophthalmologists still use it.

Goniotomy

The implementation of the De Vincentiis technique can be credited to Barkan [6], who contributed control by means of a specially designed gonioscopic lens, which has taken his name. He also studied the chamber angle in normal children and in those with congenital glaucoma.

The corneal epithelium should be transparent and free of edema, or otherwise, a few drops of alcohol 70% should be applied on the cornea [29] and then the epithelium should be removed with the edge of a knife. A pupil with drug-induced miosis should be preferred.

At the beginning, in 1949, we used the Barkan lens (Fig. 15.2), which was available in two different sizes. We subsequently adopted the different lenses specially designed by Swan (Fig. 15.3), Cardona (Fig. 15.4a), Leydhecker (Fig. 15.4b), and Worst (Fig. 15.5). We have obtained better results with the Worst lens, and, in our opinion, this is the safest. The Worst lens for chamber angle microsurgery is available in two sizes, according to the size of the eye to operate (Fig. 15.5a, b).

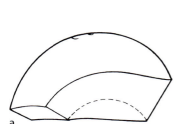 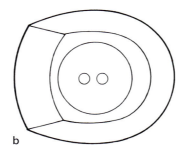 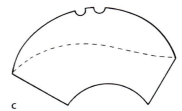

a   b   c

Fig. 15.2a–c The Barkan gonioscopic lens. **a** Profile; **b** view from above; **c** section

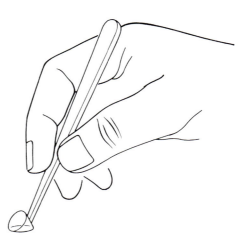

Fig. 15.3 The Swan gonioscopic lens

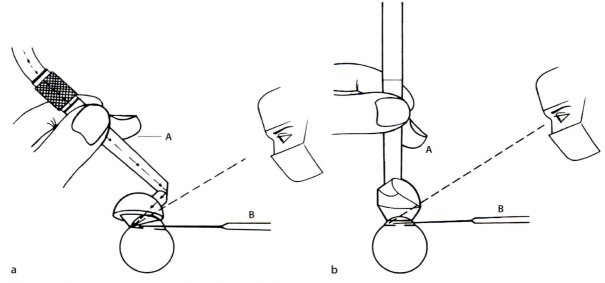

Fig. 15.4 **a** The Cardona gonioscopic lens. **b** The Leydhecker gonioscopic lens

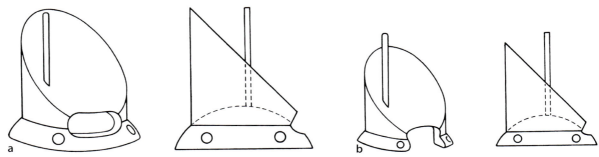

Fig. 15.5a,b The Worst gonioscopic lenses for goniotomy with surgical microscope. Two models in their actual sizes in perspective and section views. The tube enters the lens through its upper part and allows the passage of serum to prevent the formation of air bubbles during the procedure. In **a** and **b**, different sizes depending on the dimensions of the eye to be operated

Figure 15.6 shows the appropriate position for the patient, microscope, and surgeon. The anteroposterior axis of the infant's head should be 45° to the horizontal plane, since this gives perfect visualization of the chamber angle. In Fig. 15.6, gonioscopy is being performed in the nasal area of the chamber angle. The visual axis of the surgeon should be oblique, as shown in the figure; consequently, the axes of the microscope and of the other illumination devices should be slanted by inserting piece A (manufactured by Zeiss, Oberkochen, Germany, based on a drawing and measurements I made for this purpose), between the microscope's arm and the upper horizontal support. This piece, sketched in the upper right-hand side of the figure, is made of a rod (1) around which piece 2 turns, and in whose hole (3) the microscope's arm is placed.

The microscope's axis can thus be slanted as necessary. Some optical devices perform the same tasks by means of prisms, but their cost is higher. The most highly recommended of these was designed by Draeger, in 1970, for the Muller microscopes.

Once all the elements have been arranged, the sketch shows the two main principles of the Worst method. The contact lens has a duct connected to a syringe by means of a thin plastic tube that enables the cavity between the lens and the cornea to be filled with saline solution, thus allowing continuous visibility. The goniotomy used for sweeping the tissue (pathological mesodermal remnants) interposed between the chamber angle and the trabecular meshwork has a duct inside and a hole in its cutting edge. This duct is connected by means of a plastic tube to a bottle of

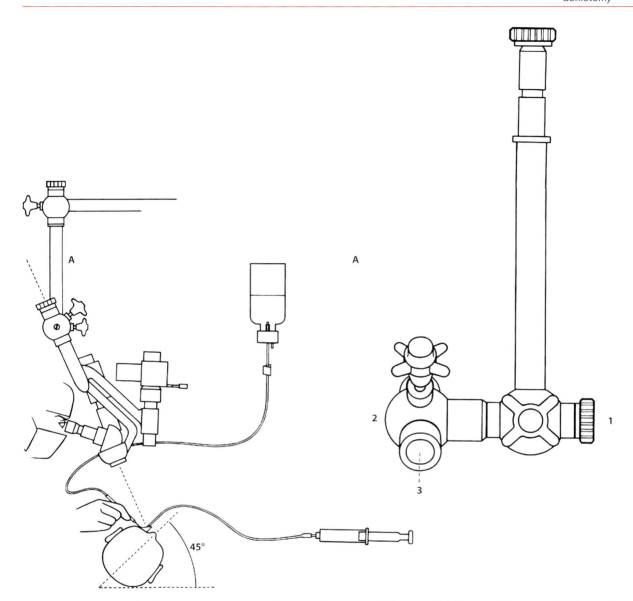

Fig. 15.6 Goniotomy. Infant's position at 45°. Using a device to tilt the microscope. A Enlarged at the angle in the top right of the figure. The device (*2*), with an arm of the microscope put into its hole (*3*), turns around the rod (*A*). The tilt is adjusted by means of the screw (*1*) (Sampaolesi, personal design and technique, 1970). The arm was specially built for this purpose by Zeiss (Oberkochen, Germany)

saline solution, which is generally kept 1 m above the stretcher, so that while the goniotomy is introduced, the chamber angle remains completely filled and well-formed and the iris is displaced slightly backward, thus leaving the chamber angle area, on which the procedure must be performed, wholly uncovered.

Briefly, the original and useful aspects of the Worst technique are the following:

1. The lens is applied and fastened to the sclera by means of stitches (Fig. 15.7).
2. The chamber angle between the lens and the cornea is liquid and permanently free of air.
3. There is continuous irrigation of the chamber angle through the goniotome, with no chamber angle loss.

Technique

1. General anesthesia
2. The Worst lens is fixed to the episcleral plane with four stitches inserted in the four holes of the scleral support of the lens (Fig. 15.7). The stitches can be more easily inserted into the holes if the contact lens is previously applied, held with the hand, and properly centered on the cornea. The opening through which the goniotome will be introduced should be located at the edge of the meridian, opposite the area chosen for goniotomy. At the same time, the areas of the sclera where each stitch will be made are well marked through the holes by means of a punch for lacrimal ducts.

The stitches are made with only one suture, as shown by Fig. 15.8. The crossing of the threads at the center

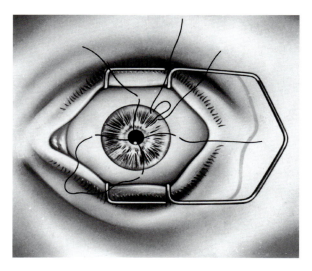

Fig. 15.7 Four stitches, at 12, 6, 3, and 9 o'clock, are passed with only one suture and with the proper, flat needles. By cutting with scissors first at the center, where the threads cross (at the level of the pupil, as shown in the figure), and second, at the lower left, four free sutures are obtained, which can be passed through the hole at the base of the Worst lens for goniotomies. The stitch at the superior temporal area is passed through the oval-shaped opening of the lens, through which the goniotome penetrates. The surgeon must pull this loop toward himself when introducing the goniotome

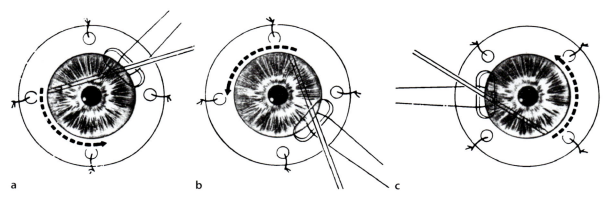

a   b   c

Fig. 15.8a–c Goniotomy performed with the Worst lens. **a** Goniotomy in the inferior nasal quadrant; the goniotome is introduced through the inferior temporal area and shifted from 9 to 6 o'clock. **b** Superior nasal goniotomy. The goniotome penetrates through the inferior temporal area and is displaced from 12 to 9 o'clock. **c** If a third goniotomy is required, it is performed in the temporal area, by inserting the goniotome into the nasal limbus at 9 and shifting it from 5 to 1 o'clock

of the cornea is held with a clamp and cut with scissors, thus leaving the four stitches ready to be passed through the holes of the scleral support of the lens in order to tie them later. As shown in Fig. 15.8a, the fifth U-shaped stitch is then passed and its two edges are inserted into the oval-shaped hole in the lens, which has been designed for inserting the goniotome. This thread allows the goniotome to be located between its two branches, so that pulling it, when introducing the goniotome, facilitates the maneuver. The goniotome is introduced, guided by the microscope, and the Barkan membrane or pathological mesodermal tissue is removed from the chamber angle. The steps to be followed are shown in Fig. 15.8.

Goniotomy is followed by a hyphema of varying degrees of severity, which indicates that the goniotomy has been performed at the appropriate place. This hyphema reverses in a few hours.

Atropine 1% eye drops are instilled and both eyes are occluded with a dressing. Twenty-four hours after surgery, the eye is examined and the occlusion removed. Generally, the hyphema is found to have disappeared.

Goniopuncture

Scheie (1961) applied the technique of goniopuncture on 36 eyes with juvenile glaucoma and 52 eyes with infantile glaucoma. His results were encouraging: IOP was normalized in 57% of eyes by one or more goniopunctures. The longest follow-up period was 11 years and the shortest 1 year.

Trabeculotomy for Chamber Angle Type I

In 1959, Dellaporta [24], studying the pathological anatomy specimens of 100 eyes subject to cyclodialysis, found that the trabecular meshwork had become detached in the area of the anterior chamber where the spatula was introduced: he therefore proposed the trabeculodialysis technique. He communicated his results to Burian [25], who, in 1960, made the first *ab externo* trabeculotomy in a case with glaucoma and Marfan syndrome. Allen and Burian [26] described the technique used experimentally in enucleated human eyes: a conjunctival flap is made with a good dissection, and then, advancing on the sclerocorneal limbus, an incision is made perpendicular to the limbus, and a stitch is passed through each margin so that it is slightly open,

thus leaving the Schlemm canal uncovered in order to channel it with a trabeculotome specially designed for this purpose.

In the same year, Smith [27, 28], in England, made a trabeculotomy canalizing the Schlemm canal by two incisions similar to those made by Burian, with a nylon thread. After passing it through, it is pulled from both ends and in this way what was an arch becomes a cord with the resulting destruction of the meshwork.

Similar techniques were used by Walter and Kanagasundaran [29] and Strachan [30], the latter using a tear-duct dilator as an instrument.

In 1966, the most important contribution to the operation was made by Harms [31–33], who made a scleral lamellar dissection (like Cairns, for the trabeculectomy procedure) in the area of the Schlemm canal, advancing slightly into the transparent cornea. With an incision perpendicular to the limbos, they revealed the Schlemm canal, sectioned its outer wall, and canalized it.

In 1969, the Lyon [34] school with Paufique, Sourdille, and Ortiz-Olmedo, presented the results of trabeculotomy with the same technique as Harms to the Ophthalmology Congress in Paris. Ortiz-Olmedo provided a complete review of trabeculotomy in his doctoral thesis.

In 1971 [35], Dannheim performed trabeculotomy on 300 eyes of adult patients with different types of glaucoma, but he also studied infants. He considered trabeculotomy to be a technique carrying quite a low risk of operative and postoperative complications in comparison with fistulizing methods. Its effect in controlling intraocular pressure is no worse than that of classical operating procedures. In these cases performed in adults, the IOP was regulated only between 20 and 24 mmHg. Today, however, to reach a target pressure, this is not sufficient to stop the damage caused by glaucoma from progressing.

From results obtained in 86 eyes, Luntz [36] considered trabeculotomy to be superior to goniotomy. In the same year, in another paper [37], he reported obtaining a success rate of 93.4% in 75 eyes of 47 children.

In 1979, Rothkoff et al. [38] performed trabeculotomy on seven eyes of five children with follow-up for periods ranging from 18 months to 4 years. They recommend trabeculotomy for both early diagnosed cases and children with late-onset congenital glaucoma. Their results, even in children over 1 year of age, are good, matching the report made by McPherson in 1973 [39].

Reasons for Trabeculotomy

Goldmann and Grant found that resistance to the outlet of the aqueous humor is mainly found in the trabecular meshwork. The idea of trabeculotomy is to open up the trabecular meshwork from the Schlemm canal to the anterior chamber to ease the penetration of the aqueous humor in the Schlemm cavity and set up its communication with the outlet venous system.

I have performed experimental trabeculotomies in cadaveric eyes and then studied them with scanning electron microscopy [40]. Figures 15.9 and 15.10 show the images obtained with light microscopy and Fig. 15.11, with electron microscopy. I made the latter immediately before enucleating an eye with retinoblastoma at age 4 months, with the parents' consent. Once the trabeculotomy was made, the eye was fixed with glutaraldehyde by intrachamber injection and the optic nerve was sectioned immediately.

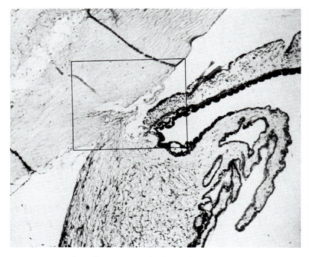

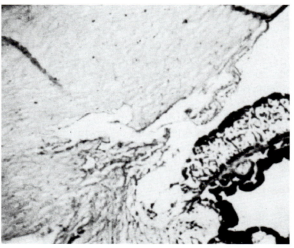

Fig. 15.9 Trabeculotomy. Pathological anatomy. Trabeculotomy made in a patient with choroid melanosarcoma, before enucleation, after an injection of glutaraldehyde in the anterior chamber, with the patient's permission. At the *left* part, the Schlemm canal can be seen in communication with the anterior chamber through the continuity solution made in the trabecular meshwork. At the *right* part, with greater magnification, the zone in the *square* in the *left* figure

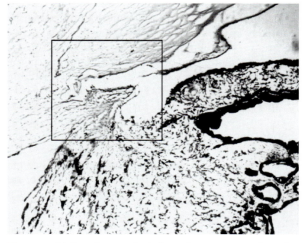

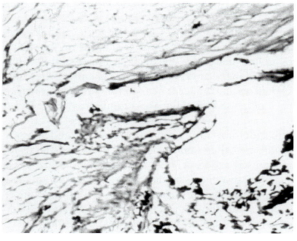

Fig. 15.10 Trabeculotomy. Pathological anatomy. In the other eye of a patient with intraocular tumor, a trabeculotomy was made before enucleation, with the patient's consent. The Schlemm canal is in communication with the anterior chamber. This is from the final part of the trabeculotomy; the point of the instrument has lifted the endothelium and the Descemet membrane at the *right* at a greater magnification

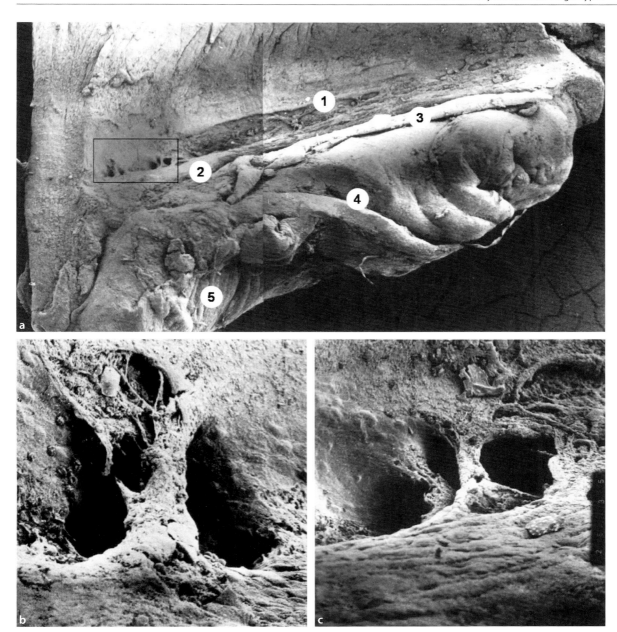

Fig. 15.11 a Piece from a 6-month-old child with unilateral retinoblastoma. The parents' consent was given to do a trabeculectomy before enucleation. When the Cocher tweezers were placed before the constriction of the optic nerve to section it, glutaraldehyde was injected intraocularly in the anterior chamber. The trabecular meshwork can be seen clearly and the internal wall of the Schlemm canal, turned and supported on the anterior face of the iris. This shows up the internal part of the external wall of the Schlemm canal. Three external collectors can be seen in this which exit toward the sclera: 1 External wall of the Schlemm canal shown by the trabeculotomy.

2 Prominent scleral spur. 3 Internal wall of Schlemm's canal and trabecular meshwork rolled up. 4 Anterior surface of the iris. 5 Ciliary processes. In the *square*, two external collectors divided by septa. **b, c** These are the external Schlemm collectors, corresponding to the *black squares* in the previous figure. In the first, there is a septum dividing them, and in the one on the right there are two. The specimen of normal and pathological (congenital glaucoma) anatomy are the first ones done and were made by Dr. R. Sampaolesi and Dr. C. Argento at the Institute of Bioneurology directed by Dr. Juan Tramesani. The technician who made the inclusion was Mrs. Isable Farias

Figure 15.11 clearly shows the trabecular meshwork and the internal wall of the Schlemm canal turned and supported on the anterior face of the iris. This method shows the internal part of the external wall of the Schlemm canal. Six external collectors can be seen here exiting toward the sclera. Figure 15.11b and c show the openings of the collectors with greater magnification.

General Points About Surgery

In order to perform a trabeculotomy, it is first necessary to experiment on cadaveric eyes in order to have a clear idea of the necessary size of the scleral flap, the positioning of the incision in relation to the surgical limbus, the difficulties in finding the Schlemm canal, and the problems canalizing it. A surgical microscope is always necessary and it is preferable to use microscopes that give 30–40 diameters or special microscopes such as the Harms microscope, developed by Zeiss (Oberkochen, Germany), which also helps greatly increase the amount of light per unit of surface.

Instruments

Harms probe is shown in Fig. 15.12a. Each arm is 0.3 mm in diameter; the arm that is not introduced is a guide for the surgeon to follow for the position of the arm introduced. Makensen added a handle to Harms trabeculotome (Fig. 15.12b).

The right and left trabeculotomes, from the Lyon school, made by Moria, are shown in Fig. 15.12c and are 0.2 mm in diameter; each of them is a conical probe with a handle that forms a 130° angle so as not to get in the way when operating with a microscope. There are special needles for intubating Schlemm's canal. Figure 15.12d shows the Beaver knife, which is very useful for dissecting the scleral flap.

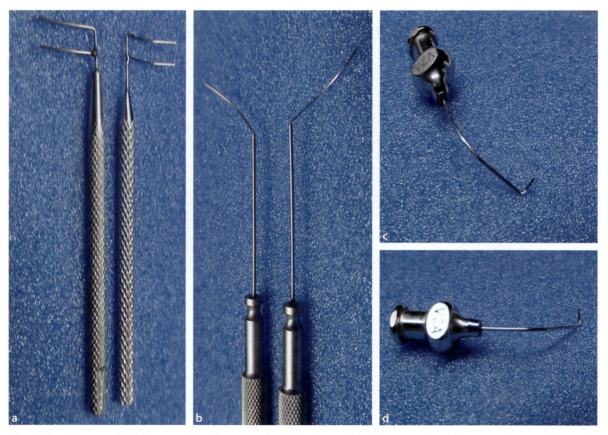

Fig. 15.12 a Harms and Mackensen trabeculotome probe. **b** Paufique trabeculotome. **c, d** Needle to introduce Healon in the Schlemm canal

Harms Technique

At first Harms dried the dissected scleral lamina to give the patients the possibility of a filtering bleb if the trabeculotomy did not work. But when it was seen that the trabeculotomy worked on its own, they stopped drying the scleral flap and sutured it.

Figure 15.13 shows the dissection of an elliptical conjunctival flap whose the ends do not reach the limbus (1); in the middle part of the flap, toward the corneoscleral limbus, the dissection enters the corneal tissue. The limits of the scleral flap incision can also be seen in this figure, made in three stages and measuring 2×3 mm. In 2, the scleral flap is already lifted and supported by two threads of virgin silk. The incision was made in the center of the bed and perpendicular to the limbus. In 3, the opening of the Schlemm duct and the Vannas scissors that penetrate and section of the outer wall of the duct can be seen. In 4, the deep arm of Harms probe penetrates the Schlemm canal. In 5, a chalazion-type curette pushes the round end of the Harms probe and presses the whole of it inside. In 6, a needle-holder takes the upper arm of the Harms probe and performs the trabeculotomy on the right side. The same is done for the left part. In 7, the stitch can be seen closing the scleral incision, and in 8, the scleral and conjunctival

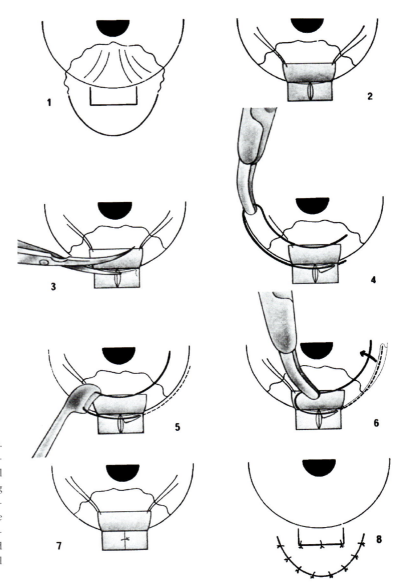

Fig. 15.13 Trabeculotomy. Harms technique. *1* Conjunctival flap. *2* Scleral flap and incision perpendicular to the limbus. *3* Scleral section parallel to the limbus, introducing one blade of the scissors in the Schlemm canal. *4* Introduction of Harms probe. *5* The probe is pushed with a curette. *6* The trabeculotomy is made turning the probe round with a needle-holder. *7* Closing the scleral plane. *8* Closing the conjunctival plane

incisions are closed. One interesting detail is that, to help introduce the probe, the point of a closed twee-zers should be used to depress the opposite lip of the incision perpendicular to the limbus.

The Lyon School Technique

Paufique, Sourdille, and Ortiz-Olmedo (1969) use the following technique (Fig. 15.14a). In 1, the conjuncti-val flap can be seen and the dissection of the small 2×4-mm scleral flap with a scleral depth two-thirds of the scleral thickness in 2. In 3, the incision perpendicular to the limbus can be seen showing the opening of the Schlemm canal, which is shown marked with a dot-ted line. Part 4 shows the Moria trabeculotome being

introduced, which is then rotated until the trabeculo-tomy is produced. The same maneuver is made on the left side. In 5, the incision to find the Schlemm canal is closed. The scleral and the conjunctival incision are being closed in 5, and both flaps in 6.

Figure 15.14b shows the series of steps for introduc-ing the trabeculotome into the Schlemm canal, break-ing the trabecular meshwork and extracting the trabe-culotome. It is fundamental that this should follow the curvature of the limbus and that the maneuver should be made in a tangential plane so that it is located at half the depth of the anterior chamber. The trabecular meshwork breaks suddenly, and so it is important that neither the cornea nor the iris be touched.

We have used both the Harms and Paufique tech-niques with the same results.

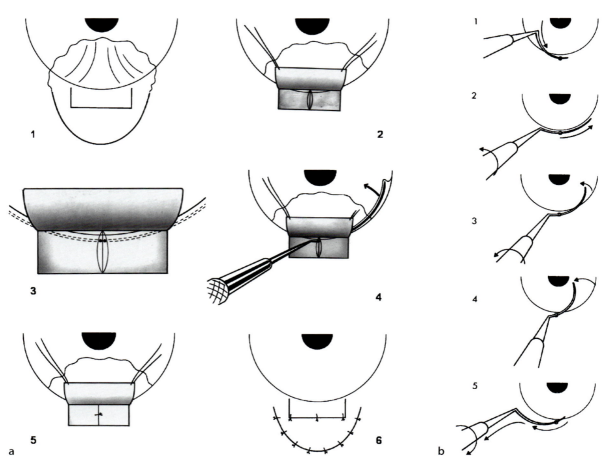

Fig. 15.14 a Trabeculotomy. The Lyon School technique. *1* Con-junctival flap. *2* Scleral flap. *3* Scleral incision perpendicular to the limbus, disclosing the Schlemm canal. *4* Introduction of the trabeculotome, then repeated on the left side. *5* Closing the scleral incision. *6* Replacement and closing of scleral and conjunctival flaps. **b** The delicate introduction of the trabecu-lotome and its extraction

Making the Scleral Flap

The small scleral flap is important in performing trabeculotomy. We make three incisions beginning with
the incisions perpendicular to the limbus, 2.5 mm in
length, and then we join them with the parallel incision. We use a Beaver handle with interchangeable
blades. This scleral flap has a rectangular shape of approximately 2.5 mm in its two incisions perpendicular
to the limbus and 4 mm in the incision parallel to the
limbus. This rectangular shape lets the trabeculotome
penetrate more easily into the opening of the Schlemm
canal. For the point to penetrate, it must be supported
on the side opposite the side it will enter, with the
sclera depressed slightly, and then it is slid to thread
the Schlemm canal.

Location of the Incision and Looking
for the Schlemm Canal

We consider it very important to use transillumination (the Minsky maneuver), supporting the transil-
luminator on the cornea protected by the conjunctival
flap (Fig. 15.15). In this way the limbus zone where the
Schlemm canal is situated can be clearly seen.

The incision is made perpendicular to the limbus in
the area indicated by the transillumination, 3–4 mm
in length. With a diamond knife or razor blade and
working with the greatest magnification, it gradually

deepens until an upper black triangle appears that corresponds to the Schlemm canal and a larger mother-of-
pearl triangle with horizontal bands, the upper part of
which corresponds to the scleral spur (Fig. 15.16a). The
trabeculotome is inserted in the upper black triangle
corresponding to the Schlemm canal (Fig. 15.16b).

The trabeculotome lifts the trabecular meshwork
without breaking it on the left side (Fig. 15.17a). The
trabeculotome enters the Schlemm canal (Fig. 15.17b)
and breaks the trabecular meshwork and enters the
anterior chamber (Fig. 15.17c). After the trabeculotomy, the anterior chamber remains perfectly formed
(Fig. 15.17d).

We close the vertical incision with a stitch of virgin
silk and the scleral flap with three stitches of the same
material, which is also used for closing the conjunctiva.

After the trabeculotomy, a small hyphema should
appear in the anterior chamber that does not reach the
edge of the pupil (Fig. 15.18). A larger hyphema means
that a cyclodialysis has been performed instead of a
trabeculotomy. A German author also described this
sign after we reported it.

The suction of the contact lens when the observation is made makes blood pass from the interior of the
Schlemm canal to the anterior chamber. This is the
proof that the operation has been performed correctly
and that the aqueous humor is in communication with
the episcleral venous system through the Schlemm canal (Fig. 15.19).

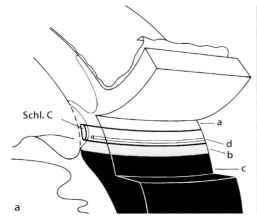
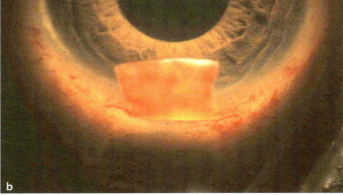

Fig. 15.15a,b The Minsky maneuver (transillumination).
a Diagram. *a* Clear zone corresponding to the trabecular
meshwork. *b* Zone of shade where the Schlemm canal must be
sought. *c* Dark zone caused by choroidal pigmentary epithelium. *d* Friedenwald artery (artery of the Schlemm canal). *Schl
C* the Schlemm canal. **b** Photograph of the Minsky maneuver
in an eye with congenital glaucoma

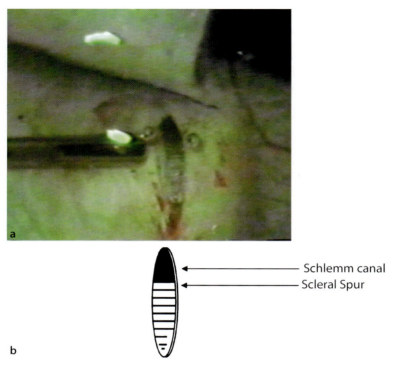

Schlemm canal
Scleral Spur

b

Fig. 15.16 a Finding the Schlemm canal. The incision is made perpendicular to the limbus in the area indicated by the transillumination. It is made 3–4 mm long using the diamond knife or razor blade and working with greater magnification, going slowly deeper until in the vertical oval left by the incision can be seen the upper black triangle, corresponding to the Schlemm canal and the lower pearly triangle with horizontal bands corresponding to the scleral spur.

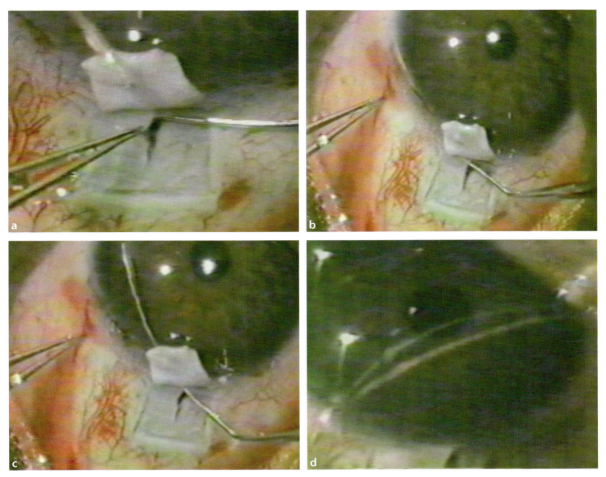

Fig. 15.17a–d The trabeculotome lifts the trabecular meshwork without breaking it on the left side (**a**), the trabeculotome enters the Schlemm canal (**b**), and it breaks the trabecular meshwork and the trabeculotome enters the anterior chamber (**c**). After the trabeculotomy, the anterior chamber remains perfectly formed (**d**)

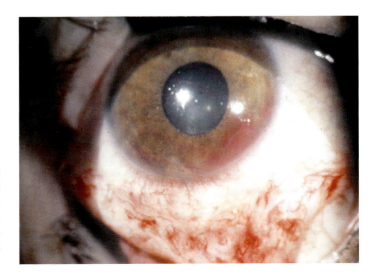

Fig. 15.18 After the whole trabeculotomy, a small hyphema should appear in the anterior chamber that does not reach the edge of the pupil. When a larger hyphema is seen, a cyclodialysis has been performed instead of a trabeculotomy. When there is no hyphema, the trabeculotomy was not made at the right place

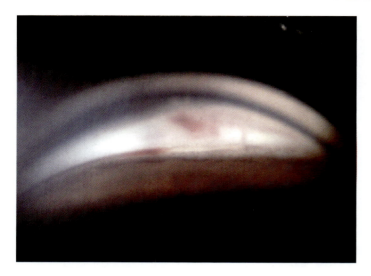

Fig. 15.19 Posttrabeculotomy gonioscopy. The suction of the contact lens when the observation is made makes blood pass from the interior of the Schlemm canal to the anterior chamber. This proves that the operation has been performed correctly and that the aqueous humor is in communication with the episcleral venous system through the Schlemm canal

Postsurgical Gonioscopy

The most frequent gonioscopic results after trabeculotomy are shown together in Fig. 15.20. These are very clear modifications to the structure of the chamber angle, which until now we had not been used to seeing in congenital glaucoma surgery.

If the trabeculotomy was done correctly, the trabecular meshwork is preserved in the point where the trabeculotome entered. The breakage of the mesh can be seen on either side of this zone, with chains of membrane with neater edges in the zone next to the Descemet membrane and more untidy edges next to the spur (1, Fig. 15.20). The spur is seen as a clearer, whiter and mother-of-pearl formation in the area of the trabeculotomy (2, Fig. 15.20). Generally, three goniosynechiae can also be seen in well-done trabeculotomies. A small central goniosynechia (3, Fig. 15.20) can be seen at the point where the trabeculotome entered, i.e., with the trabecular meshwork complete, reaching up to the spur or even to the height of the trabecular meshwork at the level of the Schlemm canal. This goniosynechia may result from the reaction of the trabecular meshwork tissue of the internal wall of the Schlemm canal against the insult suffered by the external wall. At the right and left ends of the trabeculotomy, two other triangular and wider goniosynechiae can be seen (4 and 5, Fig. 15.20), reaching up to the Schwalbe line. These may have a similar origin to the one just described and also receive the injury that the point of the trabeculotome causes to the outer wall of the angle and sometimes to the rear wall of the Descemet membrane and the endothelium. If the Moria trabeculotome is used, this problem is more common,

since there is less monitoring of its depth and, since the trabecular meshwork breaks sharply, the surgeon does not want the trabeculotome to go deeper and tends to move it upward.

In the Schlemm area, the edges of the breaking of the trabecular meshwork can be seen and, further in, the outer wall of the duct. The near edge of the Schwalbe line can always be seen more easily and the one nearer the spur is more difficult to see and sometimes does not exist.

Instead of the breakage of the Schlemm canal, it is usual to see blood deposited behind it, shaped like the duct (6, Fig. 15.20). Sometimes, when performing an early gonioscopy, a thread of blood comes out of this part, mixing with the aqueous humor (7, Fig. 15.20).

The spur can be clearly seen in all cases. It is pearly white, more obviously than in the regions that have not been operated. The trabeculotomy area in its near ends sometimes ends in a rounded shape.

The Descemet membrane in the zone of the trabeculotomy often presents small radial folds perpendicular to the Schwalbe line (Fig. 15.20). This may result from the Descemet membrane having less support when the trabecular meshwork has been broken. Sometimes these folds retain a little of the blood that came out during the surgery, which may last 15–20 days; therefore, we assume that there is slight filtration between the Descemet membrane and its adjacent parenchyma. These lamellar remains of blood are located below the Descemet membrane and remains for a long time, 6–8 months or more; we are reminded of what is seen after a cyclodialysis in which the Descemet membrane is accidentally dried with the spatula, so that blood penetrates the space. In the center of the corneal tissue,

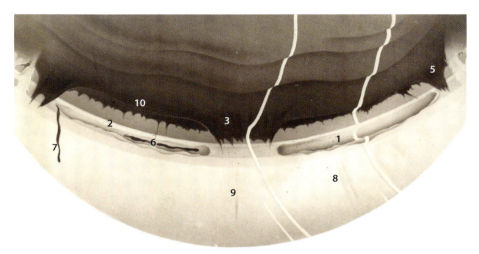

Fig. 15.20 Postsurgical gonioscopy. *1* Schlemm canal open. *2* Spur more visible than normally. *3* Central goniosynechiae, reaches the spur. *4, 5* Triangular lateral goniosynechiae, reaching the Schwalbe line. *6* Coagulated blood inside the Schlemm canal. *7* Liquid blood comes out of one end of the the Schlemm canal and mixes with the aqueous humor during gonioscopy. *8* Folds in the Descemet membrane. *9* Scleral incision showing through the cornea. *10* Retreat of the last circular fold of the iris

below the untouched trabecular meshwork, an elongated shadow can be seen (9, Fig. 15.20), corresponding to the external incision.

In the zone corresponding to the opening of the trabecular meshwork, the last circular fold of the iris retreats (10, Fig. 15.20). This element is constantly found and must be very important in the mechanism involved in the intraocular pressure decreasing. We rarely see:

1. Depigmentation of the trabecular meshwork in the breakage area, as occurs in pigmentary glaucoma.
2. Iris root dialysis.
3. Cyclodialysis.
4. Iris prolapse with large synechiae in the incision area as a result of the breakage of the internal wall of the trabecular meshwork at this point during the operation.
5. Some 5 or 6 months after doing the trabeculotomy, in a very few cases, pigmentation is seen advancing from the angle toward the posterior face of the cornea.

Figures 15.21 and 15.22 show other chamber angles after trabeculotomy.

Action of Atropine in Children After a Trabeculotomy

If atropine is instilled 15 days after surgery, the ocular pressure drops, as can be seen in Fig. 15.23a, and, looking at the chamber angle, the area of the Schlemm canal opens up and the chamber deepens (Fig. 15.23b).

Mechanism of Action of the Trabeculotomy

It is difficult to explain precisely what mechanism the operation uses, but it is clearly the breakage of the trabecular meshwork that opens the way for the aqueous humor to enter the Schlemm canal and removes its resistance. The retreat of the last circular fold of the iris that is seen in all cases is remarkable.

During trabeculotomy, Abudi and Manzitti propose an implant of amniotic membrane to prevent postoperative adhesion under the scleral flap, in order to maintain a functional bleb after surgery (V.R. Abudi and K. Manzitti, personal communication).

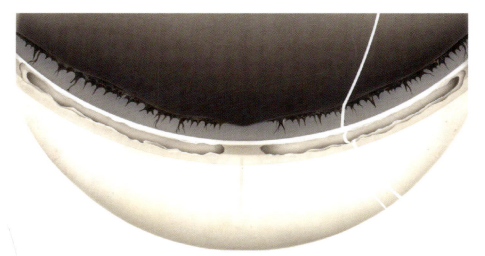

Fig. 15.21 Perfect posttrabeculotomy gonioscopy. The Schlemm canal can be seen quite open on both sides. The iris profile line passing to the corneal part dips to the level of the concavity of the outer side of the Schlemm canal

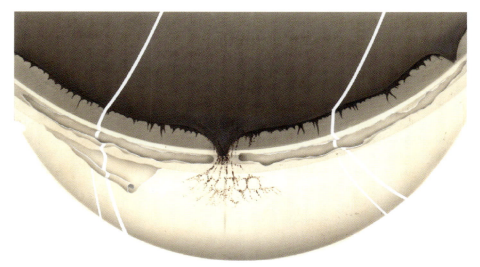

Fig. 15.22 Posttrabeculotomy gonioscopy. At the central goniosynechiae, a proliferation of pigment can be seen at the posterior face of the cornea. In the left part, when the trabeculotome entered, as well as the trabeculotomy, it lifted up the endothelium and the Descemet membrane, which rolled itself up

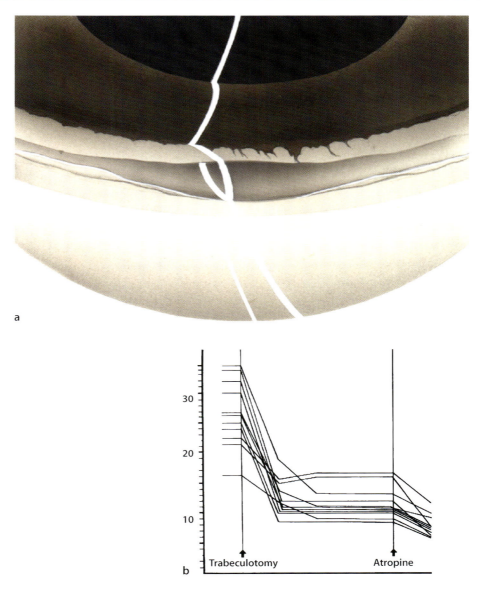

Fig. 15.23 a Trabeculotomy after surgery, 15 days after instilling a drop of atropine 1%. The way the trabeculotomy opens up can be seen clearly. **b** Graph of the drop in ocular pressure that occurs after instilling atropine in several children after trabeculotomy

Surgery for Refractory Congenital Glaucoma Type II

Combined Surgery: Trabeculotomy and Trabeculectomy for Chamber Angle Type II

Introduction

In 1971, after trabeculotomy was proposed by Harms and Paufique for congenital glaucoma, I started using the technique in primary congenital glaucomas. By 1975, 30% of congenital glaucoma patients on whom I had performed trabeculotomy had come back to my office with high IOP with pathological values and their axial length had continued to grow, as evidenced by echometry. Therefore, in 1975 I thought of the possibility of combining trabeculotomy and trabeculectomy in a single session in these refractory glaucomas. The results were successful.

When a new examination of the chamber angle was performed in those refractory glaucomas in which the first trabeculotomy had not been successful (i.e. IOP had failed to be regulated and the axial length continued to grow), I found that all these refractory glaucomas had the same type of angle (Type II) and so I changed the surgical indications.

In the second edition of my book *Glaucoma* [41] (p 754), I wrote, "I started to perform this combined technique in 1975 for congenital glaucomas which, in the first two years of age, had type 2 chamber angle (apparent high insertion of the iris), markedly increased axial length, and tears in Descemet's membrane and endothelium, since in this type of glaucoma trabeculotomy alone failed to regulate the IOP. I also extended this indication to secondary congenital glaucomas such as Axenfeld's syndrome, Rieger's syndrome, etc."

In 1988, my paper, "Congenital glaucoma. Long-term results after surgery" [42], was published, reporting 32 trabeculectomies and 29 combined surgeries, performing trabeculotomy and trabeculectomy in a single session. The follow-up after surgery ranged from 10 to 17 years.

In 1998, Mandal [43] published a paper titled "Surgical results of combined trabeculotomy-trabeculectomy for developmental glaucoma. Primary combined trabeculotomy and trabeculectomy in a single session." They reported the results obtained over 5 years in a sample of 120 patients with a follow-up of at least 6 months. They concluded that "primary combined trabeculotomy and trabeculectomy is safe, effective, and sufficiently predictable to be considered the first choice of surgical treatment in primary congenital glaucoma." In 2003, the same author [44] presented a new paper titled "Outcome of surgery on infants younger than 1 month with congenital glaucoma." It reported a sample of 47 eyes of 25 consecutive newborn patients with congenital glaucoma who underwent single-session combined trabeculotomy and trabeculectomy between 1990 and 2000. They concluded that "primary combined trabeculotomy-trabeculectomy offers a variable surgical option in infants that have cloudy corneas at birth as a result of congenital glaucoma. It is associated with favorable visual outcome and a low rate of anesthetic complications in an Indian population."

In 2000, Meyer et al. [45], in their paper, "Trabekulotomie bei Kongenitalem Glaukom. Ein Vergleich zur Goniotomie" (Trabeculotomy in congenital glaucoma. A comparison with goniotomy), reported the results obtained in 37 trabeculotomy cases in which they had to perform combined trabeculotomy + trabeculectomy 14 times in order to regulate the IOP and stop eye growth. In this article, they quote my first paper of 1988 as follows: "Sampaolesi's criteria is to do combined surgery: trabeculotomy with trabeculectomy as a standard procedure in refractory congenital glaucomas and in secondary congenital glaucomas (for example: Axenfeld's, Rieger's Syndromes, etc.). This is the reason why we thought it very important to include his criteria into this evaluation."

The paper by Kiefer et al. [46], "Correlation of postoperative axial length growth and intraocular pressure in congenital glaucoma. A retrospective study in trabeculotomy and goniotomy," concluded that "axial length measurement can help to ascertain halting or progression of congenital glaucoma and thus is considered an important parameter for congenital glaucoma follow-up. The nomogram of axial length growth over age compiles data published by Sampaolesi in a paper published in 1981: 'Ocular echometry in the diagnosis of congenital glaucoma.'" This paper presents a graph where the authors show the normal growth curve reproduced from my paper, with the pathological growth curve of the refractory congenital glaucomas of their population superimposed on it.

The population studied included 61 eyes belonging to 44 children, 26 males and 18 females, with the following features:

- 27 unilateral cases: 14 males and 13 females.
- 17 bilateral cases: 12 males and 5 females.
- 43 eyes (70%) with chamber angle type I that underwent trabeculotomy.
- 18 eyes (30%) with chamber angle type II that underwent combined surgery (trabeculotomy + trabeculectomy).
- 32 trabeculotomies and 29 combined surgeries (trabeculotomy + trabeculectomy) were performed.

Meyer et al. [45] had similar results in a population of 37 eyes:

- 23 eyes (62%) that underwent trabeculotomy.
- 14 eyes (38%) that underwent combined surgery.

In our first paper on the combined operation, the proportion between simple trabeculotomy and combined operation (trabeculotomy + trabeculectomy) was as follows: 65% trabeculotomies and 35% combined operation. Indeed, if we compare both results it is encouraging to find consistency in the results obtained in Argentina and Europe with surgical techniques for congenital glaucoma.

Combined Surgery Trabeculotomy and Trabeculectomy in the Same Surgical Session

Until 1995, I managed to find the Schlemm canal in the first phase of surgery with the Harms and Paufique technique. After creating a 4×3-mm square scleral flap, two vertical incisions were made perpendicular to the limbus and adjacent to the outer and inner margin of the scleral bed at the level of the Schlemm canal (Fig. 15.24). After trabeculotomy on the right

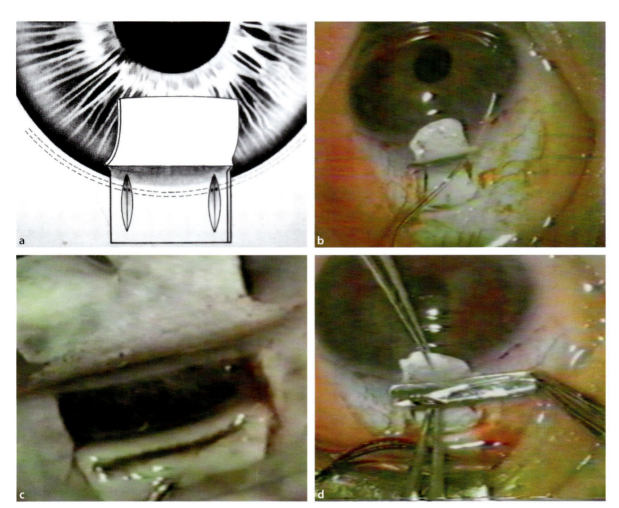

Fig. 15.24a–d Combined trabeculectomy and trabeculotomy operation. In **a** and **b**, after making the first step of the conjunctival and scleral flap, as in the common trabeculotomy operation (See Fig. 15.15, *1* and *2*), instead of making one incision to look for the Schlemm's canal, two are made, one on each side. In **c** and **d**, we look for Schlemm canal and make the right trabeculotomy through the right incision and the left one through the left incision. Then an incision is made parallel to the limbus that joins the two ends nearest the limbus of the previous incisions and the anterior chamber is entered. Then the piece of the trabecular meshwork is removed, sectioning it at the spur, the trabeculotomy piece is removed, a peripheral iridectomy is done, and we finish by stitching the scleral and conjunctival flaps

and left sides, a third incision is made parallel to the limbus above the Schlemm canal and two further incisions perpendicular to the first one in order to remove the trabeculectomy specimen, which includes the Schlemm canal in the central area, where the trabeculectomy has been made. Finally, the sclera is cut below the Schlemm canal, a peripheral iridectomy is made, the scleral flap is closed with two sutures, and the conjunctiva is secured to the limbus.

Combined Surgery with Kozlov's Technique for Finding the Schlemm Canal in the First Step

From 1995, when we were introduced to Kozlov's nonpenetrating deep sclerectomy, we changed the technique shown in Fig. 15.24 for Kozlov's modified technique. The surgical steps we follow to find the Schlemm canal are reported in the following figures [47] (Figs. 15.25, 15.26).

A second trapezoidal scleral flap is dissected (Figs. 15.27, 15.28, 15.29, 15.30). This second scleral flap is created carefully so that it includes the external wall of the Schlemm canal (Figure 15.31). In the blood of the Schlemm canal coming from the Friedenwald artery, there is a whiteness that corresponds to the aqueous humor.

Trabeculotomy on the right side (Fig. 15.32a) is the same as on the left side. The trabeculectomy piece is extracted, as are the inner wall of the Schlemm canal, the Schwalbe line, and the outermost part of the cornea (Fig. 15.32b).

The trabeculectomy piece is dissected (Fig. 15.33a). In Fig. 15.32b and c, a diagram is drawn over the piece so that the ophthalmologist can easily find the scleral spur, the inner wall of the Schlemm canal, the juxtacanalicular tissue, and the corneoscleral trabecular meshwork.

While tweezers hold the trabeculectomy piece to be extracted, we pass a trabeculotome, which shows the persistence of the Barkan membrane that has to be removed before extracting the trabeculectomy piece (Fig. 15.34). The cut must pass behind it. The scleral flap is then closed, followed by the conjunctiva.

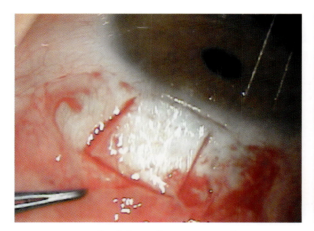

Fig. 15.25 First scleral flap. After sectioning the conjunctiva at the corneoscleral limbus, three incisions are made: two are perpendicular to the limbus and the third one, parallel to it, to obtain a 4×4-mm scleral flap

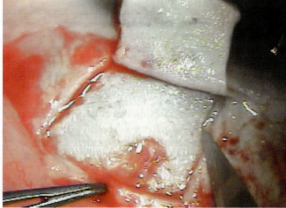

Fig. 15.26 Dissection of the first scleral flap as in a trabeculectomy

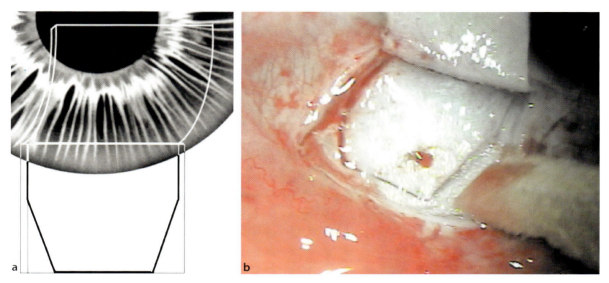

Fig. 15.27a,b Beginning of dissection of a second trapezoidal scleral flap including the external wall of the Schlemm canal

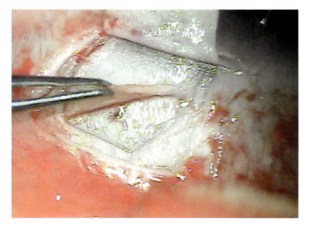

Fig. 15.28 Progression of dissection of a second trapezoidal scleral flap

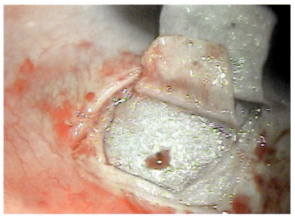

Fig. 15.29 Progression of dissection of a second trapezoidal scleral flap

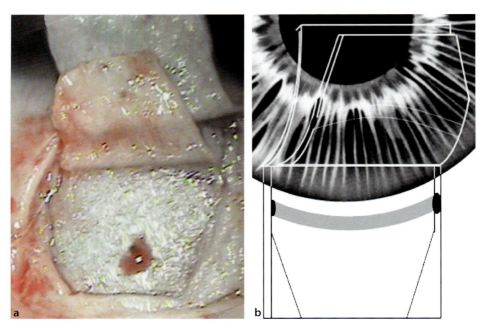

Fig. 15.30a,b Progression of dissection of a second trapezoidal scleral flap

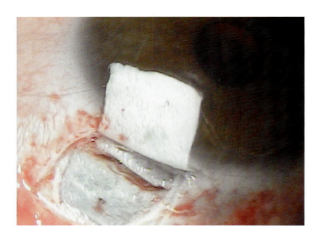

Fig. 15.31 After cutting this second scleral flap that includes the external wall of the Schlemm canal, the Schlemm canal is open with blood coming from the Friedenwald artery. There is a whiteness that corresponds to the aqueous humor

Fig. 15.32 **a** Trabeculoto-my on the right side and **b** the left side. **b** Extraction of the trabeculectomy piece, the inner wall of the Schlemm canal, the Schwalbe line, and the outermost part of the cornea. *SP* scleral spur, *I.W. Schl* inner wall of the Schlemm canal, *Schw* the Schwalbe' line

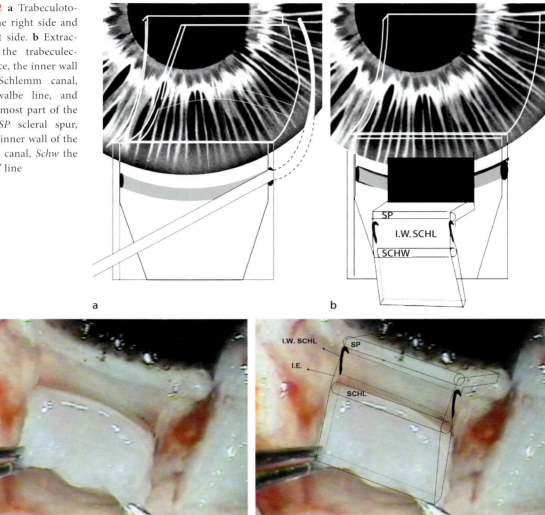

a   b

Fig. 15.33 **a** Dissection of the trabeculectomy piece. **b** Shown over the piece is a diagram so that the ophthalmologist can easily find the scleral spur, the inner wall of the Schlemm canal, the juxtacanalicular tissue and the corneoscleral trabecular meshwork. *SP* scleral spur, *I.W. Schl* inner wall of the Schlemm canal, *Schw* the Schwalbe line

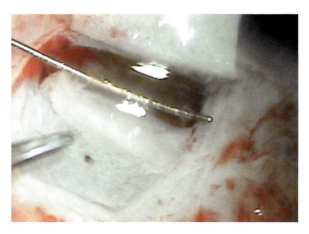

Fig. 15.34 While tweezers hold the trabeculectomy piece to be removed, we pass a trabeculotome that shows the persistence of the Barkan membrane that has to be removed before extracting the trabeculectomy piece. The cut must pass behind it

Pathology of the Specimens of the First (Trabeculectomy) Technique and the Second (Modified Kozlov) Technique

Figure 15.35 shows semiserial cuts of the pathological anatomy of a trabeculectomy piece. Figure 15.36a shows the same section as Fig. 15.35c, showing that as well as the pathological mesodermal remnants, the anterior face of the ciliary body is centripetally displaced. This displacement is also sketched in Fig. 15.39b.

We will now look at what surface electron microscopy discovers in trabeculectomy pieces. On the left of Fig. 15.37a, a normal trabecular meshwork can be seen with the trabeculae, the intertrabecular spaces, and the red blood cells passing freely through these spaces. Each trabecula is approximately 6 or 7 μm thick, and each round granule of pigment, 1–1.5 μm. Two granules can be seen in the upper trabecula below the red blood cell on the right. the Barkan membrane can be seen in b, occupying the intertrabecular spaces with some small holes. The persistence of the Barkan membrane can also be seen in c and in d.

Figure 15.38 is from a specimen obtained from a combined operation of a 2-month-old child with refractory congenital glaucoma. In Fig. 15.38a, the complete specimen of the trabeculectomy can be seen at low magnification. The zone between Fig. 15.38b–d shows the Schlemm canal opened by the trabeculotome. This zone can be seen with greater amplification in Fig. 15.38c. The black square adjacent to this zone that can be seen in Fig. 15.38a is considerably magnified in Fig. 15.38b and d.

Figure 15.39 shows the surface optical microscopy technique (Dr. Zarate's method), taken from a series corresponding to the optical image. The section becomes transparent as in an inclusion process. When it is dehydrated, it is examined with the microscope with an eosin background stain. The pathological mesodermal tissue is seen with ramifications reaching the rear face of the cornea (Fig. 15.40).

Fig.15.35 a Hematoxylin eosin stain (×40). A mesh of diffuse mesodermal remnants can be seen occupying the pretrabecular and trabecular region, ending below the ciliary muscle, which is displaced forward. **b** The same case as in the previous figure. Semiserial cuts. PAS stain (×40). The Descemet membrane (PAS-positive) stands out, reaching the point of the trabecular meshwork. The diffuse mesodermal remnants are dyed more weakly than in the Descemet membrane. **c** Semiserial cuts. Masson Trichrome stain (×40). With this technique, it is possible to clearly recognize the anomalous position of the ciliary muscle, situated above the filtration zone and the Schlemm canal. **d** Semiserial cuts in the same case. Gomori reticulin stain (×40). The diffuse mesodermal remnants are stained black with this technique because of its wealth of reticular fibers. The reticular fibers surrounding the fibers of the ciliary muscle are also stained

Fig. 15.36 a The same section as Fig. 15.34c, showing that as well as the pathological mesodermal remnants, the anterior face of the ciliary body is centripetally displaced. This displacement is sketched in **b**

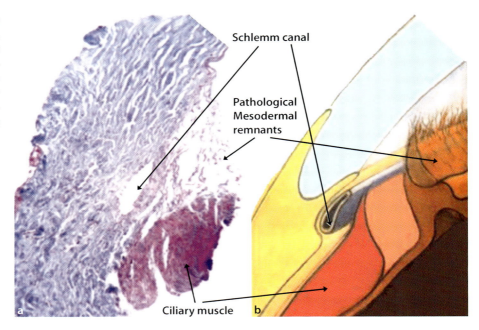

Schlemm canal

Pathological Mesodermal remnants

Ciliary muscle

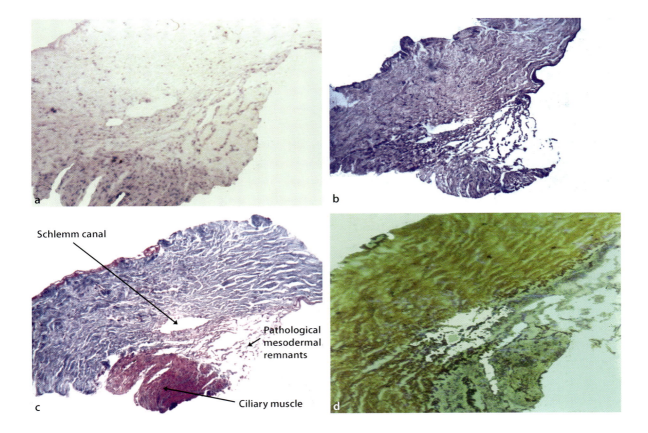

Schlemm canal

Pathological mesodermal remnants

Ciliary muscle

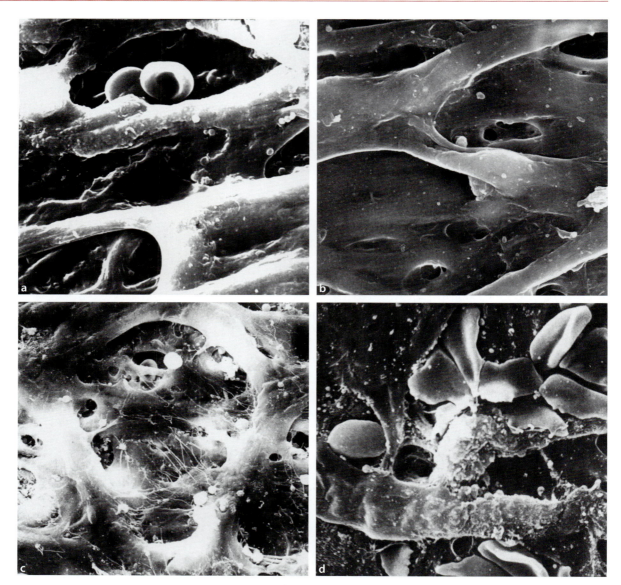

Fig. 15.37a–d Scanning electron microscopy. **a** Normal trabecular meshwork can be seen with the trabeculae, the intertrabecular spaces, and the red globules passing freely through these spaces. Each trabecula is some 6 or 7 µm thick, and each round granule of pigment, 1–1.5 µm. Two granules can be seen in the upper trabecula below the red blood cells on the right. **b–d** The Barkan membrane occupying the intertrabecular spaces with some small holes and blocking the passage of red cells

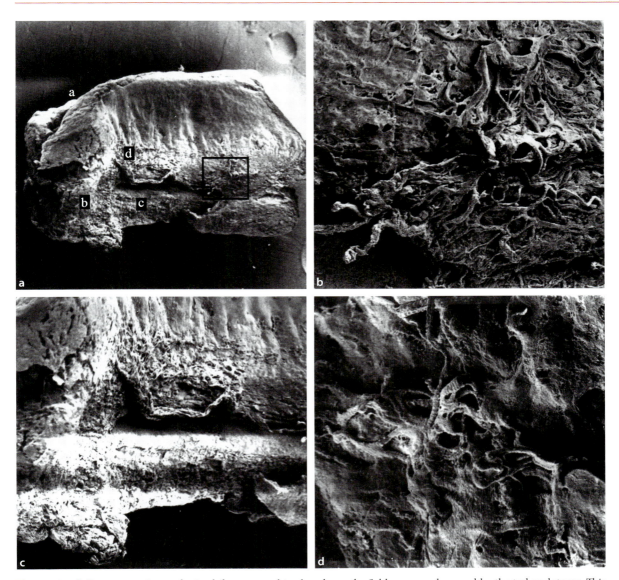

Fig. 15.38a–d From a specimen obtained from a combined operation of a 2-month-old child with refractory congenital glaucoma. **a** The complete specimen of the trabeculectomy can be seen at low magnification. The zone between *b, c,* and *d* shows the Schlemm canal opened by the trabeculotome. This zone can be seen with greater amplification in **c**. The *black* **square** adjacent to this zone that can be seen in **a** is considerably magnified in **b** and **d**

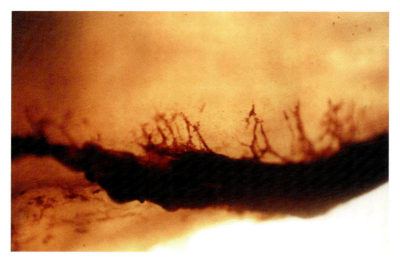

Fig. 15.39 The surface optical microscopy technique (Dr. Zarate's method), taken from a series corresponding to the optical image. The section becomes transparent as in an inclusion process. When it is dehydrated, it is examined with the microscope with an eosin background stain. The pathological mesodermal tissue is seen with ramifications reaching the rear face of the cornea

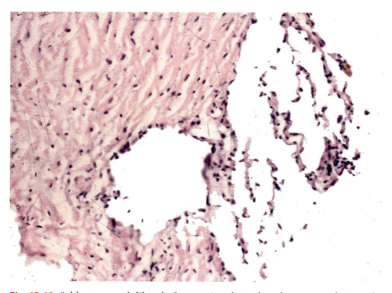

Fig. 15.40 Schlemm canal dilated after passing the trabeculotome inside it, without performing trabeculotomy, in a cadaver eye

Nonpenetrating Deep Sclerectomy for Late Congenital Glaucoma

Background

It was Krasnov [48, 49] who originally proposed the removal of the external wall of the Schlemm canal and coined the word sinusotomy for the procedure by which he removed the external wall of the Schlemm canal from 10 to 8 o'clock over 120°; the inner wall of the Schlemm canal was left untouched and then the conjunctiva was closed. Alkseev [50], proposed removing the endothelium of the inner wall of the Schlemm canal and of the juxtacanalicular tissue in sinusotomy in order to increase the permeability of the inner wall of the chamber angle.

Zimmerman et al. [51] introduced nonpenetrating trabeculectomy; Fyodorov et al. [52, 53] proposed deep sclerectomy and later together with Kozlov and others (1989), nonpenetrating deep sclerectomy; Kozlov et al. [47] perfected the method with the addition of a cylindrical collagen implant and later developed laser goniopuncture, methods that were further developed by Kozlov and Kozlova [54] and by Kozlov and Kozlova and Kozlova et al. [55, 56]. In Kozlov's technique, in addition to the resection of the external wall of the Schlemm canal, the inner wall of the Schlemm canal with the endothelium, together with the juxtacanalicular tissue and external corneoscleral trabecular meshwork are removed. In 1991, Arenas Archila [57] proposed trabeculotomy *ab externo*, by which the same tissues were removed, after removal of the external wall of the Schlemm canal, but using a microtrephine working at a speed of 800 rpm. In 1999, Stegman et al. [58] reported their results with viscocanalostomy in black African patients. Sourdille et al. [59] used a triangular reticulated hyaluronic acid implant of the same size as that of the second triangular scleral flap. We have successfully tested this technique, which, as it is currently known, is also successfully used by Demailly et al. [60]. Moreover, a very complete book has been published recently by Mermoud and Shaarawy [61], who has extensive experience in nonpenetrating surgery.

The main advantage of nonpenetrating deep sclerectomy (NPDS) lies with the high percentage of cases in which it prevents the three most severe complications of trabeculectomy: flat chamber, hyphema, and choroidal detachment. Furthermore, since neither anterior chamber opening nor iridectomy or atropine instillation into the anterior chamber are required, the postoperative period is short, with the patient preserving the preoperative visual acuity, in contrast to our experience with trabeculectomy, which has a difficult postoperative course, independently of the success of the procedure.

Moreover, the mild postoperative period, as well as the low percentage of complications, has encouraged surgeons to safely recommend this technique as early as in the preperimetric period, when damage to the optic nerve has already occurred and pharmacotherapy has failed to regulate IOP, though visual acuity and visual field are still normal. This technique is thus quite close to the ideal therapy for the prevention of serious anatomic and functional damage caused by the disease. We perform this technique only in late congenital glaucoma (see Chap. 20).

Nonpenetrating Deep Sclerectomy: Anatomical Landmarks

Figures 15.41, 15.42, 15.43, and 15.44 illustrate the anatomical landmarks.

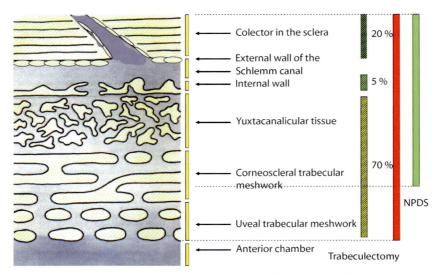

Fig. 15.41 Resistance on the conventional outflow pathway, which was removed by trabeculectomy (*vertical red line*). With NPDS (*vertical green line*) we removed the external wall of the Schlemm canal with collectors upon removing the triangular flap. Removal of the internal tissues includes internal wall of the Schlemm canal, the juxtacanalicular tissue, the external part of the corneoscleral trabecular meshwork. The internal part of the corneoscleral trabecular meshwork and the uveal trabecular meshwork, which, together with the Descemet membrane form the trabecular Descemet membrane, remain unmoved

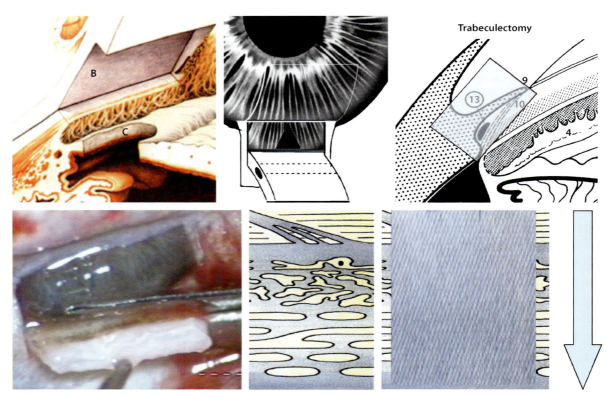

Fig. 15.42 Trabeculectomy: all tissues of the internal and external places of resistance are removed when the deep scleral flap is created

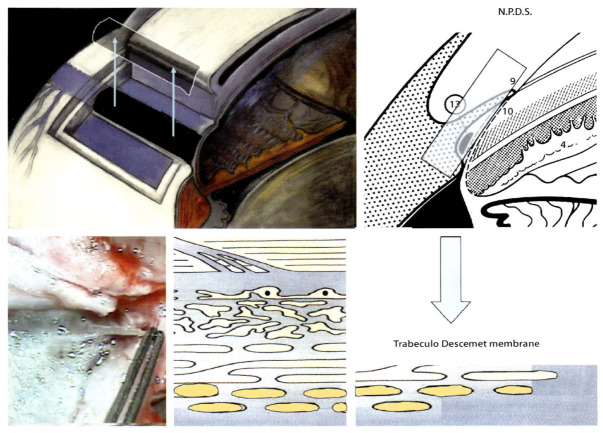

N.P.D.S.

Trabeculo Descemet membrane

Fig. 15.43 In NPDS, the external wall of the Schlemm canal is removed with the second triangular scleral flap and with the Mermoud forceps, a membrane comprising the inner wall of the Schlemm canal, the juxtacanalicular tissue, and the external part of the corneoscleral trabecular meshwork is also removed. The tissues that are left in their place are the trabec- ular Descemet membrane, made up of the internal part of the corneoscleral meshwork and the uveal meshwork. As stated by Dr. Mermoud, this membrane is strong enough to support the anterior chamber and also permeable enough to improve aqueous humor outflow with the consequent intraocular pressure reduction

Fig. 15.44 Chamber angle sections of the chamber angle. *5* Ciliary muscle, *6* ciliary body, *7* sclera, *8* limbus, *9* scleral septum and Schwalbe line, *11* iris, *12* cornea, *13* Schlemm canal, *14* lens gonioscopic image, *S. SPUR* scleral spur, *TR* trabecular meshwork, *TRSHL* trabecular meshwork of the Schlemm canal, *LSCHW*, Schwalbe line, *CB* ciliary body band, *LRI* last fold of the iris, *I PR* iris process. Optical cut, *1* profile line at the posterior corneal surface, *2* profile line at the anterior corneal surface, *3* profile line at the anterior iris surface

Chamber angle

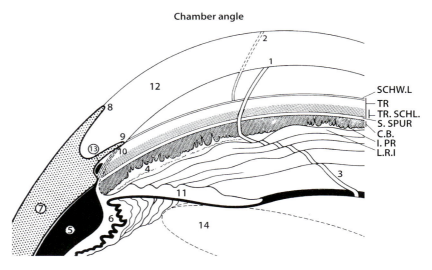

Nonpenetrating Deep Sclerectomy: Surgical Technique

After retrobulbar anesthesia with 2–4 ml of a solution of Xylocaine 4%, the conjunctiva and the Tenon capsule are opened at the upper fornix or at the limbus. With the sclera thus exposed, careful hemostasis is performed using a bipolar cautery manufactured by MIRA (MIRA Western Surgical Specialties, Uxbridge, MA, USA). A nylon suture is placed on the cornea 1 mm from the limbus, at 12 o'clock, to move the eye.

Step 1

A rectangular one-third scleral thickness limbal-based scleral flap, the same as that created for trabeculectomy, is dissected. One side of this rectangle, 5 mm in length, is parallel to the limbus, while another one is perpendicular to it and 6 mm long. Anteriorly, the scleral flap is dissected closer to the cornea than usual in trabeculectomy procedures. Corneal lamellae are dissected along 1.5 mm (Fig. 15.45).

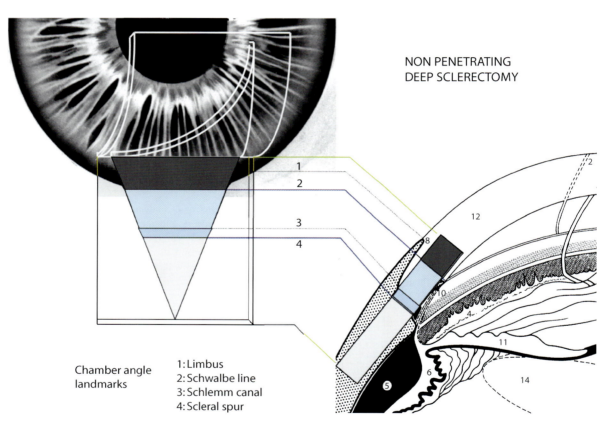

NON PENETRATING
DEEP SCLERECTOMY

Chamber angle landmarks

1: Limbus
2: Schwalbe line
3: Schlemm canal
4: Scleral spur

Fig. 15.45 The dissection has been correctly performed if three clear areas are visualized. *Dark area* (limbal area); *blue area 2* (more posterior), with its anterior limit corresponding to the Schwalbe line, and its posterior limit, to the scleral spur and the open the Schlemm canal; *white-grayish area 3* (behind the blue area), triangular, made up of scleral tissue and covering the external surface of the ciliary muscle. On the *right side* of this figure the correspondence of the surgical appearance of the three areas with the anatomical elements of the chamber angle can be seen

Step 2

A second limbal-based triangular scleral flap is then created by penetrating 1.5 mm into the corneal tissue. A useful landmark step for this dissection, which must be performed carefully, is the orientation of the scleral fibers, which, although arranged in multiple directions at the scleral level, behind this flap become neatly parallel and circular at the level of the scleral spur, thus adopting a more whitish and nacreous appearance. Aqueous humor percolation at this stage, with the anterior chamber closed, when the dissection goes from the scleral spur toward the cornea, indicates that the incision is placed in the proper plane. The triangular flap containing the external wall of the Schlemm canal, including its endothelium, is then resected. Anteriorly, the dissection should be made down to the deep corneal lamellae so that only the corneal endothelium remains. The Descemet membrane and a small layer of corneal lamellae are left. The dissection plane can generally be easily created at this final stage by pulling the vertex of the triangular flap toward the cornea with a clamp (Fig. 15.46). Figure 15. 47 shows the pathological anatomy of the external wall of the Schlemm canal.

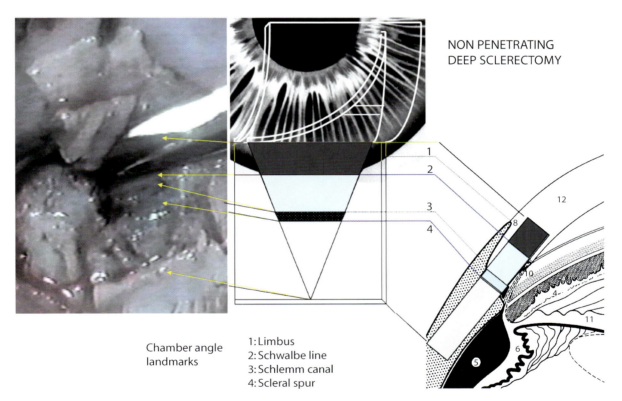

NON PENETRATING
DEEP SCLERECTOMY

Chamber angle landmarks

1: Limbus
2: Schwalbe line
3: Schlemm canal
4: Scleral spur

Fig. 15.46 Removal of the second triangular scleral flap (*left*), on which the external wall of the Schlemm canal, identified by its hazel or brown granular appearance, can be seen. *Center* and *right* correlation of this photograph with the landmarks

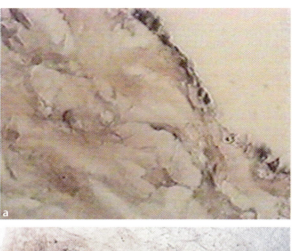

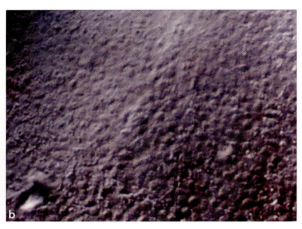

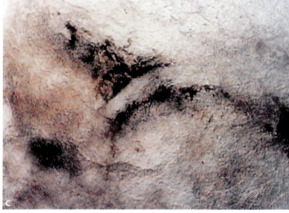

Fig.15.47 a Pathological examination of the triangular flap showing some corneal lamellae and the endothelium of the external wall of the Schlemm canal. **b** Endothelial nuclei of the external wall of the Schlemm canal (flat preparation). **c** Collector of the external wall of the Schlemm canal

Step 3

The most important step of NPDS involves the removal of the internal elements of resistance. If this membrane is not removed the intraocular pressure will fail to be regulated (Fig. 15.48).

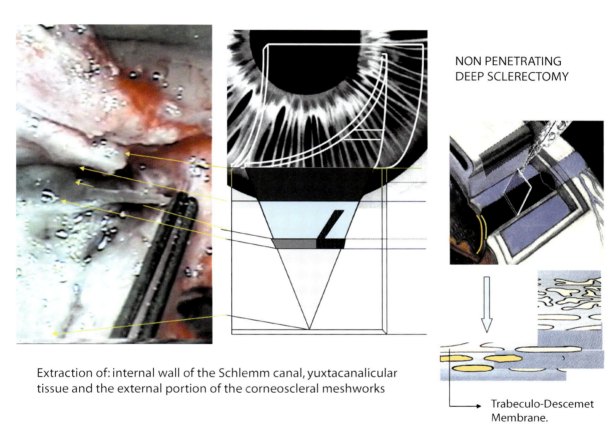

NON PENETRATING
DEEP SCLERECTOMY

Extraction of: internal wall of the Schlemm canal, yuxtacanalicular tissue and the external portion of the corneoscleral meshworks

Trabeculo-Descemet
Membrane.

Fig. 15.48 Dissection of the inner wall of the Schlemm canal with its endothelium, juxtacanalicular tissue, and the external corneoscleral trabecular meshwork (*left*). Schematic representation of the tissue removed and of its previous locations (*center*), where only the internal corneoscleral trabecular meshwork and the uveal trabecular meshwork, which, together with the Descemet membrane form the trabecular Descemet membrane, are left (*bottom right*)

Step 4

At this step, the implant is secured to the sclera with a nylon 10-0 suture (Fig. 15.49).

Implants may be made of different materials. In our first 60 patients, we used the implant manufactured by Staar Surgical AG (Nidau, Switzerland). It is a cylindrical collagen implant measuring 2.5 mm in length and 1 mm in diameter processed from lyophilized American porcine scleral collagen, which is sterilized using a radiation procedure. The water content of the hydrated device is 99%. This implant is resorbed within 6–9 months after surgery, as demonstrated by ultrasound biomicroscopy (UBM). In the last 22 cases, we used the corneal implant SKGEL 3.5 (Laboratoire Corneal, Paris, France). This implant is triangular and it is made of sodium hyaluronate.

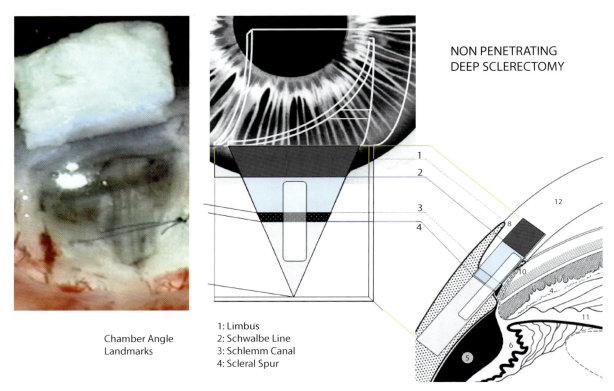

NON PENETRATING
DEEP SCLERECTOMY

Chamber Angle
Landmarks

1: Limbus
2: Schwalbe Line
3: Schlemm Canal
4: Scleral Spur

Fig. 15.49 Correctly placed implant (Staar Surgical AG, Nidau, Switzerland). After the placement of the implant, which is secured with a nylon suture, the scleral flap is closed with two nylon sutures. The photograph shows the implant once sutured

Complications of Surgery

Triangular Flap Dissected Too Superficially

The dissection of the triangular flap is not deep enough for the resection of the external wall of the Schlemm canal. The graph at the center of the figure shows the key element allowing the surgeon to find the Schlemm canal. The most posterior darker blue sector (between 3 and 4 in the blue area) indicates the location of the Schlemm canal (Fig. 15.50).

The external wall of the Schlemm canal must be dissected with a round cutting spatula specially designed for this purpose by Grieshaber (Fig. 15.51). This dissection can be made with direct illumination or under transillumination (Fig. 15.52).

To find the Schlemm canal, it is very important to view the surgical area with direct illumination and with transillumination (the Minsky maneuver). The area is transilluminated by the optical fiber of the microscope supported by the cornea, and separated from it by one of the white triangles used for drying, but embedded in physiological solution to prevent the cornea from overheating (Fig. 15.53). In Fig. 15.53a, the view is in direct illumination and in Fig. 15.53b, transillumination. Transillumination clearly reveals the location of the Schlemm canal (white arrows).

In Fig. 15.54, the external wall of the Schlemm canal of the same case has been completely removed.

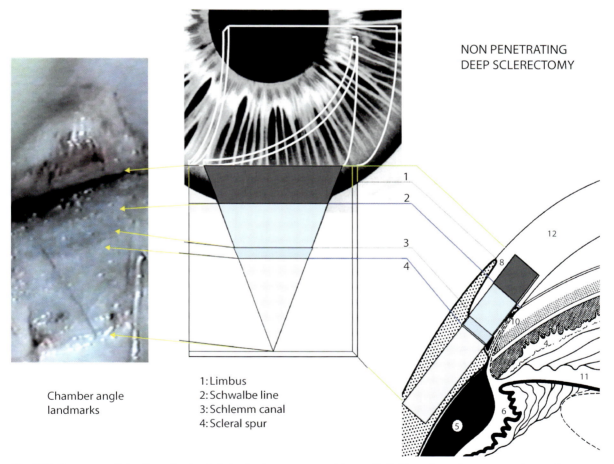

NON PENETRATING
DEEP SCLERECTOMY

Chamber angle
landmarks

1: Limbus
2: Schwalbe line
3: Schlemm canal
4: Scleral spur

Fig. 15.50 Image seen if the dissection has failed to be done on the correct plane and it is not deep enough for the resection of the external wall of the Schlemm canal by means of the triangular flap. All three areas are visible but the open Schlemm canal is not (*left*). The schematic representation at the center shows the key element for the surgeon to find the Schlemm canal: the most posterior darker blue sector (between *3* and *4*) of the *blue area*

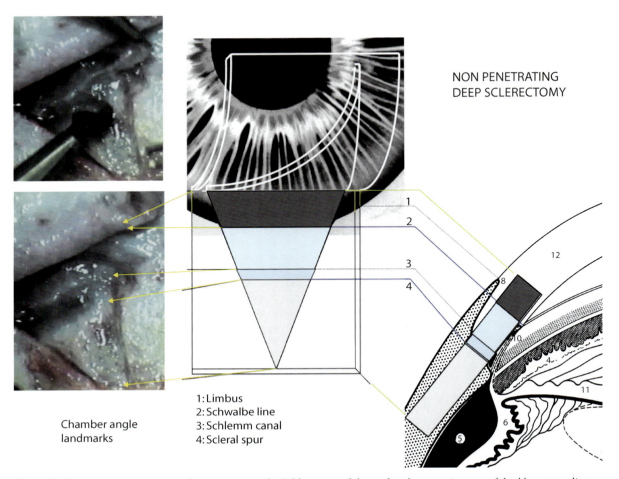

NON PENETRATING
DEEP SCLERECTOMY

Chamber angle
landmarks

1: Limbus
2: Schwalbe line
3: Schlemm canal
4: Scleral spur

Fig. 15.51 The most important surgical step is to open the Schlemm canal, located at the posterior part of the *blue area*, adjacent to the scleral spur

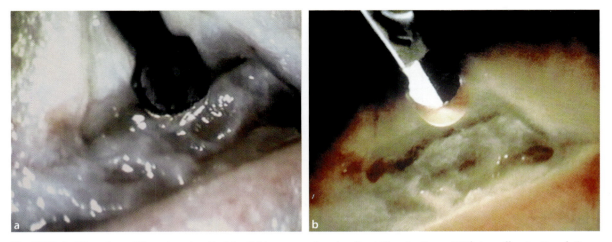

Fig. 15.52a,b Dissection of the external wall of the Schlemm canal under direct illumination. **a** With transillumination. **b** Done with an instrument specially designed for this purpose by Grieshaber

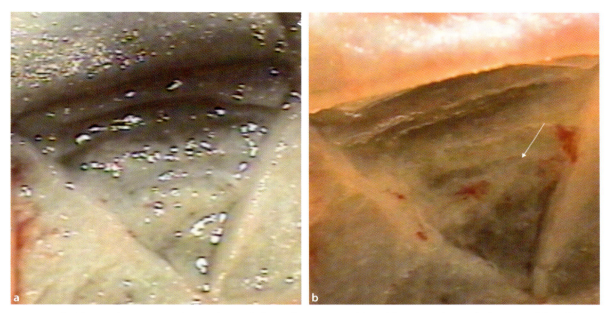

Fig. 15.53a,b The Minsky maneuver (see text). **a** With direct illumination of the Schlemm canal area, the location of the Schlemm canal cannot be seen, whereas with transillumination (**b**) this can be seen very clearly (*white arrows*)

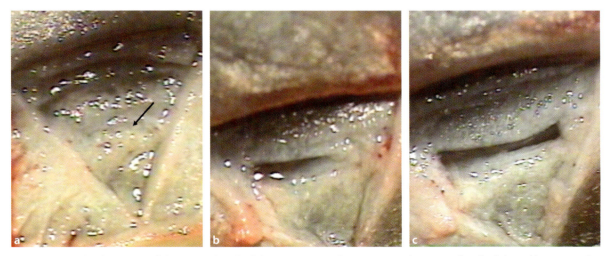

Fig. 15.54a–c The dissection of the external wall of the same case is shown in **a–c**. The external wall of the Schlemm canal is completely removed

Triangular Flap Dissected Too Deeply

In this case, when the surgeon tries to remove part of the second flap, the iris prolapses because a perforation of the internal wall has been made (Fig.15.55). If this occurs, the surgical procedure should invariably be turned into a trabeculectomy.

NPDS Pearls

The goal of step 1 (uproofing the Schlemm canal) is to remove the external wall to clearly expose the canal. This step is shown in Fig. 15.56.

In step 2, the surgeon removes the external elements with Mermoud forceps [62], as shown in Fig. 15.57a. When this step is perfectly done, the space between the scleral spur and the Schwalbe line is enlarged, and aqueous humor percolation is observed (Fig. 15.57b, c).

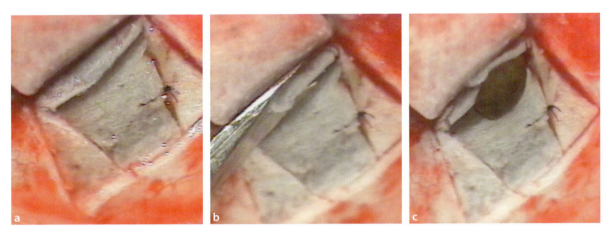

Fig. 15.55a–c In this case, when the surgeon tried to remove part of the second flap, the iris prolapsed because a perforation of the internal wall had been made (a–c). When this happens, the surgical procedure must invariably be turned into a trabeculectomy

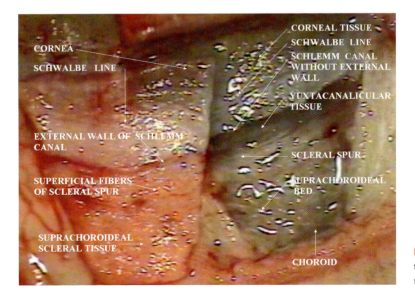

Fig. 15.56 The goal of step 1 (uproofing the Schlemm canal) is to remove the external wall of the Schlemm canal

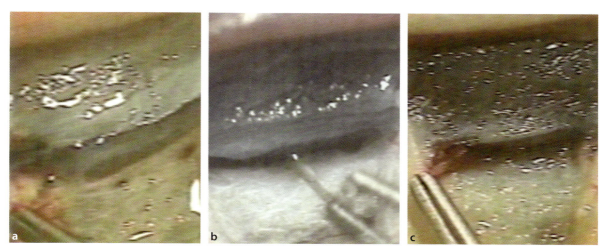

Fig. 15.57a–c The second critical step is number 2. It is necessary to remove the internal elements, internal wall of the Schlemm canal, juxtacanalicular tissue, and the external part of the corneoscleral trabecular meshwork in order to regulate the intraocular pressure. It should be kept in mind that between the internal and external part of the corneoscleral trabecular meshwork there is a natural cleavage pane

Ultrasound Biomicroscopy After Surgery

The ultrasound biomicroscopy in Fig. 15.58 shows, from left to right, the conjunctival tissue with aqueous humor, separating it from the quadrangular scleral flap, and two parallel lines behind it corresponding to the implant, where the nylon suture securing it can be seen. The implant is surrounded by aqueous humor and the scleral lake is seen behind it. The intrascleral lake and the trabeculo-Decemet membrane, 8 months later, are shown in Fig. 15.58b. The implant is reabsorbed.

Gonioscopy After NPDS

Figure 15.59 illustrates the typical appearance of the chamber angle after NPDS. The dark area (Fig. 15.59a) on the external wall of the chamber angle is the scleral lake (1), which can be clearly seen full of liquid with a fine slit cut (b). Figure 15.59a shows the Schlemm canal and the trabecular meshwork, which have become convex, raised toward the interior of the anterior chamber, because they have been displaced, and therefore, deformed, by the cylindrical implant.

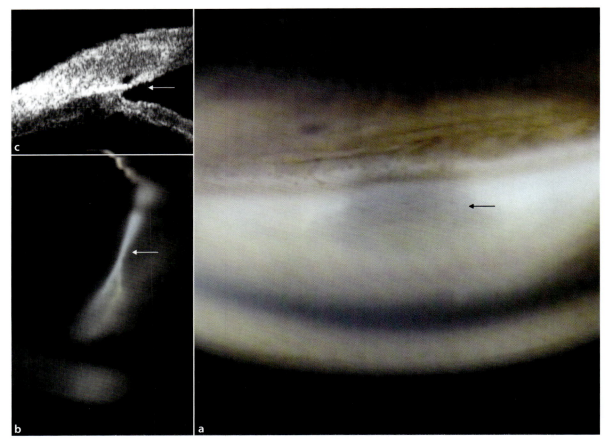

Fig. 15.58a,b Gonioscopy after NPDS

STAR IMPLANT

SUTURE

INTRASCLERAL LAKE   TRABECULO DECEMET MEMBRANE

Fig. 15.59a–c Typical appearance of the chamber angle after NPDS. The Schlemm canal and the trabecular meshwork have become convex, raised toward the interior of the anterior chamber, because they have been displaced by the cylindrical implant, which deforms them. In **a**, the *dark area* seen by diffuse illumination on the external wall of the chamber angle is the scleral lake, which, in **b**, is seen full of liquid with a fine slit cut. **c** UBM of the same case

Chamber Angle Before and After NPDS

The chamber angle studied with an optical cut made by the slit lamp shows that after NPDS that of the Schwalbe line and scleral spur where removed, and the optical cut between these two elements is concave because this is where the scleral lake is filled with aqueous humor (Fig. 15.60).

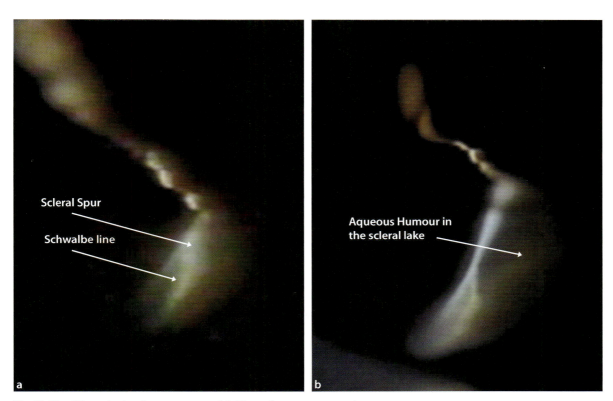

Fig. 15.60 **a** Slit cut in the place nonoperated. **b** Place where surgery was done

ND:Yag Laser Goniopuncture

In 20% of cases, YAG goniopuncture was required after surgery when the IOP in the follow-up reached values greater than 18 mmHg so that the anterior chamber would communicate with the scleral lake. The beam is focused on the trabecular Descemet membrane with a power of 2–3.5 mJ; however, sometimes higher power, 4–5 mJ, is required, but it should be kept in mind that

a power above 4 mJ may cause small hemorrhages, which can be stopped by pressing the lens firmly against the eye. A total of five to 20 shots should be made at the Schwalbe line, as well as above and below it (Fig. 15.61). In 85% of late congenital glaucoma cases, the IOP is well-regulated and its progression is stopped. Figure 15.61b shows the most important surgical instruments used in this surgery.

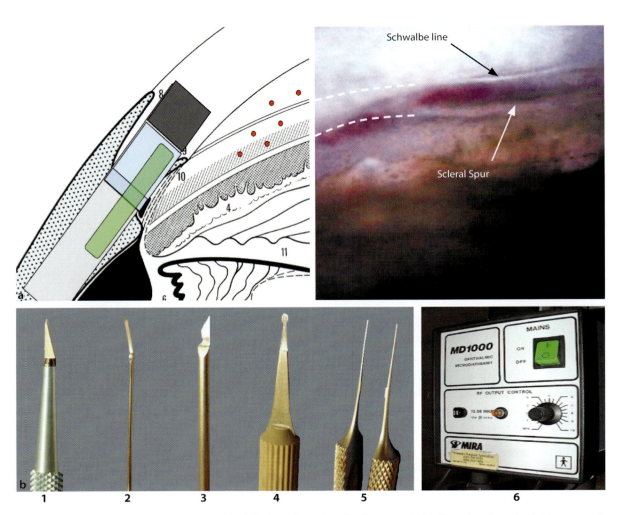

Fig. 15.61 a Nd:Yag laser goniopuncture. On the left, the right place to perform goniopuncture: at the Schwalbe line, in the posterior corneal surface and in the trabecular meshwork. On the *right*, there is a goniophotograph shows the Schwalbe line, the scleral spur, and blood coming from the Schlemm canal, after goniopuncture. **b** *1* 15° Diamond blade, *2*, NPDS spatula, *3* NPDS diamond blade, *4* NPDS uproofing blade, *5* Mermoud forceps, *6* ophthalmy microdiathermy (MIRA)

Valve Devices in Congenital Glaucomas

Introduction

The first to construct a valve was Molteno [63]. His basic idea was not only to insert a tube in the anterior chamber to extract the aqueous humor, but also to create a broad surface for its reabsorption, located in the equatorial zone of the eye at the level of the rectus muscles. The plate was made of acrylic material 8.5 mm in diameter, with an acrylic tube through which the aqueous humor flows into the sub-Tenon space. A series of valves with different designs then appeared, such as those of Brooks et al. [64], Lim et al. [65], Coleman et al. [66], Ahmed, personal communication, Krupin [67], Mermoud [68], etc.

We will discuss the indications, contraindications, surgical technique, intra- and postsurgical complications, results, and the authors' experience in valve implants for congenital glaucomas.

Indications

Implanting a valve will never be the first operation in a congenital glaucoma. It will be inserted as a first surgery only in cases of congenital aniridia. Trabeculotomies and combined operations (trabeculotomy with trabeculectomy in a single session) will always be performed. All the other congenital glaucomas, such as those associated with ocular, or ocular and somatic malformations, etc., will be treated in the same way. Two or more trabeculotomies and combined operations will be made before indicating a valve implant as the last resort.

Types of Implants

Valve devices can be divided into limited and unlimited devices: the former have mechanisms that at least partially prevent prolonged hypotony after surgery, while the latter lack this mechanism and may lead to the complication more frequently.

Even though the manufacturer, New World Medical, Inc. (Rancho Cucamonga, CA, USA), has a special pediatric model (FP8), we prefer to insert the valve model S3 made of polypropylene, designed for adults, in children with refractory congenital glaucoma, because we have never had any allergic reactions and above all because in all cases the eye of a child with congenital glaucoma is larger than that of an adult.

The most commonly used state-approved valve in our area is the Ahmed valve (Fig. 15.62). Until now we have used the Ahmed valve for adults in its classic version and not the silicone pediatric valve.

Child or adolescent eyes are generally phakic, and it should be remembered that, in many cases, these eyes, being type II refractory glaucomas, are myopic, with a

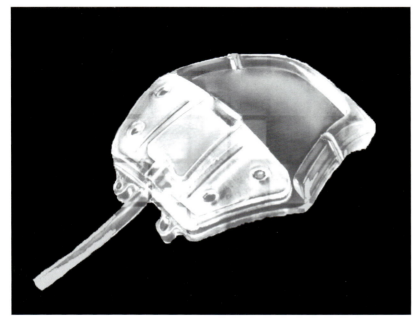

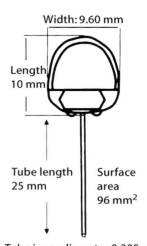

Width: 9.60 mm

Length 10 mm

Tube length 25 mm

Surface area 96 mm^2

Tube inner diameter 0.305 mm
Tube outer diameter 0.635 mm

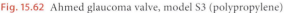

Fig. 15.62 Ahmed glaucoma valve, model S3 (polypropylene)

substantial increase in their axial length and therefore with thinner walls and a much thinner sclera than in the adult. It should also be mentioned that eyes in children will grow with time, and this should also be taken into account. This is why the surgical technique varies from the technique routinely used with older patients. It involves a change in the location of the tube in the anterior chamber and a change in the technique used to cover the tube.

The implant technique retains some points used in adults: for example, the preferred locations will be, in this order: temporal superior, nasal superior, temporal inferior, and nasal inferior.

In adults, there are three ways of situating Ahmed valve tubes so that they do not extrude: below a scleral flap fashioned within the patient's own sclera, guided by a needle through an intrascleral tunnel, or covered with a patch of donor sclera.

In congenital glaucoma cases, scleral thinning can at times even lead to zones of real scleromalacia; therefore the technique of choice is to cover with a donor patch of sclera, so as not to use the patient's own sclera, which would only lead to greater thinning.

The tube in the anterior chamber should be slightly longer than is usual in adults. This is because the eye

is going to continue growing naturally, and if the glaucoma should decompensate, it may grow even more. We have even seen cases where the tube comes out of the anterior chamber because of normal eye growth. Leaving a long section inside the anterior chamber thus prevents this complication.

Lastly, since these eyes are in general phakic, the tube is not usually located radially to the pupil, but paracentrally and peripherally (Fig. 15.63), which means that the tube should be placed parallel to the pupil, leaving it completely outside the pupil area, without pointing toward it. This prevents the point of the tube from touching the lens, thus preventing cataract formation in children, who are more prone to injury than adults.

The surgical steps are the following:
1. Opening of the conjunctiva;
2. Scleral flap;
3. Puncture of the anterior chamber with a 26-gauge needle;
4. Insertion of the valve;
5. Fixation of the valve with two sutures;
6. Cutting of the tube;
7. Introduction of the tube;
8. Suture of the tube at 1.5 mm outside the scleral flap.

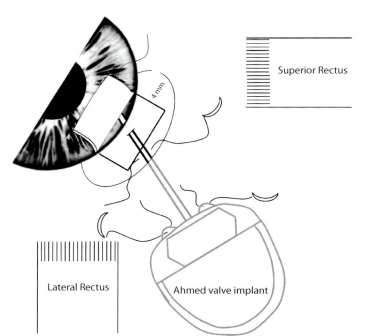

Superior Rectus

Lateral Rectus

Ahmed valve implant

4 mm

Fig. 15.63 Ahmed valve implant in its place

Photographs of the Surgical Steps

Photographs of the different surgical steps in a patient with three previous interventions whose IOP had risen to 52 mmHg, in refractory congenital glaucoma are shown in Figs. 15.64, 15.65, 15.66, 15.67, and 15.68.

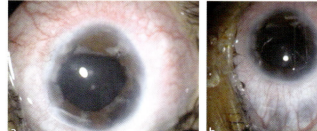
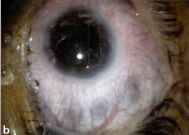
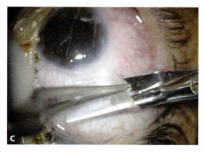

Fig. 15.64 **a** Rieger's mesodermal dysgenesis. **b** Location of the corneal traction point formed with an 8-0 silk suture. **c** Fornix-based conjunctival opening and the posterior scarification of the Tenon and episclera to prepare the bed

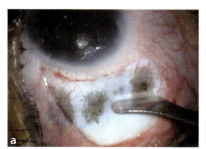
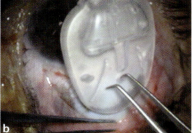
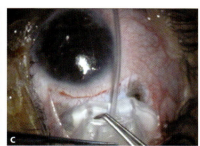

Fig. 15.65 **a** The Tenon is removed to prevent the later formation of cysts. **b, c** The valve is introduced below the conjunctival flap, i.e., in the subconjunctival space.

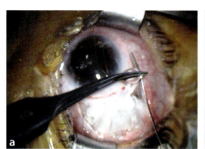
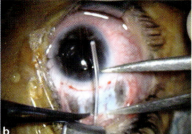
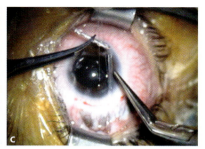

Fig. 15.66 **a** Permeability test. **b** A gauge is used to measure and ensure that the base of the valve is 8.00 mm from the sclero-corneal limbus. **c** The tube cut with the level upward

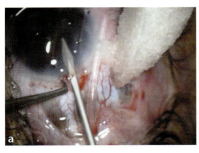
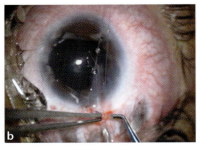
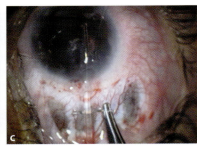

Fig. 15.67 a The moment of making the paracentesis in a para-pupillary direction and not radial to the pupillary axis; inject-ing light viscoelastic in the anterior chamber. **b** Introduction of the tube in the anterior chamber, checking where the point is, its relation with the visual axis and its anteroposterior posi-tioning, confirming that it is not in contact with the iris or the cornea. **c** A nylon stitch is made to fix it in the episclera

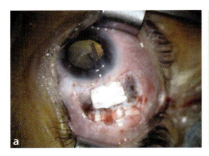
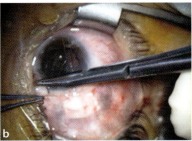
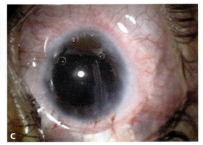

Fig. 15.68 a The first stitch to fix the donor scleral patch. **b** The conjunctival closing with absorbable 8-0 silk suture. **c** After testing the bleb with physiological solution, on the right can be seen the final position of the tube in the anterior chamber. The lower temporal filtering corresponds to the injection of gen-tamicin and corticoids

Postsurgical Biomicroscopy in Valve Implants

As we have mentioned, implanting the tube is rather different than in adults. The tube must remain in a parapupillary position, above the iris and not radial to the visual axis. In the anteroposterior direction, it should also be situated between the cornea and the iris, leaving a space between the tube and these structures. Lastly, as far as possible, its intrachamber portion should be somewhat longer than usual for later growth of the ocular globe, with the bevel, as in other cases, toward the front.

It is also important during check-ups to see how the bleb maintains its shape, without seeing the edge of the valve body. When the conjunctiva surrounds the valve and shows its edge, it is because the bleb has formed a cyst and is not filtering properly (Fig. 15.69, 15.70, 15.71).

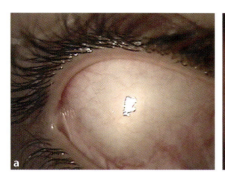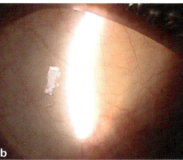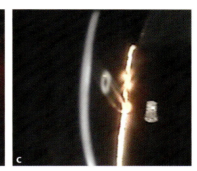

Fig. 15.69a–c The normal appearance of the filtering bleb over the valve body can be seen on the *left*; the beam of the slit-lamp can be seen in the *middle the section*. On the *right*, with the same beam, the correct position anteroposteriorly, with no contact with the cornea or iris

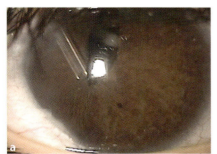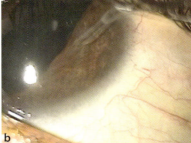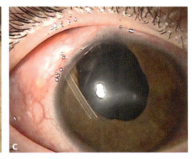

Fig. 15.70a–c Three cases can be seen in which the tube, contrasting with adult cases, has been placed outside the pupil edge, and in general with a more extended piece inside the chamber

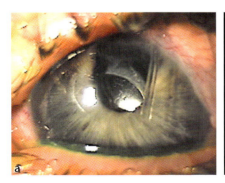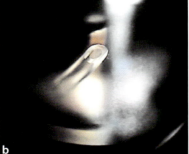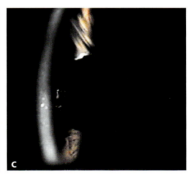

Fig. 15.71a–c The valve implant in congenital glaucoma with posterior pseudophakia is shown on the *left*; in the *center*, the correct location of the tube in the anterior chamber as observed with gonioscopy. On the *right*, the usual position used in adults, in which it reaches the pupil border, almost radially in a pseudophakic eye

Complications of Valve Implants

The most common complications in valve implants in young people are the appearance of inflammatory granulomas, traumatic extrusion, spontaneous extrusion, corneal decompensation from the tube touching the endothelium, cataract produced by the tube touching the crystalline lens, the tube leaving the anterior chamber because of the growth of the ocular globe, unregulated normal IOP for the child's age, loosening of the valve body from its original placement, and cyst formation of the valve body by the Tenon capsule.

Other less frequent complications are blebitis and endophthalmitis. Even though valve implants tend to have fewer infections than perforating surgery, these have been described. It should be made clear that, as has already been shown, the use of antimetabolites associated with the valve implant does not increase their hypotensive efficacy, and so they should not be used in this surgery.

Results

Even though we have much greater experience in trabeculectomy and trabeculotomy, in cases in which we have decided to use valve implants, pressures have nearly always been between the 10 and 15 mmHg that a newborn requires. Mean IOPs achieved were 14.5 ± 5 mmHg, so that in 40% of the cases, medication was needed to help to regulate ocular pressure correctly. It should be clarified here that in general these were reoperations for the second, third, or fourth time (see Figs. 15.72, 15.73, 15.74, 15.75, 15.76).

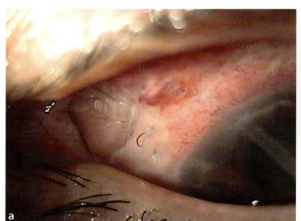 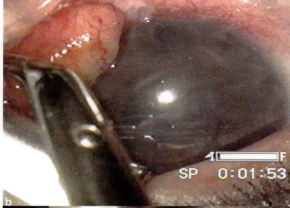

Fig. 15.72a,b The spontaneous extrusion of an Ahmed valve implant with a loosening of the valve body (nylon point near the limbus) can be seen on the *left*. The increase in the section of the tube in the anterior chamber can also be seen, resulting from inward movement of the implant. An inflammatory granuloma can be seen on the *right* that obliged the removal of the valve implant

Clinical History No. 1

This boy, first seen in 1965 at the age of 3 months, has been followed up for over 40 years (Figs. 15.72, 15.73). Another ophthalmologist performed two goniotomies without results.

Conclusion of Clinical History No.1

Congenital glaucoma operated for the first time at the age of one, then later on, two times at the right eye and four times at the left eye. Plus surgery for retinal detachment in the right eye and Ahmed valve in the left eye, and finally cataract surgery in both eyes. At the age of 40 years good visual field and a visual accuity of 20/20 in both eyes.

This is a good example of how the ophthalmologist must not be descoraged, and has to reoperate when necessary. This young man supports today his mother and is on the way of becomming a well known writer.

	Right eye	Left eye
Surgery	**Goniotomy (I)**	**Goniotomy (I)**
IOP	26 mmHg	28 mmHg
Axial length	?–15 D	?–15 D
Cornea	Edema	
Chamber angle	Type II	Type II
	Goniosynechia	Goniosynechia
Surgery	**Iridencleisis (II)**	**Iridencleisis (II)**
1965–1974	**Normal IOP: 11–16 mmHg**	Normal IOP: 11–16 mmHg
1974 (age 9)		Traumatic glaucoma (hit by ball)
IOP		40 mmHg (treatment with Ocusert)
1978 (age 13)	**Retinal detachment (surgery III)**	
Visual acuity	–30, finger counting at 2 m	–27, 0.3
1994 (age 29)		**Trabeculotomy (1 hs) (III)**
2002 (age 37)		**Ahmed valve (IV)**
Axial length, 2005	34.33 mm	**34.26 mm**
2006 (age 41)	**Cataract surgery (IV)**	**Cataract surgery (V)**
	(Intraocular lens 1 D)	(Intraocular lens 1 D)
IOP	16 mmHg	18 mmHg
Visual acuity	Sph. –2.5: 20/40	Cyl. –3.5 108: 20/200 (far)
	Sph. + 2.5: 20/20	Sph. + 2.5: 20/20

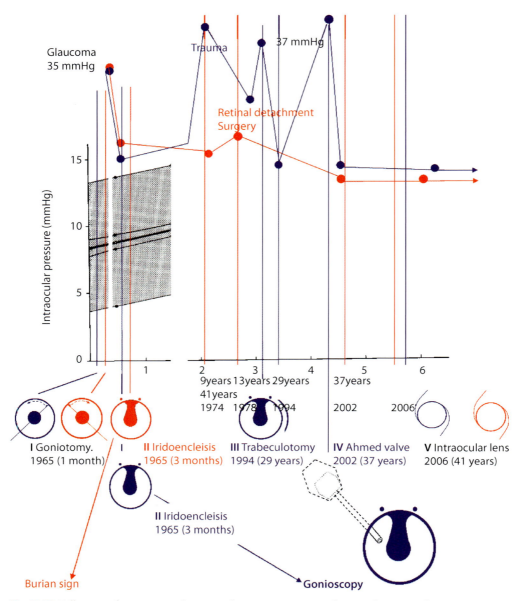

Fig. 15.73 Follow-up of case no. 1 with intraocular pressures, ages, and types of surgeries done

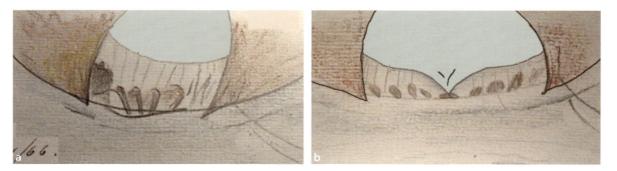

Fig. 15.74a,b Drawing of gonioscopy after iridectomy showing the ciliary processes and the capsule of the lens of case no. 1

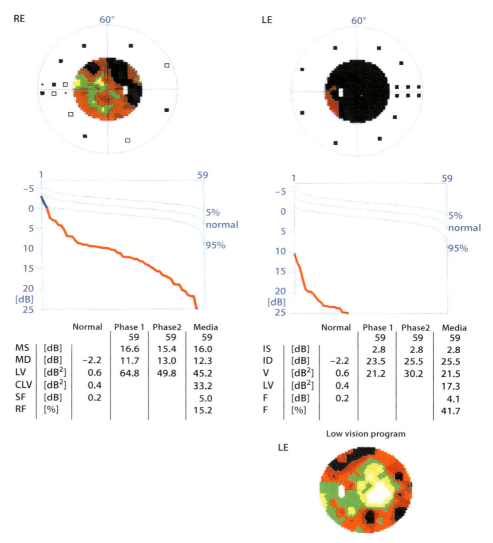

		Normal	Phase 1	Phase2	Media
			59	59	59
MS	[dB]		16.6	15.4	16.0
MD	[dB]	−2.2	11.7	13.0	12.3
LV	[dB²]	0.6	64.8	49.8	45.2
CLV	[dB²]	0.4			33.2
SF	[dB]	0.2			5.0
RF	[%]				15.2

		Normal	Phase 1	Phase2	Media
			59	59	59
IS	[dB]		2.8	2.8	2.8
ID	[dB]	−2.2	23.5	25.5	25.5
V	[dB²]	0.6	21.2	30.2	21.5
LV	[dB²]	0.4			17.3
F	[dB]	0.2			4.1
F	[%]				41.7

Low vision program

LE

Fig. 15.75 Visual field, *right* and *left* eyes, with Octopus Program G2, low on the *right* visual field of the *left* eye with Octopus Program low vision

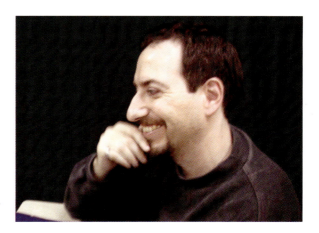

Fig. 15.76 Photograph of patient, case no. 1. The writer presenting his book

Annex

Trabeculectomy

Purpose of Trabeculectomy

Trabeculectomy has been a great success in the history of glaucoma surgery. It has replaced all the fistulizing operations done until then and is accepted worldwide.

John Cairns made the first trials in 1967 in Cambridge. In 1968 [69], he published the surgical technique for the first time.

Barkan [70] was the first to introduce the term "trabeculectomy." Explaining its goniotomy, he said that, depending on the case, it could be called trabeculotomy or *ab externo* trabeculectomy.

About the same time, Vasco-Posadas [71] described a similar surgery that he called protected filtering. A little later, Fronimopoulos and Christakis [72], Watson and Barnett [73], Nesterov et al. [74], and Krasnov [75] published modifications to Cairns's original technique. The purpose of this surgery is to remove an approximately 4×2-mm piece of trabecular meshwork, including the spur, the Schlemm canal, the Schwalbe line, and juxtacanalicular meshwork to make way for the aqueous humor to flow out freely through the Schlemm canal, "without subconjunctival drainage of the aqueous humour," as Cairns said. However, in most cases, a good filtering bleb is formed.

Surgical Technique Steps

Conjunctival Flap

A limbus- or fornix-based conjunctival flap is formed.

Coagulation of the Vessels

At the insertion of the Tenon capsule, 3 or 4 mm behind the limbus, there are small vessels that have to be coagulated along the entire edge of the insertion of this capsule. We perform the coagulation with equipment made by MIRA (Uxbridge, MA, USA), which uses bipolar microdiathermy with two electrodes in the point itself. This equipment was recommended to us by Dr. Alvarado and we particularly recommend it. Its point is very fine, and the intensity of the coagulation can be regulated in great detail. It can be used for coagulating the major arterial circle of the iris, the blood vessels of the ciliary body band, etc. Dr. Alvarado states that, by preventing hemorrhage at this level, not only is

blood flow interrupted, but also activator hormone escape is stopped, which causes intense scarring, which, when there is a filtering bleb, leads to surgical failure. Dr. Alvarado, personal communication, conducted a study on wound scarring in general and wound scarring occurring in glaucoma after fistulizing operations such as this, and divided them into three stages: the first includes the surgical trauma and necrosis with hemorrhage. The second produces fibrovascular scarring through the fibroblasts, macrophages, and the formation of new vessels. The third stage occurs when scarring stops and the tissue oxygenates normally. He therefore provided recommendations so that the healing process takes place and is not modified, leading to limited fibrous scarring of the bleb in its environment, fibrosis, and reduction of the bleb until it flattens and disappears. To prevent all this, he advises not cutting the conjunctival and Tenon blood vessels, a rapid cauterizing of the vessels, and finally, attempting to obtain the vascular part of the operated tissues to return to the presurgical state as soon as possible.

He then goes on to dissect the conjunctiva and sclera Tenon with scissors until he reaches the insertion of the upper rectus. A strabismus hook with a hole can be passed, as we described earlier, or a loop can be passed directly on the upper rectus before the incision. In this way, the eye remains well fixed for the maneuvers that follow, which are much more delicate and precise.

Dissection of the Scleral Flap

Figure 15.77 shows that before starting the scleral flap, a needle with an 8-0 Biosorb suture is passed in the corneal part of the sclerocorneal limbus to fix the eye. After dissecting the conjunctival flap, the dissection of the scleral flap is begun, which is a rectangle with one side 5 mm long, parallel to the limbus, and two vertical incisions joining it to the limbus.

Excision of the Trabeculectomy Piece

After dissecting the scleral flap (Fig. 15.78a), two incisions are made perpendicular to the limbus (1, 2), which are 0.5 mm inside the incisions of the primitive scleral flap. While doing this, it is helpful to use transillumination of the Minsky maneuver (Fig. 15.78b, d) to locate the anatomic elements that are to be excised.

It is very important to respect these measurements to obtain a good trabeculectomy piece. On the left of Fig. 15.79, the correct dimensions can be seen, and on the right, what should not be done.

Fig. 15.77 Fixation of the eye with Biosorb 8-0 (Alcon) and drawing of the scleral flap with its measurements

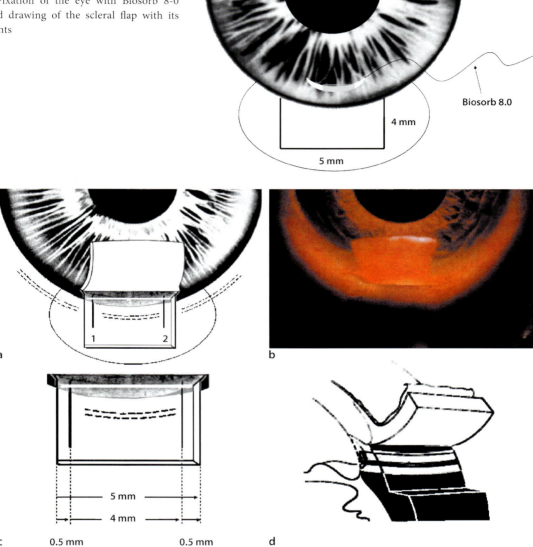

Fig. 15.78 a Two incisions perpendicular to the limbus. b Minsky manoeuvre. c Distance between the first and second scleral flap. d Position of Schlemm canal

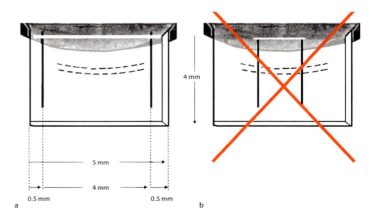

Fig. 15.79 a The correct size for the second flap. b The wrong size for the second flap

Figure 15.80 shows the third incision that joins the two perpendicular incisions (1, 2). It should be noted carefully that it goes 0.5 mm beyond the perpendicular incisions. This is most important because the surgeon can thus take the trabeculectomy piece with small forceps.

Incision 3 is deepened until the anterior chamber is opened and, using angled Vannas scissors made by Storz or Katena, the incision is completed. The last two cuts correspond to the segment passing the vertical incisions.

At this point, so that the iris does not come into the incision, it is necessary to empty the anterior chamber. This is done by introducing a delicate iris spatula in the anterior chamber parallel to the iris and rotating it 90° so that it opens the sides of the incision. The aqueous humor comes out and, in order to empty the chamber completely, triangular sponges should be placed over the incision to absorb it. This maneuver has to be repeated several times; once the chamber is completely emptied, the iris does not prolapse. Then the two vertical incisions are completed until they reach the vertex of the angle.

Figure 15.81a shows the flap to be removed, which has the Schlemm canal in its center, 15.81b shows the iridectomy, 15.81c, the trabeculectomy piece removed.

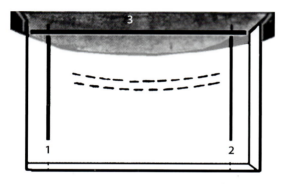

Fig. 15.80 The third incision that joins the two perpendicular incisions

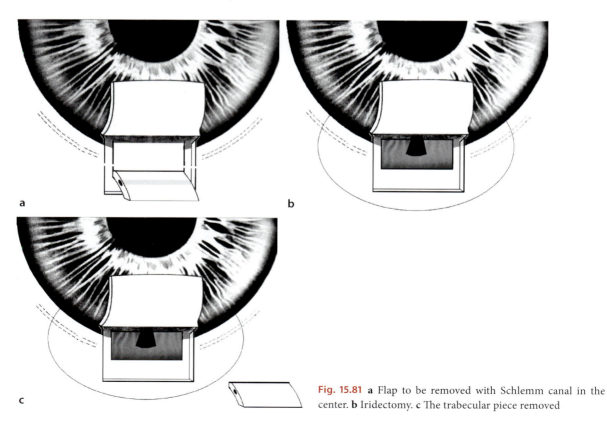

Fig. 15.81 a Flap to be removed with Schlemm canal in the center. **b** Iridectomy. **c** The trabecular piece removed

Iridectomy

If the iris tends to introduce itself into the wound, the anterior chamber is emptied again with the spatula, before going on to perform the iridectomy. We then use forceps that are not overly fine-toothed to take all the layers of the iris, for example, the Hoskin #22. In this way, the iris is taken with the left hand, pulling gently; the surgeon sees the pupil stretch, without the sphincter coming out through the trabeculectomy, and with De Wecker scissors, held between the index finger and thumb of the right hand, performs the iris cut. If a round iridectomy is desired, the blades of the scissors must be parallel to the limbus; if a triangular iridectomy is planned, they must be perpendicular to it. For the latter maneuver, a Barraquer model specially designed for the microscope is very useful, in which the cutting blades form a 90° angle with the body of the scissors.

After performing the iridectomy, we instill 1% sterilized atropine on the wound itself. The iridectomy is cleaned so that no iris remains stuck in the wound, deforming the pupil. An iris spatula, no longer than 1–2 mm, is introduced gently from right to left in the anterior chamber, in the ends of the incision, taking care not to touch the crystalline lens.

Figure 15.82 shows that the iridectomy must not be made very peripheral, as the major arterial circle of the iris passes there and, if cut, will cause a profuse hemorrhage. The cut in that part of the trabeculectomy piece to be removed must pass the scleral spur. It contains the scleral spur, the Schlemm canal, and the Schwalbe line.

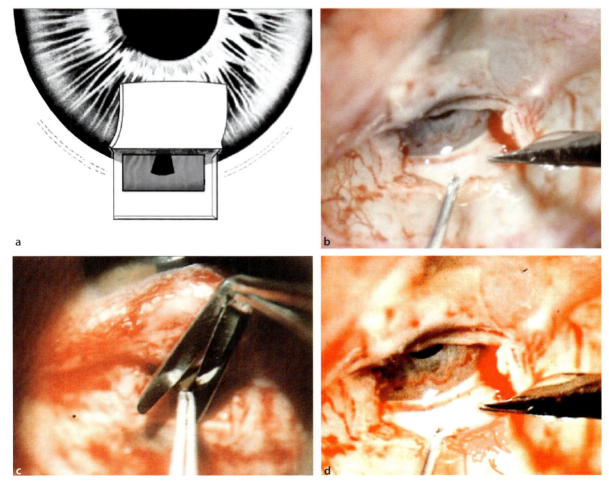

Fig. 15.82 a Drawing of the iridectomy. **b** Photograph, the iridectomy must not be very peripheral as the major arterial circle of the iris passes there, and if cut it will cause a profuse hemorrhage. **c** Photograph of the cutting of the iridectomy. **d** The incision of the trabeculectomy piece to be extracted must pass the scleral spur. *e,f see next page*

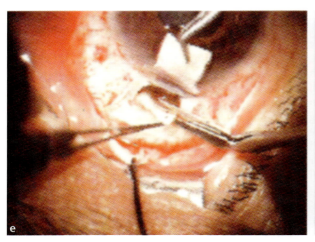
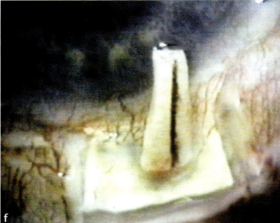

Fig. 15.82 (*continued*) **e** Cutting at the level of the scleral spur. **f** The trabeculectomy piece excised shows a very pigmented Schlemm canal in a case of pigmentary glaucoma

Suture of the Scleral Flap and the Conjunctiva

The scleral flap is folded back, putting it in its place, and two stitches are made with 10-0 nylon suture in its ends. Nylon is used to avoid the granulomas that we saw when we used virgin silk, which, in the case of a filtering bleb, can limit it and make the operation fail. If the conjunctival flap is fornix-based, we put two virgin silk stitches at 9 and 3 o'clock, in such a way that the conjunctiva covers the entire limbus and overlaps the cornea 1 mm. If it is a limbus-based flap, we carefully make separate silk stitches that take the conjunctiva and the Tenon capsule as well as each lip of the wound. A continuous suture can be made with cross-stitching in its ends so that it does not loosen. Figure 15.83 shows the most important surgical instruments used.

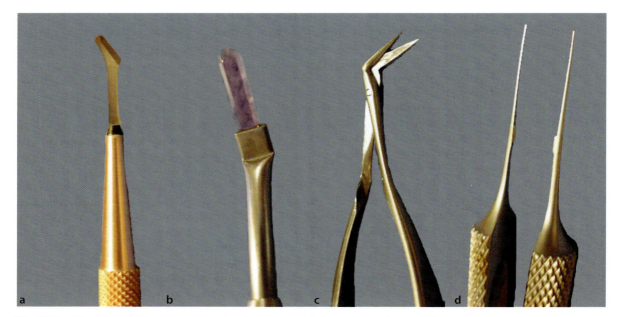

Fig. 15.83 **a** Desmaress, **b** Huco crescent blade, **c** Vannas angulated scissors, **d** Mermoud forceps

References

1. Taylor U (1891) Sulla incisione dell'angolo irideo (contribuzione all cura del glaucoma). Ann Ottalmol; 20: 117–127

2. Taylor U (1894) Sulla incisione dell'angolo irideo. Lav Clin Ocul Napoli 4:197

3. De Vincentiis C (1893) Incisione dell'angolo irideo nel glaucoma. Ann Ottalmol 22:540–541

4. De Vincentiis C (1895) Sulla Cosidetta: "sclérotomie interne". Lav Clin Ocul Napoli VI:227–235

5. Scalinci N (1900) La incisione del tessuto dell'angolo irideo nell'idroftalmo. Ann Ott 29:324

6. Barkan O (1936) New operation for chronic glaucoma: restoration of physiological function by opening Schlemm's canal under direct magnified vision. Am J Ophthalmol 19:951–966

7. Barkan O (1949) Techniques of goniotomy for congenital glaucoma. Arch Ophthalmol 41:65–68

8. Barkan O (1942) Operation for congenital glaucoma. Am J Ophthalmol 25:552–568

9. Barkan O (1938) Glaucoma: classification, causes and surgical control. Am J Ophthalmol 21

10. Barkan O (1945) Goniotomy. Am J Ophthalmol 28:1133–1134

11. Barkan O (1953) Surgery of congenital glaucoma. Am J Ophthalmol 36:1523–1533

12. Barkan O (1964) Pathogenesis of congenital glaucoma. Am J Ophthalmol 40:1–11

13. Worst JGF (1964) Goniotomy: an improved method for chamber-angle surgery in congenital glaucoma. Am J Ophthalmol 57:185–189

14. Broughton WL, Parks MM (1981) Analysis of treatment of congenital glaucoma by goniotomy. Am J Ophthalmol 91:566–572

15. Haas JS (1955) End results of treatment. Trans Am Acad Ophthalmol Otolaryngol 59:333–340

16. Morgan KS, Black B, Ellis FD, Helveston EM (1981) Treatment of congenital glaucoma. Am J Ophthalmol 92:799–803

17. Clothier CM, Rice NS, Dobinson P, Wakefield R (1979) Amblyopia in congenital glaucoma. Trans Ophthalmol Soc UK 99:427–431

18. Lister A (1966) The prognosis in congenital glaucoma. Trans Ophthalmol Soc UK; 86:5–18

19. Anderson JR (1939) Hydrophthalmia or congenital glaucoma. Cambridge University Press, Cambridge

20. Shaffer RN (1967) New concepts in infantile glaucoma. Can J Ophthalmol 2:243–247

21. Litinsky SM, Shaffer RN, Hetherington J, Hoskins HD (1971) Operative complications of goniotomy. Trans Am Acad Ophthalmol Otolaryngol 83:78–79

22. Cooling RT, Rice NS, McLeod D (1980) Retinal detachment in congenital glaucoma. Br J Ophthalmol 64:417–421

23. Lockie P, Elder J (1987) Spontaneous resolution of primary congenital glaucoma. Aust N Z J Ophthalmol 17:75–77

24. Dellaporta A (1959) Evaluation of anterior and posterior trabeculodialysis. Am J Ophthalmol 48:294–309

25. Burian HM (1960) A case of Marfan's syndrome with bilateral glaucoma. With description of a new type of operation for developmental glaucoma (trabeculotomy ab externo). Am J Ophthalmol 50:1187–1192

26. Allen L, Burian H (1962) Trabeculotomy ab externo. A new glaucoma operation. Technique and resultants of experimental surgery. Am J Ophthalmol 53:19–26

27. Smith R (1960) A new technique for opening the canal of Schlemm: preliminary report. Br J Ophthalmol 44:370–373

28. Smith R (1962) Nylon filament trabeculotomy. Trans Ophthalmol Soc UK 82:439–454

29. Walker WM, Kanagasundaran CR (1964) Surgery of the canal of Schlemm. Trans Ophthalmol Soc UK 84:427–442

30. Strachan JM (1967) A method of trabeculotomy with some preliminary results. Br J Ophthalmol 51:539–546

31. Harms H (1966) Glaukom-Operationen am Schlemm'schen Kanal. Sitzungsbericht, des 114 Versammlung des Vereins Rhein-Westf, Augenärzte

32. Harms H, Dannheim R (1970) Trabeculotomy. Results and problems. Microsurgery in glaucoma, 2nd International Symposium on Ophthalmology, Microsurgery Study Group. Bürgenstock, 1968. Adv Ophthalmol 22:121–131

33. Harms H (1970) Trabeculotomy. Results and problems. Adv Ophthalmol 27:95–96

34. Paufique L, Sourdille PH, Ortiz-Olmedo AH (1969) Technique et résultats de la trabeculotomie ab externo dans le traitement du glaucome congénital. Bull Mem Soc Fr Ophthal 82:54–65

35. Dannheim R (1978/1979) Long-term follow-up after trabeculotomy in open angle glaucoma. An Inst Barraquer 14:124–131

36. Luntz MH (1979) Congenital, infantile and juvenile glaucoma. Ophthalmology 86:793–802

37. Luntz MH, Livingston DG (1977) Trabeculotomy ab externo and trabeculectomy in congenital and adult-onset glaucoma. Am J Ophthalmol 83:174–179

38. Rothkoff L, Blumenthal M, Biedner B (1979) Trabeculotomy in late onset congenital glaucoma. Br J Ophthalmol 63:38–39

39. McPherson SD (1973) Results of external trabeculotomy. Am J Ophthalmol 76:918–920

40. Sampaolesi R, Argento C (1977) Scanning electron microscopy of the trabecular meshwork in normal and glaucomatous eyes. Invest Ophthalmol Vis Sci 16:302–314

41. Sampaolesi R (1991) Glaucoma, 2nd edn. Editorial Medica Panamericana, Buenos Aires

42. Sampaolesi R (1988) Congenital glaucoma. Long-term results after surgery. Fortschr Ophthalmol 85:626–631

43. Mandal AK (1996) Surgical results of combined trabeculotomy-trabeculectomy for developmental glaucoma. Pri-

mary combined trabeculotomy and trabeculectomy in a single session. Ophthalmology 105:974–983

44. Mandal AK (2003) Outcome of surgery on infants younger than 1 month with congenital glaucoma. Ophthalmology 110:1909–1915

45. Meyer G, Schwenn O, Grehn F (2000) Trabekulotomie bei Kongenitalem Glaukom. Ein Vergleich zur Goniotomie. Ophthalmologe 97:623–628

46. Kiefer G, Schwenn O, Grehn F (2001) Correlation of postoperative axial length growth and intraocular pressure in congenital glaucoma. A retrospective study in trabeculotomy and goniotomy. Graefes Arch Clin Exp Ophthalmol 239:893–899

47. Kozlov V, Bagrov SN, Anisimova SY, et al (1990) Nonpenetrating deep sclerotomy with collagen. IRTC Eye microsurgery. RSFSR Ministry of Public Health Moscow 4:62–66

48. Krasnov MM (1966) Glaucoma surgery in the region of the outer and inner wall of Schlemm's canal. In: Proceedings of the III Congress of Ophthalmology of the USSR, vol. I, Volgograd, Meditsina, p 200–210

49. Krasnov MM (1968) Externalization of Schlemm's canal (sinusotomy) in glaucoma. Br J Ophthalmol 52:157–161

50. Alekseev BN (1978) Microsurgery of the internal wall of Schelmm's canal. Vestn Oftal 4:4–14

51. Zimmerman TJ, Kooner KS, Ford VJ et al (1984) Trabeculectomy vs. non penetrating trabeculectomy. A retrospective study of two procedures in phakic patients with glaucoma. Ophthalmic Surg 15:734–740

52. Fyodorov SN, Sarkizova MB, Kurasova TP (1984) Deep sclerectomy: technique and mechanism of a new glaucomatous procedure. Glaucoma 6:281–283

53. Fyodorov SN, Kozlov VI, Timoshkina NT et al (1989) Non-penetrating sclerectomy in open-angle glaucoma. IRTC Eye Microsurgery. RSFSR Ministry of Public Health Moscow pp 52–55

54. Kozlov VI, Kozlova TV (1996) Non-penetrating deep sclerectomy with collagen draimage implantation (abstract 9-02). 5th Congress and the Glaucoma Course of the European Glaucoma Society, June 1996, Paris

55. Kozlov IV (1996) Analysis of complications of non-penetrating deep sclerectomy with collagen implant (abstract 9-02.1). 5th Congress and the Glaucoma Course of the European Glaucoma Society, Paris

56. Kozlova TV, Shaposhnikova NF, Scobeleva VB, Sokolovskaya TV (2000) Non-penetrating deep sclerectomy: evolution of the method and prospects for development. Ophthalmosurgery 3:39–53

57. Arenas Archillas E (1991) Trabeculectomy ab externo. Highlights Ophthalmol Lett XIX:9

58. Stegman R, Pienaar A, Miller D (1999) Viscocanalostomy for open-angle glaucoma in black African patients. J Cataract Refract Surg 25:316–322

59. Sourdille P, Santiago PY, Ducournau Y (1999) Chirurgie non perforante du trabeculum avec implant d'acide hyaluronique réticulé. Pourquoi, comment, quels résultats ? J Fr Ophtalmol 22:794–797

60. Demailly P, Jeanteur-Lunel MN, Berkani M et al (1996) Non-penetrating deep sclerectomy associated with collagen device in primary open angle glaucoma: middle-term retrospective study. J Fr Ophtalmol 19:659–666

61. Mermoud A, Shaarawy T (eds) (2001) Non-penetrating glaucoma surgery. Martin Dunitz, London

62. Mermoud A, Karlen ME, Schynder CC et al (1999): Nd:Yag goniopunture after deep sclerectomy with collagen implant. Ophthalmic Surg Lasers 30:120–125

63. Molteno CB (1969) New implant for drainage in glaucoma. Clinical trial. Br J Ophthalmol 53:609–615

64. Brooks SE, Dacey MP, Lee MB, Baerveldt G (1994) Modification of the glaucoma drainage implant to prevent early postoperative hypertension and hypotony: a laboratory study. Ophthalmic Surg 25:311–316

65. Lim KS, Allan BD, Lloyd AW, Mira A, Khaw PT (1998) Glaucoma drainage devices; past, present and future. Br J Ophthalmol 82:1083–1089

66. Coleman AL, Mondino BJ, Wilson MR, Casey R (1997) Clinical experience with the Ahmed Glaucoma Valve implant in eyes with prior or concurrent penetrating keratoplasties. Am J Ophthalmol 108:605–613

67. The Krupin Eye Valve Filtering Study Group (1949) Krupin eye valve with disc for filtration surgery. Ophthalmology 101:651–648

68. Mermoud A (2005) Ex-PRESS implant. Br J Ophthalmol 89:396–397

69. Cairns JE (1968) Trabeculectomy: preliminary report of a new method. Am J Ophthalmol 66:673–679

70. Barkan O (1938) Microsurgery in chronic simple glaucoma. Am J Ophthalmol 21:403–405

71. Vasco-Posadas J (1967) Glaucoma: esclerectomia subscleral. Arch Soc Am Oftal Optom 6:235

72. Fronimoupoulos J, Christakis C (1975) Goniotrepanation (Gotrep) and further observations on this operation for chronic glaucoma. Albrecht Von Graefes Arch Ophthalmol Klin Exp Ophthalmol 193:135–145

73. Watson PG, Barnett F (1975) Effectiveness of trabeculectomy in glaucoma. Am J Ophthalmol 79:831–845

74. Nesterov AP, Fedorova NV, Batmanov YE (1972) Sinus trabeculectomy, preliminary results of 100 operations. Br J Ophthalmol 56:833–839

75. Krasnov MM (1974) A modified trabeculectomy. Ann Ophthalmol 6:178–182

Contents

We have analyzed the postoperative anatomical and functional outcome in a sample of 138 patients with pediatric glaucoma. These cases were divided into three groups:

1. Congenital glaucomas operated once (glaucoma was almost reversed with a single procedure: trabeculotomy).
2. Congenital refractory glaucomas (one or more re-operations were required).

Percentage of Trabeculotomy and Combined Surgery in the Study Group

In 98 cases (70%), we performed trabeculotomy and in 38 cases (30%) combined surgery, Other authors have done the procedure in the same proportions, for example: Meyer et al. [1]. Their frequency in 37 cases was trabeculotomy, 62%, and combined surgery, 38%.

The number of cases studied was:
- Trabeculotomy: 90 patients (70.3%);
- Combined surgery: 38 patients (29.7%).

Follow-up lasted:
- In trabeculotomy: 12–40 years after surgery;
- In combined surgery: 7–35 years after surgery.

A number of parameters were studied before and after surgery:
- Intraocular pressure (IOP) in a single spot check at 9 a.m., with applanation) (Table 16.1);

Table 16.1 Intraocular pressure before and after surgery: spot check pressure and diurnal pressure curve

	Before surgery	After surgery
Trabeculotomy	24.5 mmHg	14.2 mmHg
Combined surgery	28.3 mmHg	17.8 mmHg

After surgery the daily pressure curve was normal in all cases.
- Daily pressure curve with applanation, in bed at 6, 9, 12, 15, and 18 o'clock: after surgery (Chap. 15[45, 46]);
- Median (M) and standard deviation: variability (V), normal M, not more than 19 mmHg, V not more than 2.1 mmHg;
- Axial length: measured with echometry (Fig. 16.1, Table 16.2);
- Refraction after surgery (Fig. 16.2, Table 16.3);
- Visual acuity (Fig. 16.3, Table 16.4);
- Correlation between axial length and visual acuity (Fig. 16.4);
- Optic nerve;
- Visual field.

The last two parameters are studied in Chaps. 17 and 18.

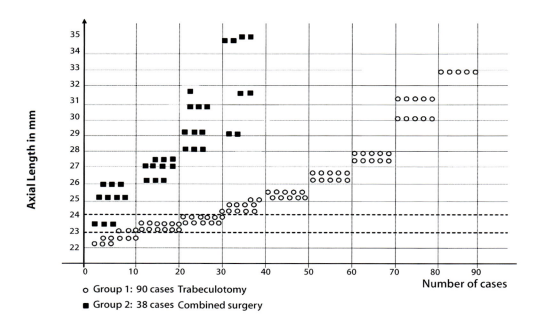

o **Group 1: 90 cases Trabeculotomy**
■ **Group 2: 38 cases Combined surgery**

Fig. 16.1 Axial length in millimeters after surgery

Table 16.2 Axial length before and after surgery

Before surgery	Mean axial length	Range
Trabeculotomy	24 mm	25–33 mm
Combined Surgery	28 mm	23.5–35 mm

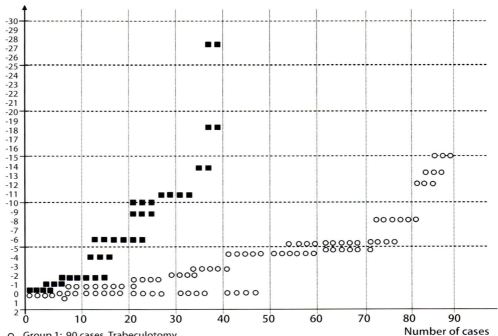

Fig. 16.2 Refraction after the surgery

Table 16.3 Refraction after surgery

After surgery	Refraction of both group	Range
Trabeculotomy	−3 D	0– −14 D
Combined Surgery	−6.6 D	0– −27 D

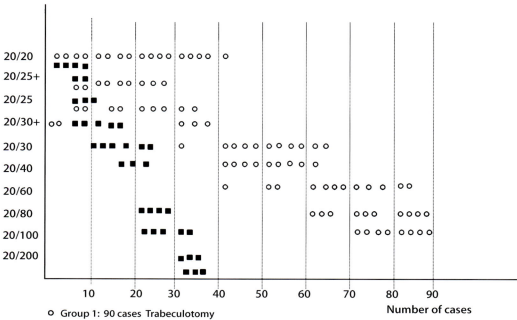

Fig. 16.3 Visual acuity in the two groups after surgery

Table 16.4 Visual acuity of both groups

After surgery	Mean visual acuity	Range
Trabeculotomy	20/30 +	20/20 to 20/200
Combined Surgery	20/60 −	20/20 to 20/200

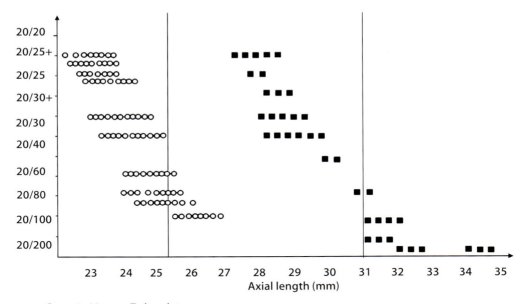

○   Group 1: 90 cases Trabeculotomy

■   Group 2: 38 cases Combined Surgery

Fig. 16.4 Correlation between axial length and visual acuity after the surgery

The figure above shows the correlation between visual acuity and axial length in 90 cases of trabeculotomy and 38 cases of combined surgery. The limit at which visual acuity drops below 20/40 is 25.5 mm and 31 mm for the trabeculotomy and combined-surgery groups, respectively. In both groups, visual acuity of less than 20/40 is due to breakage of the central Descemet's membrane, macular alterations, amblyopia, and corneal opacities.

To prevent myopia-related reduction of vision it is necessary to carry out frequent check-ups of the child's vision from immediately after surgery, using the preferential looking test.

There has been a major change in the prognosis of congenital glaucoma over the past 40 years, so that nowadays, if a corrected, well-indicated surgery is carried out, the result is good or very good. If we look at the literature, 68 years ago J. Ringland Anderson [2], in his classic monograph "Hydrophthalmia or congenital glaucoma, its causes, treatment, and outlook," described glaucoma as a disease with the worst prognosis that leads to blindness, but his son, Douglas R. Anderson [3], in his complete review published in Survey, shows us that this prognosis has since changed completely.

References

1. Meyer G, Schwenn O, Grehn F (2000) Trabekulotomie bei Kongenitalem Glaukom. Ein Vergleich zur Goniotomie. Ophthalmologe 97:623–628

2. Anderson R.J: Hydrophthalmia or congenital glaucoma (Cambridge University Press, London, 1939).

3. De Luise V.P and Anderson D.R: Primary infantile glaucoma (congenital glaucoma). Surv Ophthalmol 1983; 28: 1–19.

Optic Nerve

Contents

The Glaucomatous Optic Nerve Staging System with Confocal Tomography

History of the Optic Nerve Examination

Since the first images of the fundus were obtained with an ophthalmoscope, created by Helmholtz [1] in 1950, examination methods have continued to improve. First, examination with direct ophthalmoscopy was used, followed by examination with binocular indirect ophthalmoscopy, optic disc drawings, optic disc stereophotographs, planimetry, Takamoto and Schwartz's stereophotogrammetry, neuroretinal rim measurements, Airaksinen and Tuulonen's evaluation of the retinal nerve fiber layer, optic disc pallor measurements, angiofluoresceinography of the optic disc, image analyzer (Rodenstock Optic Nerve Head Analyzer, Topcon Analyzer), laser scanning ophthalmoscope, and Lotmar and Goldmann's stereochronoscopy. All these methods are extensively explained in the useful book The Optic Nerve in Glaucoma, by Varma and Spaeth [2].

Of these methods, we still find retinofluoresceinography particularly useful. We no longer use stereoscopic photographs of the optic nerve in adults, because of the significant interobserver variation in interpretation of results, as reported in the literature [3–5]. However, stereoscopic photographs are useful for optic nerve examinations in children under 2 years of age because, due to their flat corneas, we have failed to obtain good images with confocal tomography. In Boston, we learned about Schwartz and Takamoto's stereophotogrammetry [6], a very reliable method whose results are consistent with those obtained with the Heidelberg Retina Tomograph (HRT; Heidelberg Engineering, Heidelberg, Germany). However, it is a time-consuming method. We later performed neuroretinal rim measurements using Airaksinen et al.'s [7] method, which we were able to put into practice based on Dannheim and Airaksinen's personal communications. This turned out to be the most useful method. We also tried Lotmar and Goldmann's optic disc stereochronoscopy [8]. All these methods require pupil dilation.

The above-mentioned methods, and particularly the measurement of optic disc parameters (area, cup area, neuroretinal rim), required the formula introduced by Littman in 1982 [9] to obtain the dimensions (length, surface) of any observable object in the fundus (exudates, tumors, foreign bodies, optic discs, vessels, etc.). Images of these elements can be observed with considerable magnification produced by the ocular system.

This morphometric magnification was corrected to provide true values with the Littman formula. Littman was an engineer who worked for Zeiss whom we met in Buenos Aires. Since 1982, his formula has allowed us to obtain true measurements in millimeters or square millimeters of a body or structure on the retina. Corneal curvature, measured with an ophthalmometer, axial length, measured by echometry, and refraction are very important for this formula. Corneal thickness, its posterior curvature, lens face curvatures, the depth of the anterior chamber, and lens thickness are not required because even if they varied, their influence on the measurement is minimal. This formula does not apply for aphakia, pseudophakia, and refraction changes caused by lens opacity.

Finally, in 1990, the HRT was introduced by Heidelberg Engineering [10], and it was with this device that we started our extensive research in 1991, with more than 20,000 tomographies examined to date.

In this chapter, we cover what we believe is a very important topic: the HRT parameters used for optic nerve staging in glaucoma, as well as the follow-up of optic nerve damage [11]. The tomographic classification is mainly based on the volumes of these structures, and only secondarily on surfaces and other parameters, because stereometric and three-dimensional analyses are now available. The advantage provided by volume measurements over area measurements is that the former are raised to the third power, while the latter are only raised to the second power (whenever a change occurs, no matter how slight, there is a greater variation if the value is raised to the cube than if it is raised to the square).

Table 17.1 Parameters used for classification

Rim volume
Cup volume
Rim area
Cup area
Cup shape measure
Mean RNFL thickness
Height variation of contour line
Area between curve and plane

Parameters Used for Glaucoma Staging

As stated in the previous section, the main parameters used for the classification were volumes, followed by areas, thickness, and slope. The volumes taken into consideration are the neuroretinal rim volume and cup volume. The most important is neuroretinal rim volume; cup volume is also taken into account since a decrease in neuroretinal rim volume produces an increase in cup volume; this is a cause-effect relationship. The same occurs with area: the cup area (red) increases as the rim area (green and blue) decreases (Fig. 17.1).

The most important parameters used for the classification are listed in Table 17.1 and are illustrated in

Fig. 17.1, where the parameters belonging to the optic disc are separated from those analyzed in the contour line graph. These latter parameters are mean retinal nerve fiber layer (RNFL) thickness, height variation of the contour line and the area enclosed by the contour line, and the reference plane in the contour line height variation diagram (RNFL cross-sectional area). The reference plane is an important basis for and closely related to all other parameters. Therefore, its position must always be verified and, when performing a longitudinal study, one must check that it always remains at the same level.

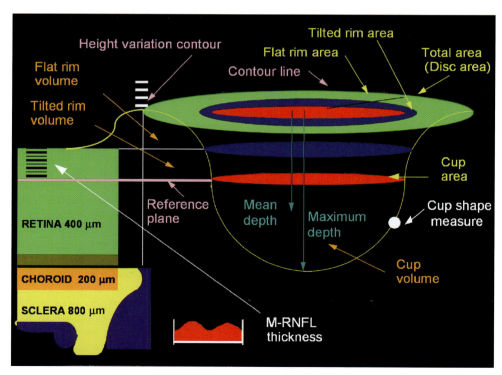

Fig. 17.1 Parameters of the HRT

Concept and Limits of Normality

The concept of normality is based on all the optic disc parameters being normal. Nevertheless, in clinical practice, one or two parameters may sometimes not be within the normal range, which does not indicate pathology. The concept and limit of normality are outlined in Fig. 17.2.

The limits of normality were obtained in a study of 108 normal volunteers [12]. Table 17.2 lists the most important limits, for example, for neuroretinal rim volume; the normal lower limit (3.20 mm^3) and not the normal upper limit is given, since this is mainly used to differentiate a large neuroretinal rim from an optic disc edema.

In some patients, a neuroretinal rim smaller than 320 mm^3 may be found during the first tomography, which is considered borderline in the classification. Nevertheless, the progression of these patients does not always involve optic nerve damage, but they remain stable for years, which indicates a physiological or normal decrease in the neuroretinal rim in this group of patients.

Progression Phases

Glaucomatous optic disc progression has been classified into the following groups:
- Normal
- Phase I
- Phase II
- Phase III
- Phase IV
- Phase V

Phases are separated from one another by more than two standard deviations, rendering the separation into the various groups more significant. Only parameters meeting this requirement are mentioned, since most of those remaining parameters have no significant differences between the various progression phases.

Normal optic discs (Table 17.3) are characterized by a barely visible Elschnig ring, except in the temporal area. Both poles have important fiber bundles, which correlate with the two camel humps displayed by the contour line diagram (Fig. 17.3).

Table 17.2 Limits of normality

Rim volume	Min.	3.20 mm^3
Cup volume	Max.	0.12 mm^3
Rim area	Min.	1.37 mm^2
Cup area	Max.	0.60 mm^2
Cup shape measure	Max.	−0.15
Mean RNFL thickness	Min.	0.17 mm
Height variation of contour line	Min.	0.27 mm
Area between curve and plane	Min.	0.87 mm^2

Table 17.3 Normal optic discs

Rim volume	>0.32 mm^3
Cup volume	<0.12 mm^3
Rim area	>1.37 mm^2
Cup area	<0.60 mm^2
Cup shape measure	<−0.15
Mean RNFL thickness	>0.17 mm
Height variation of contour line	>0.27 mm
Area between curve and plane	>0.87 mm^2

Normal visual field

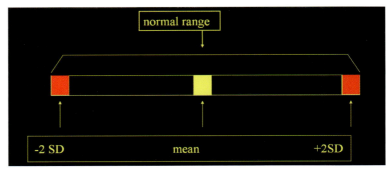

Fig. 17.2 Statistic Normal range mean and ±2 SD

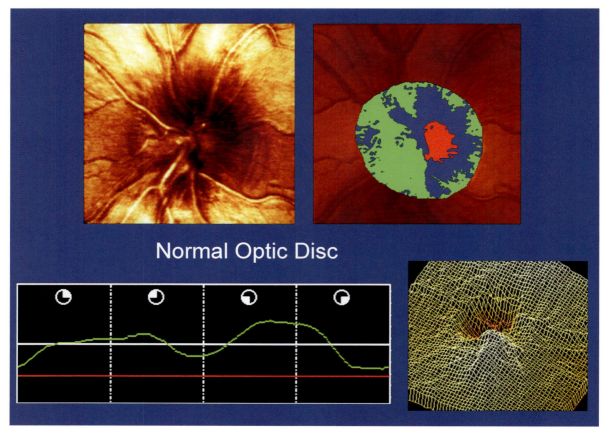

Normal Optic Disc

Fig. 17.3 HRT normal optic disc

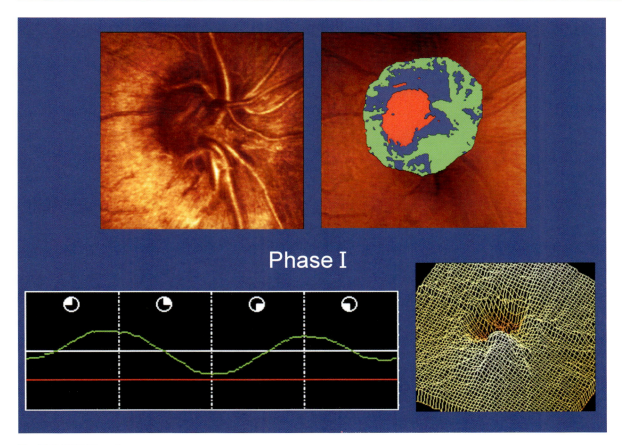

Fig. 17.4 HRT Phase I

In Phase I optic discs (Table 17.4), neuroretinal rim volume is normal on measuring the entire disc, but if the rim volume is analyzed by octants and quadrants, there is a decreased value in one of these sectors. The decrease in neuroretinal rim volume in this phase does not affect the entire optic disc. It corresponds with Burk's pseudonormal optic disc, in which the humps remain unchanged and there is a slight neuroretinal rim loss. With the exception of the cup increase, no parameters are altered, which is seen less frequently (Fig. 17.4).

Table 17.4 Phase I

Rim volume	>0.32 mm³
Cup volume	<0.12 mm³
Rim area	>1.37 mm2
Cup area	<0.60 mm2
Cup shape measure	<−0.15
Mean RNFL thickness	>0.17 mm
Height variation of contour line	>0.27 mm
Area between curve and plane	>0.87 mm²
Normal visual field	

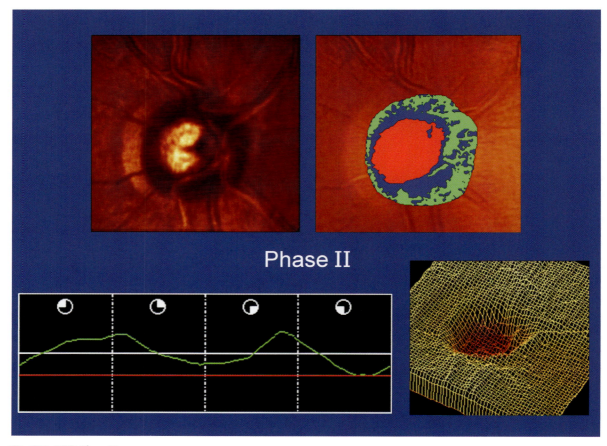

Fig. 17.5 HRT Phase II

Phase II optic discs (Table 17.5) are characterized by a generalized decrease in retinal thickness that can be seen in the contour line diagram as an approximation between the contour line proper and the reference plane. At the same time, a decrease in the height of the camel humps, which correlates with the loss of fiber bundles (see three-dimensional presentation) and with the fact that the Elschnig ring is more visible than before, can be seen (Fig. 17.5).

Table 17.5 Phase II

Rim volume	0.32–0.30 mm^3
Cup volume	0.12–0.24 mm^3
Rim area	1.37–1.20 mm^2
Cup area	0.60–1.00 mm^2
Cup shape measure	0.15–0.12
Normal visual field	

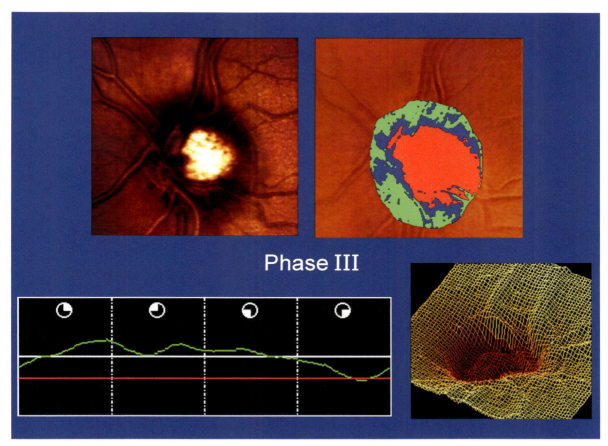

Fig. 17.6 HRT Phase III

Phase III optic discs (Table 17.6) already have a loss of up to 50% of the total retinal nerve fibers. The disappearance of both humps, which correlates with a substantial cup increase that invades the superior and the inferior poles, can be seen. The mean RNFL thickness, preventing the contour line from approaching the reference plane, remains unchanged (Fig. 17.6).

Table 17.6 Phase III

Rim volume	0.30–0.20 mm³
Cup volume	0.24–0.48 mm³
Rim area	1.20–0.80 mm²
Cup area	1.00–1.50 mm²
Cup shape measure	−0.12 to 0.12

Beginning of visual field defects

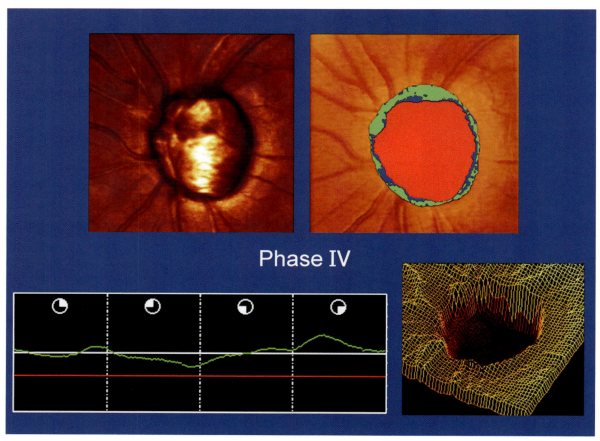

Fig. 17.7 HRT Phase IV

Phase IV optic discs (Table 17.7) are characterized by a substantial decrease in mean RNFL thickness, which causes the contour line to approach the reference plane (when localized defects occur, the contour line reaches the reference plane in the damaged areas). The summation image allows the bottom of the cup and the Elschnig ring to be seen to their full extent. The cup surface covers almost the entire optic disc surface. The neuroretinal rim persists like a thin halo around it (Fig. 17.7).

Table 17.7 Phase IV

Rim volume	0.20–0.10 mm³
Cup volume	0.48–0.96 mm³
Rim area	0.80–0.40 mm²
Cup area	1.50–1.80 mm²
Cup shape measure	−0.70 to −0.20
Moderate visual field defects	

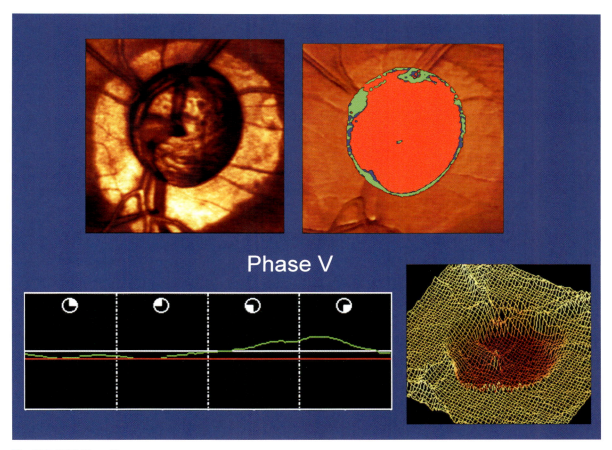

Fig. 17.8 HRT Phase V

Phase V optic discs (Table 17.8) are characterized by a final decrease in retinal thickness, where the contour line is parallel to the reference plane and, in the places where there is no neuroretinal rim left, the contour line height variation diagram is below the reference plane. This correlates with the appearance of white areas in the analysis of the surfaces and with the presence of absolute visual field defects (Fig. 17.8).

Table 17.8 Phase V

Rim volume	0.10–0.0 mm³
Cup volume	>0.96 mm³
Rim area	0.40–0.0 mm²
Cup area	>1.80 mm²
Cup shape measure	0/+

Visual field in stage 3 or 4 (terminal)

All six phases are summarized in Figs. 17.9 and 17.10. In normal optic discs, as well as in the phase I disc, the Elschnig ring can only be seen in the temporal sector, whereas in all other phases, it can be seen almost to its full extent, due to fiber atrophy. The bottom of the cup can be more clearly seen from phase III onward. When the brightness of the retina is observed in each section, it can be seen that this decreases steadily from normal to phase V. Cup shape measure changes rapidly. In phase III, the cup slope is almost perpendicular, while in phases IV and V bayonet-shaped vessels are revealed. The small vessels become more and more evident and their contours are more clearly visible as they become more definite (because of atrophy of the retinal nerve fibers). Nevertheless, at first sight, the condition of the optic disc in phase V may seem better than in phase IV. Also, the time elapsed between the normal and the phase I optic disc, or between phase I and phase II optic discs may seem the same. This is easily solved with stereometric analysis of the surfaces.

Figures 17.9 and 17.10 show the six phases together in the "Measure" menu of the HRT software, with the color-coded analysis of the surfaces. In normal optic discs, the cup is surrounded by a large neuroretinal rim and not centered in the optic disc. This occurs in normal conditions because of the substantial infiltration of fibers at the superior and inferior poles. In phase I optic discs, it is possible to see how the surface of the cup increases to the detriment of a decrease of the rim area. Simultaneously, the cup becomes central and its area invades the tilted neuroretinal rim area, thus reducing its separation from the flat neuroretinal rim. In phase II optic discs, the cup continues to increase and gets closer to the flat neuroretinal rim, leaving a thin separation covered by the tilted neuroretinal rim. The total surface of the neuroretinal rim decreases mark-

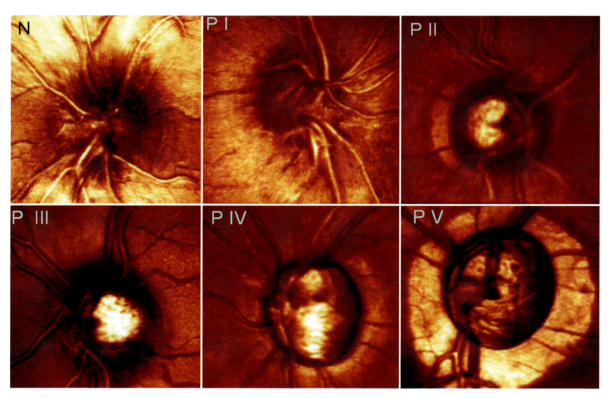

Fig. 17.9 HRT from normal to Phase V

edly. In phase III optic discs, the cup increases considerably and starts to become slightly excentric, and the tilted rim disappears completely in these regions. Consequently, the cup surface borders the flat rim surface. This can sometimes cause localized defects and, together with the diffuse atrophy of the rest of the retina, it correlates with the onset of the visual field defects in this phase. In phase IV optic discs, the cup surface almost covers the complete optic disc region. The tilted rim has almost completely disappeared. Only a thin flat rim margin separates the cup from the external optic disc margin. This small volume of neuroretinal rim keeps the visual function unchanged; this is correlated with the rapid visual field loss produced when the remaining neuroretinal rim is damaged. In phase V optic discs, the cup occupies almost the entire optic disc surface and, in some sectors, where the neuroretinal rim has been completely destroyed, the cup touches the

external optic disc margin, making the total absence of the neuroretinal rim evident in that sector. White regions can occur in phase V, which are caused by the retinal surface being below the level of the reference plane in the most severely damaged sectors. These lesions produce absolute optic disc defects with a poor prognosis. In Fig. 17.11 shows a chart of the five phases described above. In the left part and in the center is the rim volume corresponding to each phase, so that the phase diagnosis can be quickly made. On the right are the values that Burk obtained for these phases, which agree fully with our own. In the lower part are all the parameters of each phase so that, observing the values in computed tomography, the phase diagnosis can be made.

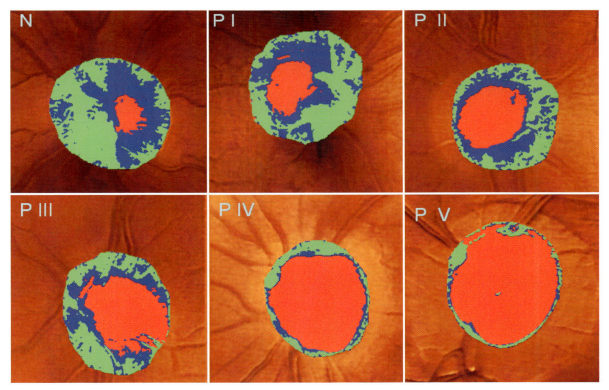

Fig. 17.10 HRT from normal to Phase V

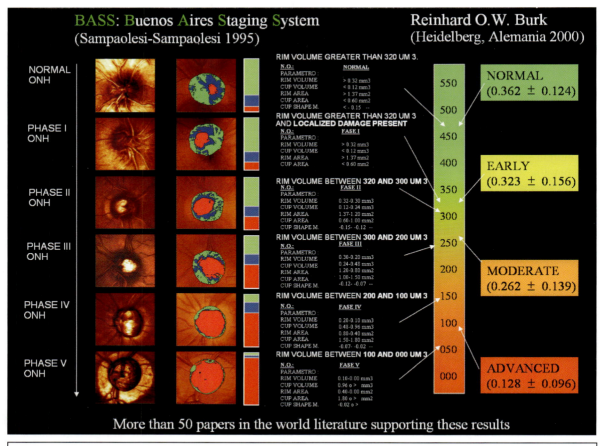

N.O. Parametro:	Normal	N.O. Parametro:	Phase III
Rim volume	> 0.32 mm^3	Rim volume	0.30-0.20 mm^3
Cup volume	< 0.12 mm^3	Cup volume	0.24-0.48 mm^3
Rim area	> 1.37 mm^2	Rim area	1.20-0.80 mm^2
Cup area	< 0.60 mm^2	Cup area	1.00-1.50 mm^2
Cup shape m.	< - 0.15	Cup shape m.	- 0.12 – - 0.07
N.O. Parametro:	Phase I	N.O. Parametro:	Phase IV
Rim volume	> 0.32 mm^3	Rim volume	0.20-0.10 mm^3
Cup volume	< 0.12 mm^3	Cup volume	0.48-0.96 mm^3
Rim area	> 1.37 mm^2	Rim area	0.80-0.40 mm^2
Cup area	< 0.60 mm^2	Cup area	1.50-1.80 mm^2
		Cup shape m.	- 0.07 – - 0.02
N.O. Parametro:	Phase II	N.O. Parametro:	Phase V
Rim volume	0.32-0.30 mm^3	Rim volume	0.10-0.00 mm^3
Cup volume	0.12-0.24 mm^3	Cup volume	0.96 o > mm^3
Rim area	1.37-1.20 mm^2	Rim area	0.40-0.00 mm^2
Cup area	0.60-1.00 mm^2	Cup area	1.80 o > mm^2
Cup shape m.	- 0.15 – - 0.12	Cup shape m.	- 0.02 o >

Fig. 17.11 Five phases of evolution of the Optic Disc study with HRT and the values of the parameters of each phase

Optic Nerve in Congenital Glaucoma

In order to study the optic nerve in congenital glaucoma we have developed the protocol described in the following sections.

Material

We have studied three different populations with pediatric glaucomas during childhood [6–9]. The first group (19 eyes) consisted of primary congenital glaucomas operated only once. The IOP was regulated and the axial length of the eyes stopped its enlargement after surgery. Surgery was successful.

The second group (12 eyes) consisted of children with primary glaucomas in which the IOP was regulated and the axial length of the eyes stopped its enlargement after 2–6 reoperations.

The third group (29 eyes) consisted of late congenital glaucoma, goniodysgenesis, or juvenile open angle glaucoma. As these diseases manifested later, generally between 4 and 6 years of age, the axial length of the eyes did not grow despite ocular hypertension because the sclera was no longer elastic. The intraocular pressure was regulated with medical therapy or surgery (Table 17.9).

Method

We studied the optic discs in three groups with the Heidelberg Retina Tomograph (HRT). Three images were acquired for each eye and the mean topography was obtained. The standard deviation of the mean topography must always be lower than 30 μm.

In addition to the study of the optic disc parameters, the profiles of the optic discs of each group were studied to scale.

Parameters

We will now explain the alterations found in each parameter for each group, compared to the parameters of a group of 110 normal subjects, ranging from 5 to 25 years of age [3].

One-way analysis of variance (ANOVA) was used for overall comparison among the four groups and post hoc comparisons were done with the Tukey test. Data was considered as statistically significant if $p<0.05$. All tests were performed with the Graph Pad InStat software (version 2.5). Table 17.10 shows the differences between groups 1, 2, and 3, while Table 17.11 shows the differences of each group with the control (normal group).

Figure 17.12 shows the analysis of the parameters disc area and cup/disc area ratio. Figure 17.13 shows the analysis of the parameters related to the mean cup depth, maximum cup depth, cup area, and cup volume. Figure 17.14 analyzes the parameters rim volume and rim area. Figure 17.15 shows the cup shape measure and contour line height variation. In each parameter, the difference between the three groups (Table 17.10) and the difference between each group and the normal group (Table 17.11) were analyzed.

Table 17.9 Three different groups studied and its control group

Material	Cases	Follow-up (years)	Male	Female
Group 1: Primary congenital glaucoma operated once	19	12–28	13	6
Group 2: Reoperated primary congenital glaucoma (refractory CG)	12	7–22	10	2
Group 3: Late congenital glaucoma (goniodysgenesis	29	11–23	15	14
Total	60	7–28	38	22
Control group: normal individuals (25) (aged 5–25 years)	110		50	60

Table 17.10 Differences between the groups

Variable	P	Differences between groups		
		1 vs 2	1 vs 3	2 vs 3
Disc area	<0.001	*	NS	**
Cup/disc area ratio	<0.001	***		
Mean cup depth	<0.001	***	NS	***
Maximum cup depth	<0.001	***	NS	***
Cup area	<0.001	***	*	**
Cup volume	<0.001	***	NS	***
Rim volume	<0.001	*	***	NS
Rim area	<0.01	NS	**	NS
Cup shape measure	<0.02	*	NS	*
Height variation of the contour	<0.05	NS	NS	NS

P represents the results obtained with the ANOVA, including normals.
* p<0.05, ** p<0.01; *** p<0.001
NS not significant

Table 17. 11 Differences with normal group

Variable	P	Differences with normal group		
		Group 1	Group 2	Group 3
Disc area	<0.001	NS	***	NS
Cup/disc area ratio	<0.001	NS	***	***
Mean cup depth	<0.001	***	NS	***
Maximum cup depth	<0.001	***	NS	***
Cup area	<0.001	NS	***	***
Cup volume	<0.001	NS	***	***
Rim volume	<0.001	**	***	NS
Rim area	<0.01	NS	***	*
Cup shape measure	<0.02	NS	**	NS
Height variation of the contour	<0.05	NS	NS	NS

P represents the results obtained with the ANOVA, including normals.
* p<0.05, ** p<0.01; *** p<0.001
NS not significant

Disc Area

In the three groups, statistically significant differences were found between groups 1 and 2 (p<0.05) and between groups 2 and 3 (p<0.01). No significant difference was found between groups 1 and 3. Compared to the normal group, significant differences were found only for group 2 (p<0.001) (Fig. 17.12a).

Cup/Disc Area Ratio

In the three groups, statistically significant differences were found between groups l and 2 (p<0.001) and between groups 1 and 3 (p<0.01). No significant differences were found between groups 2 and 3. Compared to the normal group, significant differences were found for groups 2 and 3 (p<0.0001) (Fig. 17.12b).

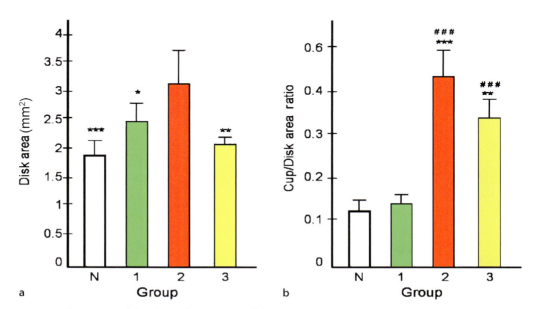

Fig. 17.12a,b Disc area (**a**) and cup/disc area ratio (**b**). Bars are mean + SEM
(**a**) *, **, ***: *p*<0.05, *p*<0.01 and *p*<0.001 vs group 2:
(**b**) **. ***: *p*<0.01 and *p*<0.001 vs group 1: ###: *p*<0.00.1 vs normal group

Mean Cup Depth

The difference between the three groups was statistically significant only between groups 1 and 2 and between groups 2 and 3 (p<0.001). Compared to the normal group, all three groups were significantly different (p<0.001) (Fig. 17.13a).

Maximum Cup Depth

As with the previous parameter, the differences were statistically significant only between groups 1 and 2 and between groups 2 and 3 (p<0.001). All three groups were significantly different from the normal group (p<0.001) (Fig. 17.13b).

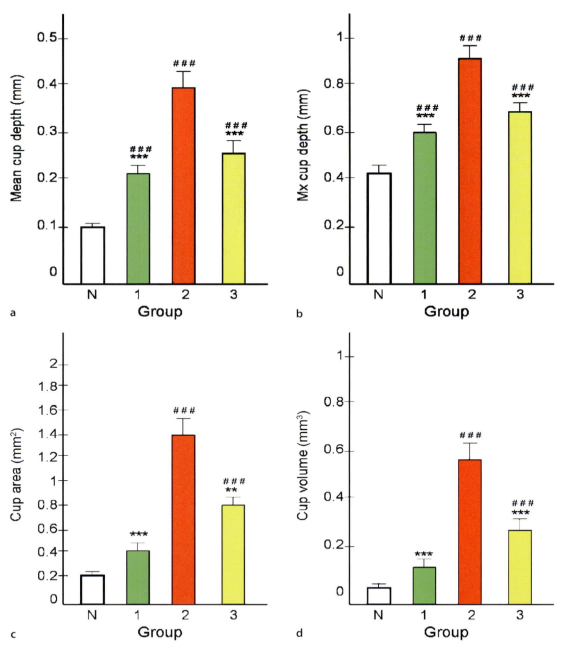

Fig. 17.13a–d Mean cup depth (**a**), maximum cup depth (**b**), cup area (**c**), and cup volume (**d**). Bars are mean + SEM
(**a**), (**b**) and (**d**) ***: *p*<0.001 vs group 2; ###: *p*<0.001 vs normal group;
(**c**) **, ***: *p*<0.01 and *p*<0.001 vs group 2; ###: *p*<0.001 vs normal group

Cup Area

In the three groups, statistically significant differences were found between groups 1 and 2 (p<0.001), between groups 1 and 3 (p<0.05), and between groups 2 and 3 (p<0.01). No significant difference was found between groups 2 and 3. Compared to the normal group, significant differences were found for groups 2 and 3 (p<0.001) (Fig. 17.13c).

Cup Volume

In the three groups, statistically significant differences were found only between groups 1 and 2 and between groups 2 and 3 (p<0.001). Compared to the normal group, significant differences were found only for groups 2 and 3 (p<0.01) (Fig. 17.13d). In group 2, the cup volume was larger than in group 1, group 3, and in normal eyes.

Rim Volume

In the three groups, statistically significant differences were found only between groups 1 and 2 (p<0.05) and between groups 1 and 3 (p<0.001). Compared to the normal group, a significant difference was found only for group 1 (p<0.01) (Fig. 17.14a). The rim volume was larger in group 1 (glaucomas operated only once) than in group 2 (reoperated congenital glaucomas).

Rim Area

In the three groups, a statistically significance difference was found only between groups 1 and 3 (p<0.01). Compared to the normal group, a significant difference was found only for group 3 (p<0.05) (Fig. 17.14b). The smallest rim areas were found in eyes belonging to group 3.

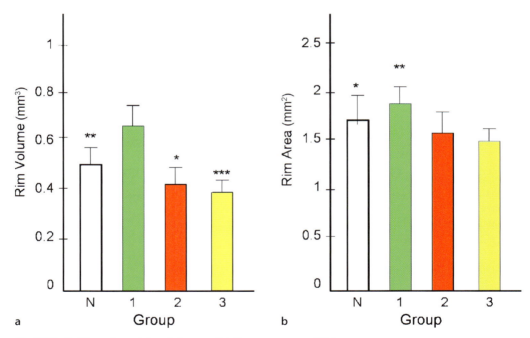

Fig. 17.14a,b Rim volume (**a**) and rim area (**b**). Bars are mean + SEM
(**a**) *, **, ***: *p*<0.05, *p*<0.01, and *p*<0.001 vs group 1;
(**b**) *, **: *p*<0.05 and *p*<0.01 vs group 3

Cup Shape Measure

In the three groups, statistically significant differences were found only between groups 1 and 2 and between groups 2 and 3 ($p<0.05$). Compared to the normal group, a significant difference was found only for group 2 ($p<0.01$) (Fig. 17.15a).

Height Variation Contour

The differences between the three groups were statistically significant. Compared to the normal group, a significant difference existed only for group 2 ($p<0.05$) (Fig. 17.15b). This indicates that even though in congenital glaucomas there is a reduction in the number of nerve fibers, there is no localized depression in any quadrant or octant, as it occurs in adults. Therefore, in children there are no disc notches or scotomatous defects.

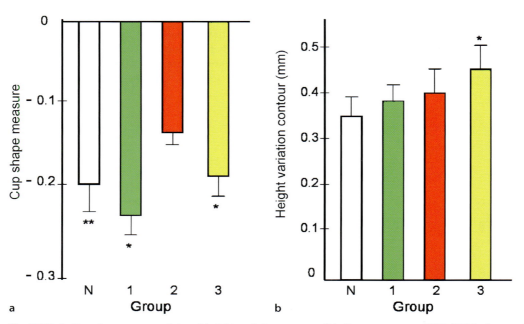

a   b

Fig. 17.15a,b Cup shape measure (a) and height variation contour (b). Bars are mean + SEM (SEM of normal group N in (a) is 0.007)
(a) *, **: $p<0.05$ and $p<0.01$ vs group 2;
(b) *: $p<0.05$ vs normal group

Cup Profiles

Chamber Angle Type I

In addition to these parameters, we computed the mean profile of the optic nerve head in each group with Turbocad software (version 2.0). In order to compare the profiles to the mean profile of a normal disc, we studied a control group of 101 normal individuals between 5 and 25 years of age.

Figure 17.16 shows the mean profile of group 1 as compared to a normal mean profile. They are almost identical, because as surgery succeeded in regulating the intraocular pressure quickly, the optic nerve did not suffer.

Comparing their surfaces, it can be observed that the increase in the cup area is due to an increase in the total disc area and not to a reduction of the neuroretinal rim area. Upon its distension, the Elschnig ring becomes larger and therefore the total disc area becomes larger than in normal eyes.

Figure 17.17 shows the image of an optic disc belonging to group 1, as obtained with the HRT.

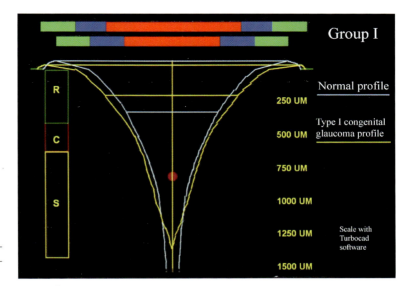

Fig. 17.16 Group 1 in *blue*, normal profile in *yellow*, profile of optic disc belonging to type I congenital glaucoma

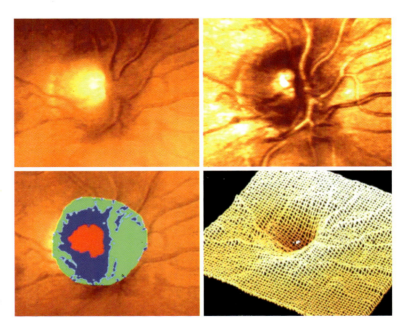

Fig. 17.17 HRT of a child with type I congenital glaucoma

Figure 17.18 shows the mean profile of group 2, which differs significantly from the normal mean profile. It also shows a great reduction in the volume of the neuroretinal rim and a great increase in the cup volume.

With regard to the surface, there is a great increase in the cup area and a reduction in the neuroretinal rim area. The total disc area is greatly enlarged by the disten-

sion of the Elschnig ring. It should be kept in mind that this cup increase occurs at the expense of a reduction of the tilted neuroretinal rim (in blue), while the flat neuroretinal rim (in green) remains almost unchanged.

Figure 17.19 shows the image of an optic disc belonging to group 2, obtained with the HRT.

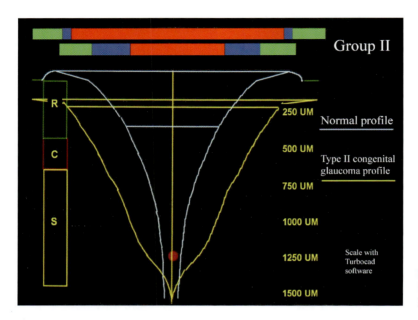

Fig. 17.18 In *blue*, normal profile, in *yellow* profile of optic disc belonging to type II congenital (refractory) glaucoma

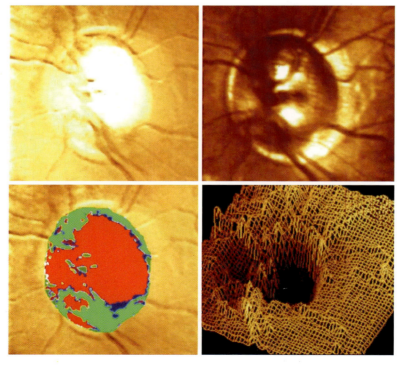

Fig. 17.19 HRT of a child with type II congenital glaucoma

Figure 17.20 shows the mean profile of group 3, which is almost the same as the normal profile. Unlike in groups 1 and 2, the total disc area is the same as in the normal group. This correlates with the fact that there is no distension of the Elschnig ring because ocular hypertension affects the eye only after 5 years of age. This behavior is the same as in adult glaucomas, where the cup area enlargement is proportional to the neuroretinal rim area reduction.

Figure 17.21 shows an optic disc belonging to group 3, obtained with the HRT. The red point of each profile graph indicates the end of the cup and the beginning of the hyaloid duct (according to histopathologic determinations, it starts when the cup surface is less or equal to 62 μm²) In group 3, unlike in groups 1 and 2, the end of the cup remains almost at the same depth as in the normal disc, since in this group the eye is no longer elastic. In the other groups, the end of the cup is considerably displaced posteriorly.

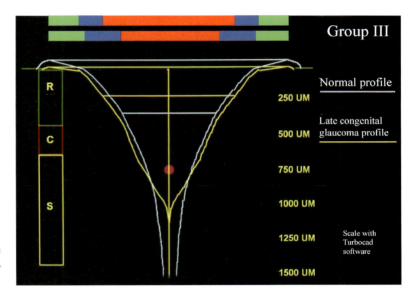

Fig. 17.20 In *blue*, normal profile, in *yellow* late congenital glaucoma profile, group III

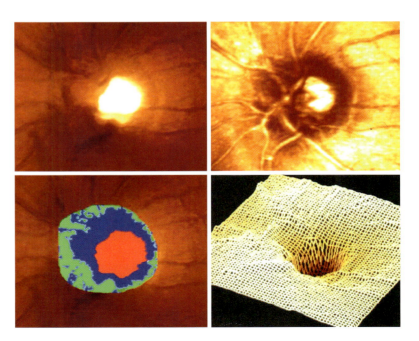

Fig. 17.21 HRT of a child with late congenital glaucoma, group III

Megalopapilla: Large Optic Nerve Heads, or Megalodiscs

One of the most common diagnostic mistakes in daily practice is caused by megalopapilla. Direct ophthalmoscopy or biomicroscopy of a megalopapilla reveals marked pallor and great cupping. We have examined children between 4 and 14 years of age who were ready to undergo surgery for congenital glaucoma. Upon thorough study, these cases had normal axial length and corneal diameter and if perimetry was possible, there was normal visual field and no signs of congenital glaucoma.

Franceschetti and Bock [14] originally coined the term "megalopapilla" for enlarged optic discs not associated with any other morphological anomalies. Megalopapilla may present with either of two phenotypic features:

1. Normal configuration with an abnormally large optic disc, high cup/disc ratio, disc surface pallor, neuroretinal rim pallor due to the presence of axons spread over a large surface, usually round or horizontally oval-shaped optic disc cup and absence of nasalization of vessels at their point of origin (usually bilateral and congenital).
2. The cup is displaced toward the top and thus obliterates the adjacent neuroretinal rim [15]. This is less common.

The appearance of the megalopapilla thus resembles that of glaucomatous neuropathy. It is indeed a pseudoglaucomatous disc. Most cases of megalopapilla may be merely a statistical variant of normality. Megalopapilla may occasionally result from altered optic axonal migration early in embryogenesis in children with basal encephalocele [16]. Basal encephalocele is often associated with other midline anomalies such as hypertelorism, broad nasal root, cleft lip, and cleft palate. Optic disc anomalies, such as pallor, dysplasia, optic disc pits, coloboma, and megalopapilla have been reported [17]. Caprioli has described an association between basal encephalocele and morning glory syndrome [18].

Our experience has shown that megalopapilla may be divided into congenital and acquired forms. Acquired megalopapilla is associated with type II congenital glaucomas (refractory congenital glaucomas, reoperated congenital glaucomas) [19]. Grimson and Perry [20] described an orbital glioma case that in children can lead to progressive enlargement of a previously normal-sized optic disc.

Collier [21] described four cases of megalopapilla associated with pulverulent cataract and suggested that this finding may be explained by the development of the epithelial primitive disc during the 2nd month of gestation and of the pulverulent cataract in the 3rd month of gestation.

Hirokane et al. [22] described megalopapilla in eight eyes of four children. The disc with glaucomatous-like cupping was so large that the macular diameter (DM) (measured from the center of the disc to the macular edge) to disc diameter ratio (DD) (DM/DD) was lower than 2.2. Although the cup/disc ratio and the appearance of the disc margin and the disc vessels in these cases were the same as those of glaucomatous eyes, the population they reported showed absence of rim pallor notch and nerve fiber layer defects typically present in glaucomatous eyes. These findings demonstrate the importance of determining the DM/DD ratio to differentiate megalopapilla from glaucoma in children with large optic cups.

Jonas [23] published an interesting paper on pseudoglautomatous physiologic large cups in megalopapilla using planimetric analysis of stereoscopic optic disc photographs. Upon studying 21 cases of megalopapilla, he concluded that "here are individuals with abnormally high cup/disc ratio but no pathologic findings." It was possible to identify intrapapillary and juxtapapillary characteristics that may be helpful in the differentiation of glaucomatous eyes and normal eyes with high cup/disc ratios.

Maisel et al. [24] studied 141 native adults from the Marshall Islands. In this genetically isolated population, he found 22 eyes of 15 subjects with megalopapilla and normal IOP. Three large discs with an 18-year photographic follow-up showed no change.

Purpose

The purpose of this study is to evaluate megalopapillas in order to determine whether they constitute a different population, by showing their specific features, to find the differences between this entity and other optic nerve head neuropathies with enlarged disc area, such as congenital glaucomas, goniodysgenesis with megalopapilla, and advanced optic nerve head glaucomatous damage, and to establish the differential diagnosis between megalopapilla and pure congenital glaucomas in children.

Material

The population studied was divided into four groups:

Group 1 33 cases of congenital megalopapilla, 13 of which were not associated with any other disease, 11 were associated with goniodysgenesis, six with open-angle glaucoma, two with hypophysis nonfunctional tumors, and one with exfoliation syndrome.

Group 2 30 optic neuropathies in pure congenital glaucoma diagnosed within the 1st year of life and operated two to seven times, which became acquired megalopapilla.

Group 3 168 open-angle cases of glaucoma in the perimetric stage (with visual field defects characteristic of phase 3 or 4).

Group 4 172 normal subjects as controls.

Method

The optic nerve was evaluated with the HRT, software version 2.12 (wavelength: 680 nm). All the stereometric parameters were measured. The visual fields were examined with Octopus perimetry. Slit-lamp examination of the posterior segment, as well as daily pressure curves to obtain the mean and standard deviation were also performed.

Classification

By definition, a megalopapilla is an optic nerve head disc with a surface greater than 2.5 mm².

Type 1 Normal configuration, bilateral, high cup/disc ratio, pale disc surface, round or oval cup and congenital. This group belongs to a previous series divided into three groups:

Group 1 Primary or pure congenital glaucomas diagnosed within the first year of age successfully operated once.

Group 2 with more than one surgery required and which is the group we have further studied here.

Group 3 Late congenital glaucomas or goniodysgenesis.

Groups 1 and 2 have a significantly enlarged axial length according to echometry, while in group 3 since diagnosis was made after 5 years of age, when the eye was no longer elastic, the axial length is normal [12]

Type 2 Cup decentered to the top, unilateral, higher frequency of cilioretinal arteries, neuroretinal rim reduced in top, round cup, and congenital.

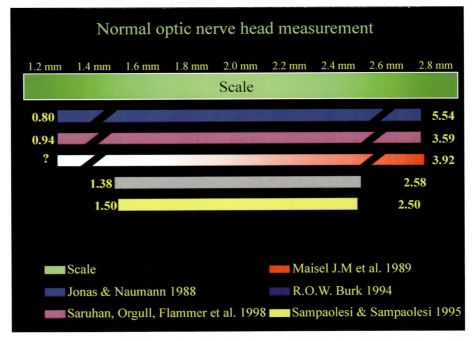

Fig. 17.22 Different measurements made by Jonas et al. [23], Maisel et al. [24], Saruhan et al. [25], Burk et al. [26], and Sampaolesi and Sampaolesi [27]

Figure 17.22 shows different measurements made by Jonas et al. [23]. Saruhan et al. [25], Maisel et al. [24], Burk et al. [26] and Sampaolesi and Sampaolesi [27].

Figure 17.23 demonstrates that normal disc areas may be present in the glaucomas as well as in the most frequent acquired neuropathies, etc.

We will now compare the optic nerve head parameters of the megalopapilla with those of normal discs, first in terms of area, then in terms of volume, and lastly in terms of the third moment.

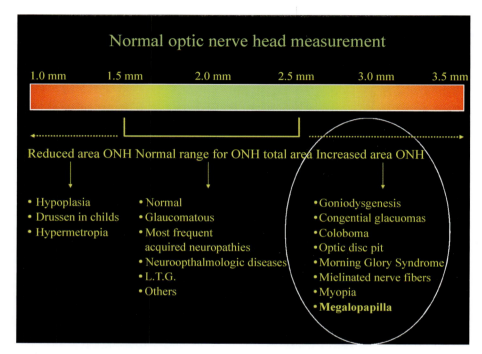

Fig. 17.23 Normal disc areas may be present in the glaucomas, as well as in the most frequent acquired neuropathies, neurophthalmologic disorders, and low-tension glaucomas, while reduced disc areas may be found in optic nerve hypoplasias, children with drusen and hyperopic cases. Increased disc areas may be found in goniodysgenesis, congenital glaucomas, optic disc colobomas, optic disc pits, morning glory syndrome, myelinated nerve fibers, myopias, and megalopapillas

Parameters of the HRT in Normal Optic Disc and Megalopapilla

The ordinates of Fig. 17.24 show the area in square millimeters, while in the abscissas, the first group compares the disc area, the second group, the rim area, and the third one, the cup area. Table 17.12 shows the static values of these comparisons, with a highly significant difference for disc area and cup area. The difference is poorly significant for rim area.

Table 17.12 Normal optic disc and megalopapilla parameters

Parameter/group	Normal	Megalopapilla
Disc area	2.05	3.07***
Rim area	1.74	1.50*
Cup area	0.32	1.57***

NS not significant; * $p<0.01$; *** $p<0.0001$. The difference is poorly significant for rim area

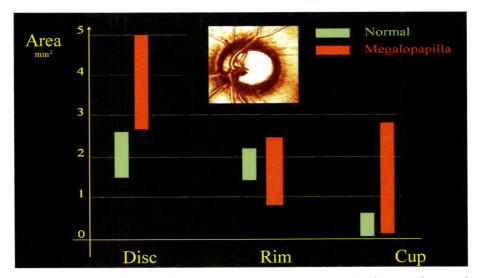

Fig. 17.24 The ordinates show the area in square millimeters. The abscissas: the first group compares the disc area, the second group, the rim area and the third, the cup area. See Table 17.12

The abscissa in Fig. 17.27 shows area values in square millimeters and in the ordinate there are six groups represented in order to make a comparison in terms of disc area, rim area, rim volume, cup area, cup volume, and cup shape measure.

When comparing the megalopapillas with advanced glaucomas, there is a statistically highly significant difference in terms of disc area, rim area, and rim volume, while the difference is less significant in terms of cup area and cup volume, and there is no significant difference as regards cup shape measure (Table 17.15).

Table 17.15 Comparison between megalopapilla and normality

Parameter/group	Normal	Megalopapilla
Disc area	2.05	3.07***
Rim area	0.20	1.50***
Rim volume	0.05	0.36***
Cup area	1.80	1.57*
Cup volume	0.96	0.59*
Cup shape M.	0.00	0.06 NS

NS not significant; * $p<0.01$; *** $p<0.0001$

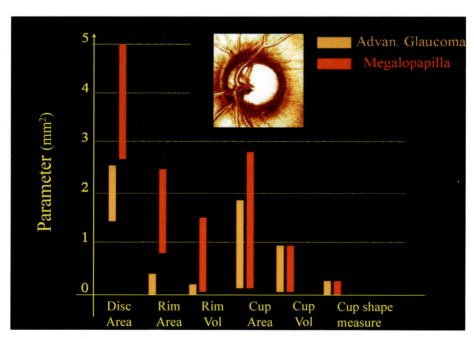

Fig. 17.27 a Values for cup shape measure. Abscissas represent the comparison between the groups studied. **b** Corresponding statistics

See Fig. 17.28 and Table 17.16 for a comparison of megalopapillas with congenital glaucomas.

In Fig. 17.28, the ordinates show parameter values either in square millimeters or cubic millimeters, and the different optic nerve head parameters are represented in the abscissa: disc area, rim area, rim volume, cup area, cup volume, and cup shape measure. The statistical difference is highly significant as regards cup shape measure, poorly significant as regards rim area, and nonsignificant in terms of disc area, rim volume, cup area, and cup volume (Table 17.16). It should be kept in mind that the cup area has the same value in the megalopapillas as in reoperated congenital glaucomas and that the mean disc area is 3 mm² in both groups. In congenital glaucomas, the axial length of the eye is large, thus enlarging the Elschnig ring and the disc in turn [19].

Table 17.16 Parameters between advanced glaucoma group with megalopapilla

Parameter/group	Normal	Megalopapilla
Disc area	3.07	3.07 NS
Rim area	1.70	1.50*
Rim volume	0.42	0.36 NS
Cup area	1.37	1.57 NS
Cup volume	0.56	0.59 NS
Cup shape M.	−0.14	0.06 ***

NS not significant; * $p<0.01$; *** $p<0.0001$

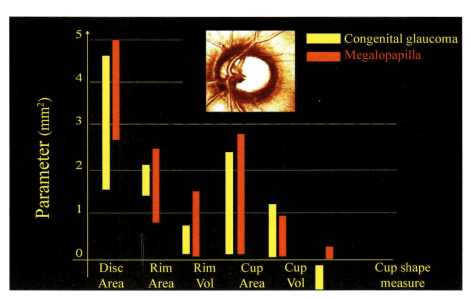

Fig. 17.28 a Comparison between the advanced glaucoma group (with visual field defect in stages III and IV) with megalopapillas. Abscissas show area values in square millimeters. Ordinate: six groups represented to compare disc area, rim area, rim volume, cup area, cup volume, and cup shape measure. **b** Statistic shows highly significant difference in terms of disc area, rim area, and rim volume, while the difference is less significant in terms of cup area and cup volume and no significant difference as regards cup shape measurement

The appearance of megalopapilla in the right eye illustrated by the HRT shown in Fig. 17.29 is almost identical to that of advanced glaucoma (left eye, same figure), thus leading to mistaken diagnosis, since upon observing megalopapilla the ophthalmologist will tend to think of congenital glaucoma first. As seen in the figure, the area of the megalopapilla is even larger.

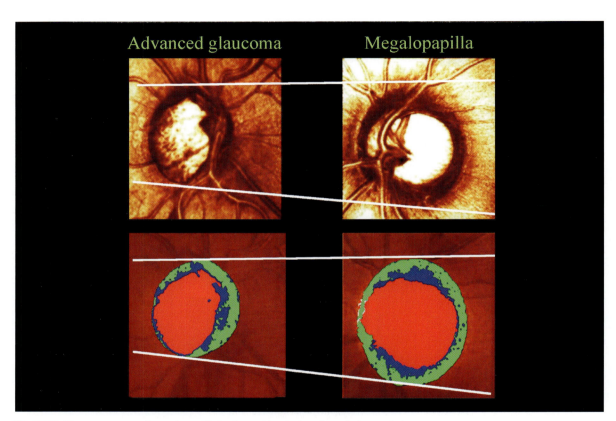

Fig. 17.29 The appearance of megalopapilla is almost identical to that of advanced glaucoma

Figure 17.30 shows three different discs:

a. A normal disc with a very small cup;
b. A glaucomatous disc with a very big cup and a lower number of fibers because many of them have died and disappeared;
c. A megalopapilla without glaucoma. This is a disc with a very big surface compared with Fig. 17.30a, b, and a very big cup. The most remarkable thing is that the number of nerve fibers that we drew in the neuroretinal rim of the megalopapilla is the same as that drawn in the normal disc.

At the bottom of Fig. 17.30a–c there is a comparison between a normal optic disc with and a glaucomatous one (Fig. 17.30a, b). The area of the disc is the same, but the area of the cup is bigger in the glaucomatous disc, and the area of the neuroretinal rim is smaller. In the normal disc (Fig. 17.30a), the slope (the third moment of cup shape measure) is smooth, but in the glaucomatous disc (Fig. 17.30b), the slope is steeper, and in the megalopapilla disc (Fig. 17.30c) the slope is also steeper. The cup shape measure, which represents the slope of the fibers, is positive in glaucomatous discs and megalopapillas, while in normal discs it is negative.

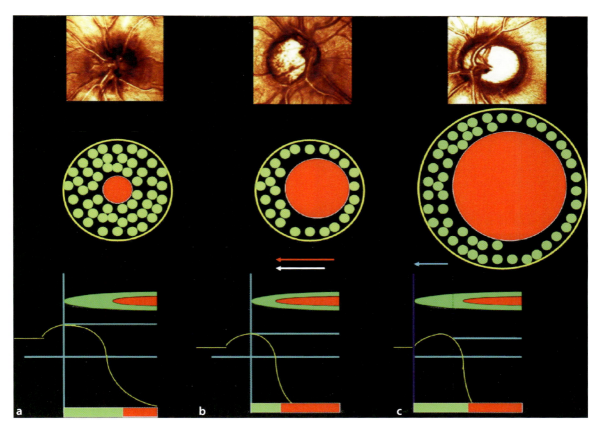

Fig. 17.30a–c Three different discs: **a** a normal disc with a very small cup, **b** a glaucomatous disc with a very big cup and a lower number of fibers because many of them have died and disappeared. **c** Megalopapilla without glaucoma. This is a disc with a very large surface compared with **a** and **b**, and a very big cup. The most remarkable thing is that the number of nerve fibers that we drew in the neuroretinal rim of the megalopapilla is the same as that drawn in the normal disc

Figure 17.31a shows the HRT of the right eye, with the following values: disc area, 3.037 mm²; cup volume, 1.011 mm³; rim volume, 0.227 mm³; cup shape measure, 0.020. The visual fields are also shown.

Figure 17.31b shows the HRT of the left eye, with the following values: disc area, 2.741; cup volume, 0.889 mm³; rim volume, 0.206 mm³; cup shape measure, 0.11. The visual fields are also shown.

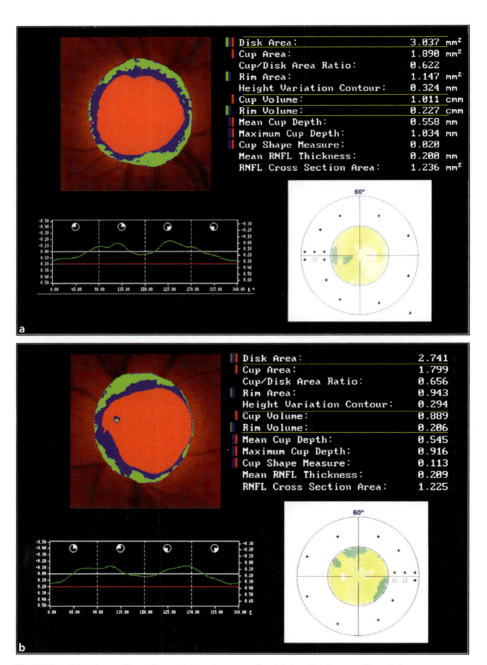

Fig. 17.31 a Megalopapilla and coexisting glaucoma; **b** with localized nerve fiber defects

The HRF of the right eye (Fig. 17.32a) shows that there is no localized perfusion defect but an increased intercapillary space and no ischemic localized zone.

In the megalopapilla case illustrated in Fig. 17.32b, there is no localized fiber layer defect at the inferior temporal area, as clearly seen both in the color and in the black and white photograph where it is signaled by two arrows, one coming from the top and the other one from the bottom. The absence of a notch in this local- ized defect, as observed in this case, is typical of mega- lopapilla. However, had this been a glaucomatous lo- calized defect with no megalopapilla, there would have been a notch. The examination with the HRF in these cases shows a clear localized nerve fiber layer defect with localized reduced perfusion, increased intercapil- lary space (black squares), and an ischemic localized zone (bright).

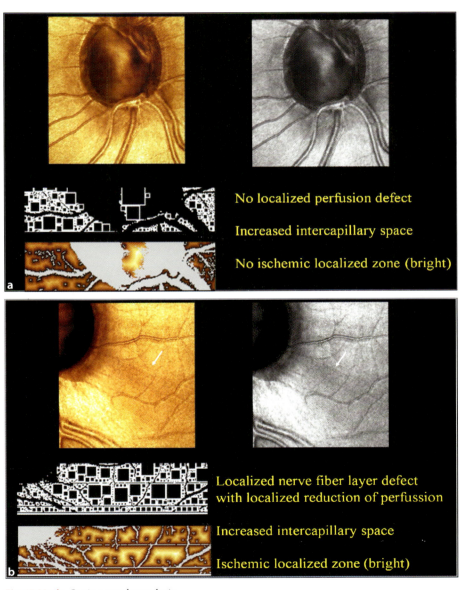

No localized perfusion defect

Increased intercapillary space

No ischemic localized zone (bright)

Localized nerve fiber layer defect with localized reduction of perfussion

Increased intercapillary space

Ischemic localized zone (bright)

Fig. 17.32a,b Optic nerve hypoplasia

Conclusions

Megalopapillas may be confused with advanced glaucomatous optic nerve head damage and other neuropathies, but they are actually a different entity, characterized by a pseudoglaucomatous disc with normal visual field and normal daily pressure curve.

The characteristics shared with glaucoma are increased cup area, cup volume, and cup shape measure. However, disc area, rim volume, and rim area are completely different.

No significant differences were found upon comparing the megalopapilla group with the congenital glaucoma group in all the optic nerve head parameters but one, cup shape measure, which is almost preserved in the congenital glaucoma group. The increase in the total area leads to an increase in the cup area, though with no decrease in the rim area, unlike what occurs in adult glaucoma.

The increase in the papillary border causes the fibers to enter almost vertically, which turns the cup shape measure values positive (pathological values). Megalopapilla is an entity that seems to have been ignored by the literature worldwide, and it is not even named in most well-known ophthalmology textbooks.

Congenital Anomalies of the Optic Nerve

Introduction

It often occurs that ophthalmologists or particularly pediatric ophthalmologists, have to examine newborns, mainly children with low vision due to congenital optic disc anomalies. There are three main references to consult: Orellana and Friedman [29], Apple and Rabb [30], and Brodsky [31].

In the last 10 years, central nervous system (CNS) defects of patients with congenital optic disc anomalies were studied by means of magnetic resonance. In this way, every type of malformation has been associated with malformation defects of the CNS.

Concepts for Diagnosis and Treatment

a. Unilaterality or bilaterality. When the anomalies are unilateral, the child generally presents esotropia during infancy, while bilateral anomalies appear earlier, as the loss of vision is accompanied by nystagmus.
b. In most cases, malformations of the CNS accompany congenital anomalies of the optic nerve. For this reason, magnetic resonance should be performed in all cases.
c. Color vision is usually maintained. This is useful for differential diagnosis because it is the opposite of what occurs in acquired optic neuropathies, where there is a marked dyschromatopsia.
d. Amblyopia usually accompanies these vision-reducing anomalies in the first years of life and during childhood. Therefore, it is important to keep this in mind, as it may be of help to the child with ocular occlusion.

CNS Malformations in Congenital Optic Disc Anomalies

When congenital optic disc anomalies occur with small optic discs, they are accompanied by malformations of the brain hemispheres, pituitary infundibulum, septum pellucidum, and corpus callosum. Those accompanied by large optic nerves, and in morning glory syndrome, present a transsphenoidal basal encephalocele, and in cases of colobomas, they are associated with congenital colobomatous syndromes.

Classification

See Tables 17.17 and 17.18 for a classification of CNS malformations in congenital optic disc anomalies.

Table 17.17 Congenital anomalies of the optic nerve

I	Hypoplasia of the optic nerve	
II	Cupped anomalies	(a) Morning glory syndrome
		(b) Optic disc colobomas
		(c) Peripapillary staphylomas
III	Megalopapilla	
IV	Optic disc pits	
V	Tilted disc syndrome	
VI	Optic nerve dysplasia	
VII	Congenital optic nerve pigmentation	
VIII	Aicardi's syndrome	
IX	Pseudopapilla	

Table 17.18 Central nervous system malformations in congenital anomalies

Small optic nerve		Brain hemispheres
		Pituitary infundibulum
		Septum pellucidum
		Corpus callosum
Large optic nerve	Morning glory syndrome	Transsphenoidal basal encephalocele
	Colomas	Systemic colobomatous syndromes

I. Hypoplasia of the Optic Nerve

Ophthalmoscopy reveals a small gray optic nerve. After studying normality, we have concluded that the mean surface of the optic nerve is 2.05 mm²; if the normal standard deviation is taken into account, micropapilla can be considered to be any optic disc with a surface under 1.59 mm² and megalopapilla, any optic disc over 2.51 mm². Regarding the micropapilla, the values we have found are quite consistent with the values obtained by Jonas: less than 1.40 mm² (mean, 2.89 mm² minus two standard deviations = 1.40 mm²) [30]. It is accompanied by a stained halo, tortuous vessels, and the double ring sign. Pathological anatomy accounts for this sign: the external ring corresponds to the place where the lamina cribrosa is continuous with the sclera and the internal ring is caused by the retina and the pigmentary epithelium abnormally extending over the lamina cribrosa [33, 34]. This double ring sign is exactly the opposite to what is observed in morning glory syndrome (see the following section).

Sometimes, hypoplasia of the optic nerve can be segmentary, superior, or inferior, with the corresponding visual field damage. Otherwise, the visual field is characterized by a general fiber constriction and defects. Hypoplastic optic nerves are accompanied by endocrine alterations, which are also congenital anomalies, such as hypothyroidism and a deficiency of the growth hormone [35–37].

Visual acuity is varied, since it ranges from light perception to 20/20, which calls for refraction correction as soon as possible.

As regards etiology, the literature makes reference to alcohol and drugs during pregnancy, insulin-dependent mothers [38], and the anomalies of the CNS that accompany small optic discs or hypoplastic optic discs, located in the brain at the pituitary infundibulum and at the septum pellucidum [39].

As for pathogenesis, hypoplastic optic discs are gestational lesions in the structures of the middle line of the CNS altering axon migration [39–42] (Fig. 17.33).

Among cupped optic disc congenital anomalies can be mentioned morning glory syndrome, optic disc colobomas, and peripapillary staphylomas.

Congenital ON Anomalies
I Optic Nerve Hypoplasia

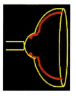

Ophthalmoscopy

- gray and small ON
Jonas < 1.40mm
Sampaolesi < 1.59mm
- Stained hale
- double ring sign
- tortuous vessels

Pathol. Anatomy

- normal external ring
- internal ring: abnormal extension R. y E.P. on the lamina cribrosa (opposite to Morning Glory)

V.A.: 20/20-light perception, refraction should be corrected!

V.F.: generalized constriction and fiber defects

Etology: Alcohol, Drugs, Insulin-Dependant Mother, Endocron Anomalies: Hypothiroidism

Pathogenesis: Gestational injuries in the structures of the mid line of the CNS altering axon migration

Segmentary Hypoplasias: Superior or inferior

Fig. 17.33 Optic nerve hypoplasia

II. Cupped Anomalies

IIa. Morning Glory Syndrome

Morning glory syndrome (MGS) is a congenital altera-tion of the eyeball manifested as a posterior mushroom-shaped cup incorporating the optic disc. It can be unilat-eral or bilateral. Visual acuity is almost always reduced, ranging from finger counting to 10/100, although cases with a visual acuity of 20/20 have been reported. It is more frequent in women. It was described for the first time by Graether in 1963 [43]; then Kindler [44] called it morning glory syndrome because of its resemblance to a violet bell-shaped flower that grows wild. Ophthal-moscopic examinations reveal a large orange or pink optic nerve with a mushroom-shaped cupping, sur-rounded in its anterior end by a thick pigmentary halo. Numerous radial vessels, more numerous than normal, where it is difficult to distinguish vessels from arter-ies, emerge from it. In the central part, there is a white, slightly prominent area that looks like a veil, which is glial tissue; sometimes this malformation involves the macula and in this case it is known as macular capture [45, 46]. In some cases, retinal detachment occurs, be-cause of small holes near the optic nerve (in 26%–38% of cases, as reported by the literature [47, 48]). In other cases, there is a communication between the vitreous body and the subarachnoid space [49].

Ultrasonography shows this syndrome as a funnel in the posterior part of the eyeball that can sometimes be qualified, and in this case it is also visible with com-puterized tomography of the orbit.

In the retinograph of MGS, the posterior cup has the appearance of a mushroom with a white veil in the cen-tral area corresponding to glial tissue. A dark adjacent area surrounded by choroidal depigmentation shows a macular sequestration with a small coloboma.

In a patient with unilateral MGS, the topographical image of confocal tomography shows protrusion of the ring as a very dark area (Fig. 17.34) and a pronounced depression in a horizontal section between the funnel area and the retina surrounding it.

Another patient had MGS in the right eye and a dou-ble optic nerve in the left eye, as described by Bonamour et al. [50], with a superior optic disc, a smaller one be-neath this one, and below it, a choroidal coloboma.

In 1963, Graether [43] was the first to describe a transient amaurosis with venous dilatation in MGS and in 1994, Ebner et al. described a transient amaurosis with arteriolar contraction depending on the sight po-sition [51].

In Brodsky's 1994 article [31], the author refers to mid-facial anomalies (hypotelorism, depressed nose, palpebral alterations) as other manifestations of this syndrome. Figure 17.35 describes the main features of MGS.

MGS manifests in the CNS as a transsphenoidal form of basal encephalocele for which surgery is con-traindicated, and rarely as absence of chiasma, agen-esis of the corpus callosum, and dilatation of the lateral ventricles. It is sometimes also accompanied by a her-niation of the hypothalamic structures (palate clefts, bone defects in the base of the skull). Brodsky also re-ports that sometimes there is a rhinorrhea attributable to basal obstruction caused by a polyp, the extraction of which could be lethal. An interesting paper by an Argentine author, Dr. Alezzandrini, describes RFG al-terations in detail [52].

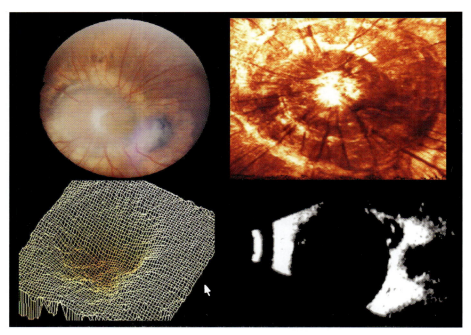

Fig. 17.34 Cupped optic nerve congenital anomalies. Morning glory syndrome

Cupped optic nerve congenital anomalies
IIa Morning Glory

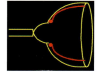

- Handmann 1929, Kindler 1970
- Very big, orange and pink
- Surrounded by a choroid-retinal pigment hale
- Central fungiform cupping (ultrasonography, A.C.T.)
- Increased number of vessels and difficult to distinguish veins from arteries
- White central veil (glia)
- Macular capture/retinal detachment, small holes near the ON
- Communication between vitreous body and subarachnoid space

- Graether (1963):

  Transient amauosis with venous dilatation

- Ebner, Sampaolesi J.R. (1994):

  Transient amauosis with arteriole contraction according to sight position

Fig. 17.35 Morning glory syndrome

IIb. Optic Disc Colobomas

Ocular manifestations can show an abnormal coaptation of the proximal area of the optic vesicle slit. The optic disc is enlarged, with sharp borders and a bright white color with a deep cup. The cup is decentered toward the bottom, making the neuroretinal rim disappear there. This defect generally presents a choroidal coloboma at the deepest part of the optic disc, and it is sometimes associated with a coloboma of the iris.

Ultrasonography and computerized tomography show a posterior pole cup of the eye as in morning glory syndrome and, contrary to this syndrome, it is generally bilateral.

Visual acuity depends on the integrity of the papillomacular bundle. The retinal vessels are normal. They are sometimes accompanied by a macular serous detachment.

Systemic manifestations include optic disc colobomas may be accompanied by Charge's syndrome [53, 54], Walker-Warburg's syndrome [55], Aicardi's syndrome [56, 57], or the linear Nevus sebaceous syndrome [58]. Sometimes the coloboma has an atypical connection with an orbital cyst [59].

In optic disc colobomas, as already said, a choroidal coloboma equal or larger in size than the optic disc in its inferior part is usually present. Sometimes there is no optic disc coloboma but this small inferior coloboma is present. One of these cases is shown on the vertical section of both depressions at the bottom of the optic disc, as well as on a tridimensional representation, the measurement of the optic disc area and of the area of the coloboma (Fig. 17.36). The main features are described in Fig. 17.37.

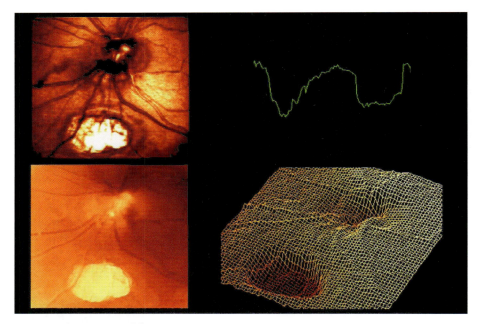

Fig. 17.36 Optic nerve colobomas

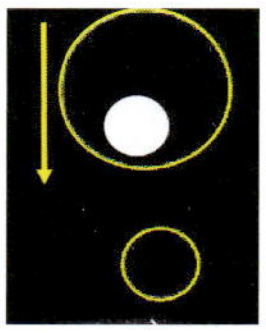

Cupped optic nerve congenital anomalies

IIb Optic nerve colobomas

Ocular Manifestations

- abnormal coaptation of the proximal part, optic slit
- Bib ON, definite edges, white, deep cupping
- Cup decentered towards the inferior part
- Absent NNR at the inferior part
- Inferior extension: "Chorodial Coloboma"and/or iris coloboma
- Posterior pole cuppng (=M.Glory), Ultrasonography, A.C.T.
- Bilateral (≠M. Glory)
- The V.A. depends on the integrity of the papillo-marcular bundle
- Serous macular detachment/Normal retinal vessels

Systemic anomalies

- Charge Syndrome (Walker-Warburg Syndrome)/Goltz focal dermal hypoplasia/ Aicardi Syndrome/Goldenhar Syndrome/Linear sebaceous nervus Syndrome/ Conection with an orbital cyst

Fig. 17.37 Optic nerve colobomas

IIc. Peripapillary Staphyloma

This is a very infrequent condition, which is unilateral and is manifested by a deep cup surrounding the optic disc, especially in its inferior part. The cup is surrounded by a pigmentary halo and, conversely to what occurs in morning glory syndrome, there is no central glial white veil. The visual acuity may be normal or reduced, and in the visual field there is a centrocecal scotoma. It is often associated with a coloboma of the iris, the retina, and the ciliary body, and only very rarely does a basal encephalocele appear, as a manifestation of the CNS [60].

In a highly myopic case combined with glaucoma, we have observed a staphylomatous depression around the optic disc in the center of which there was a flat glaucomatous optic disc. Figure 17.38 shows the pertinent confocal tomographies. Figure 17.39 shows the main characteristics.

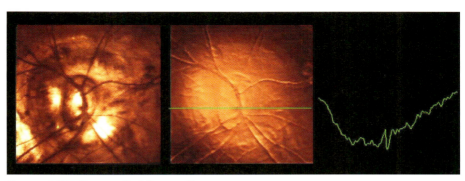

Cupped ON Congenital Anomalies

IIc   Peripapillary Staphyloma

Ophthalmoscopy:

- Deep cupping sumunding the ON (specially inferior) Surrounded by a pigment hale, (= M./Glory). There is no central glical white veil.
  Unfrequent
  Unilateral

Visul acuity:

- Very reduced, though normal sometimes
- Usually associated with iris, retinal and ciliary body colobomas

Systemic Manifestations:

- Unfrequent basal encephalocele

Fig. 17.38 Peripapillary staphyloma

III. Megalopapilla

When the optic disc surface is greater than 2.5 mm², megalopapilla is diagnosed. There are two types of megalopapilla:

1. Type I: the optic disc bears a normal configuration and the condition is bilateral. The cup/disc ratio is high, which must be kept in mind when making the differential diagnosis with low-tension glaucoma (cup/disc ratio: mean, 0.16 + 2 SD = 0.6 mm maximum). The whole optic disc surface is pale, and the cup is either round or oval.
2. Type II: this is characterized by a cup decentered toward the top of the optic disc, i.e., the contrary to what occurs in optic nerve colobomas, where the cup is decentered toward the bottom. The cilioreti-nal arteries are more common in megalopapilla [61]. The neuroretinal rim is reduced or has almost completely disappeared in the top part. It usually occurs unilaterally. Many megalopapillas appear in normal subjects with a normal visual field. It is one of the wide range of optic discs [62].

It should be kept in mind that megalopapilla may develop in congenital glaucomas, mainly in reoperated cases. This megalopapilla is acquired because as the sclera distends, with the consequent axial length and ocular volume increase, the Elschnig ring enlarges, and therefore so does the whole optic disc surface. Figure 17.38 shows the images, and their characteristics are shown in Fig. 17.40.

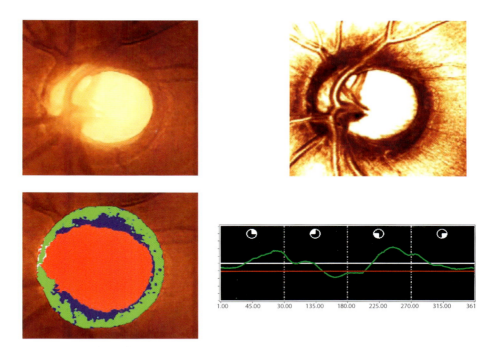

Fig. 17.39 Megalopapilla

Optic nerve congenital anomalies
III Megalopapilla

Type I:

- Surface > 2.5mm^2
- Normal configuration/higher cup/disc ratio
- Pale NRR
- Bilateral

Type II:

- Surface > 2.5mm^2
- Superior decentered cupping
- Bigger NNR at the iferior part
- Unilateral

It occurs in normal subjects with normal V.F. "it is just one of a wide range of optic discs"

Fig. 17.40 Megalopapilla

IV. Optic Disc Pits

On ophthalmoscopy, the optic disc manifests as a round or oval, gray, white, or yellow depression, usually located in the temporal area. It is accompanied by peripapillary pigmentary changes and in 50% of cases, one or two cilioretinal arteries come from the pit [63]. It is generally unilateral.

The visual field defects correlate with the position of the pit, depending on the fibers crossing the area. There is a blind spot enlargement and arcuate scotomas are the most common defects. We have sometimes found central scotomas.

As for the retina, in 25%–75% of cases macular serous edema [64, 65] leading to macular detachment occurs. Lincoff et al. [66] have studied this subject in depth and proved that the retinal separation is similar to a retinoschisis and that a retinal hole of the external layers of the macula leading to a central scotoma may develop. The retina around the macular hole is detached. Gas injections and laser photocoagulation are recommended in these cases.

Retinofluoresceinography shows that an early hypofluorescence and a late hyperfluorescence of the pit usually take place. There is no fluorescein passage to the vitreous or to the macula.

The pathological anatomy reveals that the dysplastic retina is herniated inside a pocket or cavity that extends toward the back, frequently inside the subarachnoid space through a defect of the lamina cribrosa [67, 68] (Figs. 17.41, 17.42).

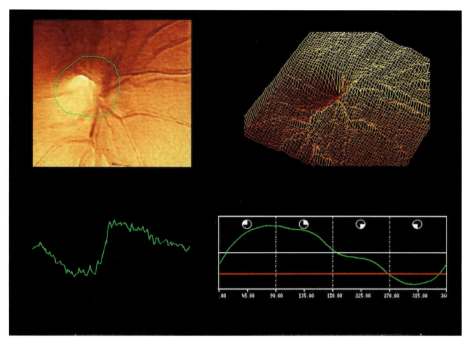

Fig. 17.41 Optic disc pits

Optic nerve congenital anomalies
IV   Optic disc pits

Ophthalmoscopy
- Round or oval depression, grey, white or yellow
- Temporal location
- Peripapillary pigmentary changes
- One or two cilioretinal arteries start at the pits
- Genarally unilateral, (15% bilateral)

Visual Field
- The defects correlatewith the pits position
- Arcuate scotoma, central scotoma

Retinal detachment
- The macular serous detachment is related to the pit
- Macular hole, sometimes, with a retinal detachment surrounding it

R.F.G.
- Early hypofluorescence and late pits hyperfluorescence

Pathological anatomy
- The retina extends over the subarachnoid space through a defect of the lamina cribrosa.
  Posterior wall at different levels.

Fig. 17.42 Optic disc pits

V. Tilted Disc Syndrome

Tilted disc syndrome is a bilateral condition where the superior temporal part of the optic nerve is elevated and the inferior nasal part is shifted in a posterior direction. This gives the optic disc an oval shape with its greater axis in an oblique position.

On ophthalmoscopy, the optic disc has its greater axis in an oblique position. There is a situs inversus of the optic disc vessels with an inferonasal congenital conus and retinal epithelium and choroid thinning in the inferonasal area that may be accompanied by inferonasal albinism.

The visual field presents a bitemporal hemianopsia or a superior quadrantanopsia. This visual field defect is a refractive scotoma secondary to a localized regional myopia in the inferotemporal retina. If a −4-D lens is used, the scotoma disappears and in this way its refractive nature is confirmed. Consequently, there is a myopic astigmatism with the greater axis parallel to the ectasia [69]. In my opinion, tilted optic disc syndrome is related to nasal ectasia of the fundus. This syndrome was described by Riise [70]. See the article by Argento and Mayorga [71] (Figs. 17.43, 17.44).

VI. Optic Nerve Dysplasia

VII. Congenital Optic Nerve Pigmentation

This is gray in albinism due to late myelinization.

VIII. Aicardi Syndrome

There is depigmented lacunae around the optic disc with pathological anatomy: lack of choroid and of pigmentary epithelium in the lacunae. Sometimes, congenital optic disc alteration. Lethal in males.

Systemic Manifestation (CNS)
Corpus Callosum Agenesia

Other ocular manifestations include microphthalmos, retrobulbar cyst, pseudoglioma, bifid spine, detachment of the macular retina, pupillary membrane, iris synechiae, and iris colobomas.

Other general manifestations include spina bifida; scoliosis, microcephalia, muscular hypotonia, and mental retardation.

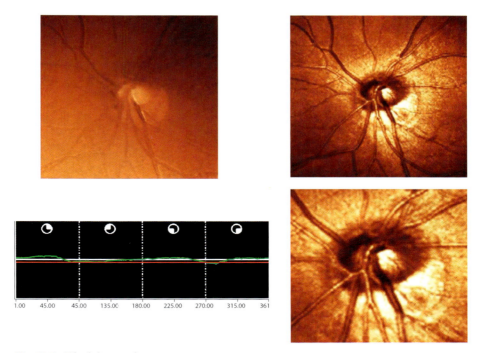

Fig. 17.43 Tilted disc syndrome

Optic nerve congenital anomalies
V Tilted disc syndrome

Ophthalmoscopy
- Superonasal overelevated ON
- Inferonasal ON with posterior displacement
- Oblique major axis
- Situs Inversus of the papillary vessels
- Congenital inferonasal conus
- Retinal epithelium and inferonasal choroid thinning
- Inferonasal albinism

Visual Vfield
- Bitemporal hemianopsia or superior quadrantopsia. It does not respect the mid line. This defect is a refractive scotoma secondary to a regional myopia localized at the inferotemporal retina. It disappear with a–4D–lens.
- The bitemporal hemioanopsia bitemporal is related to the fundus nasal ectasia.

Refraction
- Myopic astigmatism, major axis parallel to the fundus inferior and to the optic nerve ectasia

Fig. 17.44 Tilted disc syndrome

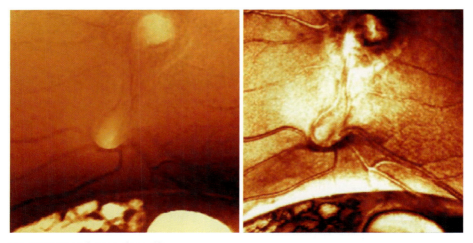

Fig. 17.45 Vascular pseudopapilla

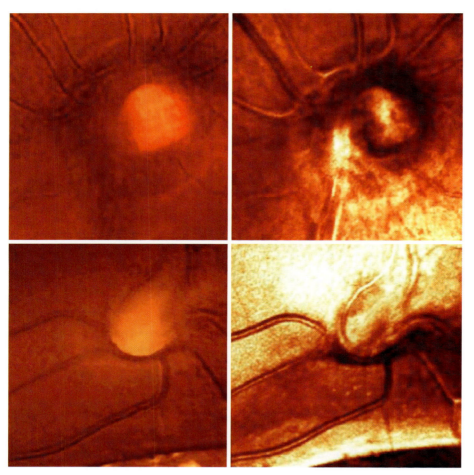

Fig. 17.46 Pseudopapilla. Both discs are displayed separately; the real optic disc is at the *top* of the image and pseudopapilla is at the *bottom*

IX. Pseudopapilla

A 20-degree tomography of pseudopapilla is shown in Fig. 17.45, which contains both discs (the papilla and the pseudopapilla) [71]. In Fig. 17.46 both discs are displayed separately, in two 10-degree field examinations (the real optic disc is at the top of the image and pseudopapilla is at the bottom). The main features of pseudopapilla are described in Fig. 17.47.

IX   Pseudopapilla

Hervouet, 1958: Hypothesis: It is feasible for a double optic nerve to develop if there is a doubling of the optical pediculum, with the dichotomization of the hyaloid artery.

Ocular Manifestations

There are 2 clinico-ophthalmoscopic forms:

a) Optic discs joined by the vertical meridian: where the supernumeric optic disc joins the inferior part of the main optic disc Vascularisation is shared

b) Optic disc doubling: the requuirements are:
   - existence of a double optic contour
   - existence of double vascularization of a central type
   - existence of two joined discs without pigmentary elements between them [43]

c) Vascular pseudopapilla: There is no actual second optic disc, but just a colobomatous scar through which retinal veins enter and choroidal arteries emerge.*

Fig. 17.47 Pseudopapilla

Clinical Cases

Case 1:
Congenital Glaucoma Type I
17 years of follow up

The clinical doctor told the parents to wait until the age of 8 months in order to unblock the lacrimal passages. The pediatric specialist suspected glaucoma and sent him to the ophthalmologist.

We were able to follow up this male patient for 17 years after surgery with six visual field examinations, eight confocal tomographies of the optic nerve, six daily pressure curves, and one HRF. His vision is 20/25 in the operated eye, and his visual field is normal with Octopus 101 and with doubling frequency technology. He has excellent grades in high school and is an outstanding soccer player.

After trabeculotomies (Chap. 16), three goniosynechiae appeared: a central one, where the trabeculotome enters, and two peripheral goniosynechiae through which it exits to the anterior chamber. The open Schlemm canal at each side of this with pigment can be seen on the goniophotograph, as well as the central goniosynechia. In the left part, the Descemet membrane can be seen detached by the trabeculotome.

That is, in this case I kept the trabeculotome very close to the cornea and detached the Descemet membrane (Figs. 17.48, 17.49, 17.50, 17.51, 17.52, Table 17.19).

	Right eye	Left eye
1988		
Axial length	22.06 mm	25.98 mm
IOP	10 mmHg	20 mmHg
Corneal diameter	13 mm	14.5 mm
Chamber angle	Normal	Type I
Surgery 1988	–	Trabeculotomy
2005		
Axial length	23.81 mm	24.85 mm
Visual acuity	−0.50 180° = 20/20	−0.50 180° = 20/20
IOP	16 mmHg	13 mmHg
Daily pressure curve	Normal	Normal
Optic nerve (HRT)	Normal	Normal

Table 17.19 Case 1. HRT 2005

Left eye		Right eye	
Parameters	Global	Parameters	Global
Disc area (mm²)	2.276	Disc area (mm²)	3.029
Cup area (mm²)	0.453	Cup area (mm²)	0.660
Rim area	1.823	Rim area	2.370
Cup/disc area ratio	0.199	Cup/disc area ratio	0.218
Rim/disc area ratio	0.801	Rim/disc area ratio	0.782
Cup volume (mm³)	0.084	Cup volume (mm³)	0.189
Rim volume (mm³)	0.272	Rim volume (mm³)	0.520
Mean cup depth (mm)	0.159	Mean cup depth (mm)	0.240
Maximum cup depth (mm)	0.606	Maximum cup depth (mm)	0.784
Height variation contour (mm)	0.212	Height variation contour (mm)	0.331
Cup shape measure	−0.311	Cup shape measure	0.285
Mean RNFL thickness (mm)	0.140	Mean RNFL thickness (mm)	0.207
RNFL cross-sectional area (mm²)	0.749	RNFL cross-sectional area (mm²)	1.278

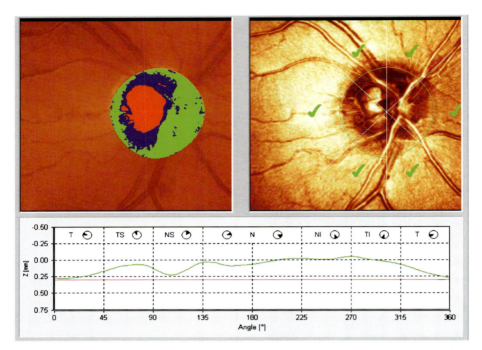

Fig. 17.48 HRT of the right eye

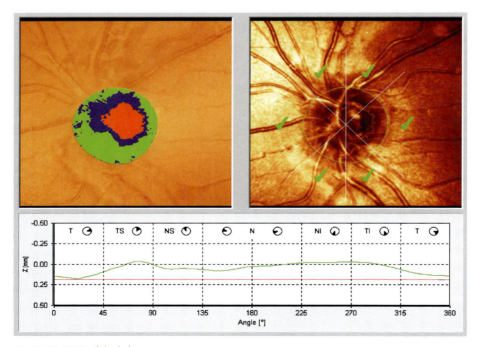

Fig. 17.49 HRT of the left eye

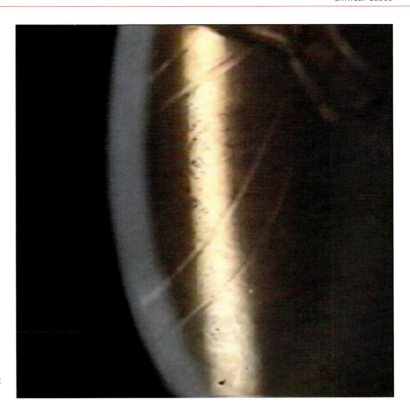

Fig. 17.50 Peripheral ruptures of Descemet membrane (Haab striae)

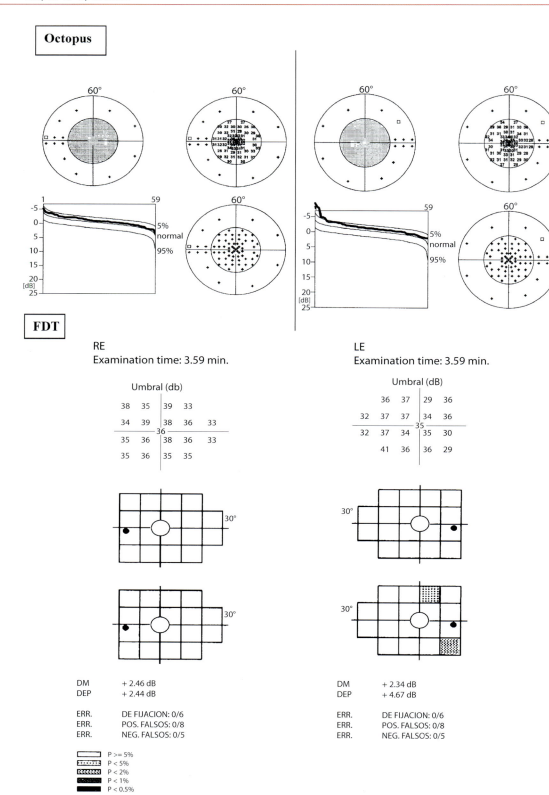

Fig. 17.51 Visual field with Octopus in FDT of right and left eyes

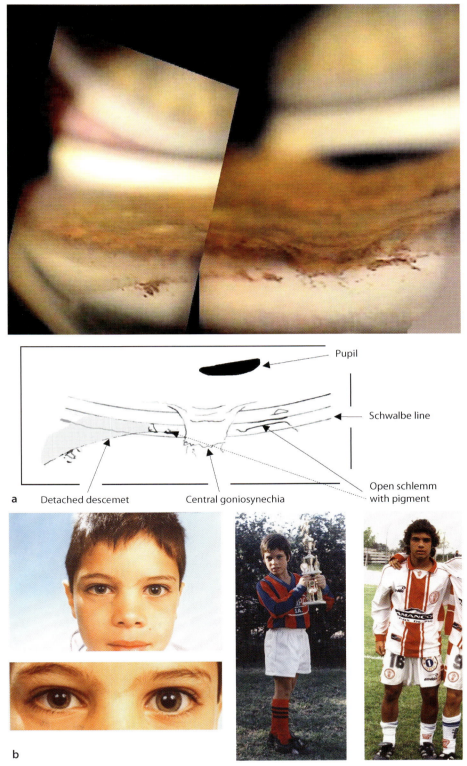

Pupil

Schwalbe line

a   Detached descemet   Central goniosynechia

Open schlemm
with pigment

b

Fig. 17.52 **a** Goniophotograph and drawing after surgery. **b** Photograph of the eyes of the patient and the same patient as a soccer player

Case 2:
Congenital Glaucoma Type I (Unilateral)
35 years of follow up

This child was treated until 5 months for dacryocystitis. At 10 months, the right eye was seen to be much larger and 5 days later corneal edema appeared in this eye. Nonetheless, it was not operated until the age of 1 year and 8 months (Figs. 17.53, 17.54, 17.55, 17.56, 17.57, 17.58).

The fact that the parents waited 1 year and 3 months to decide to operate the right eye and that the glaucoma in the left eye appeared later gave rise in the first eye to glaucoma alterations of the optic nerve and the visual field and a reduction in visual acuity of 20/80.

	Right eye	Left eye
1970		
Axial length	24.32 mm	22.6 mm
IOP	25 mmHg	9 mmHg
Corneal diameter	13.5 mm	11.5 mm
Chamber angle[a]	Type I	Normal
Surgery 1970	Trabeculotomy	–
2005	(35 years later)	
Axial length	25.4 mm	24.46 mm
Visual acuity	Sph + 2, Cil. +1.50 140° = 20/80	20/20
Optic nerve (HRT)	Phase II	Normal
Visual field		
Octopus 101 G2	Stage 2	Normal
FDT	Stage 3	Normal
IOP	16 mmHg	13 mmHg
DPC	Normal	Normal

[a]Persistence of pathological mesodermal remains and Barkan's membrane. The ciliary body band is visible

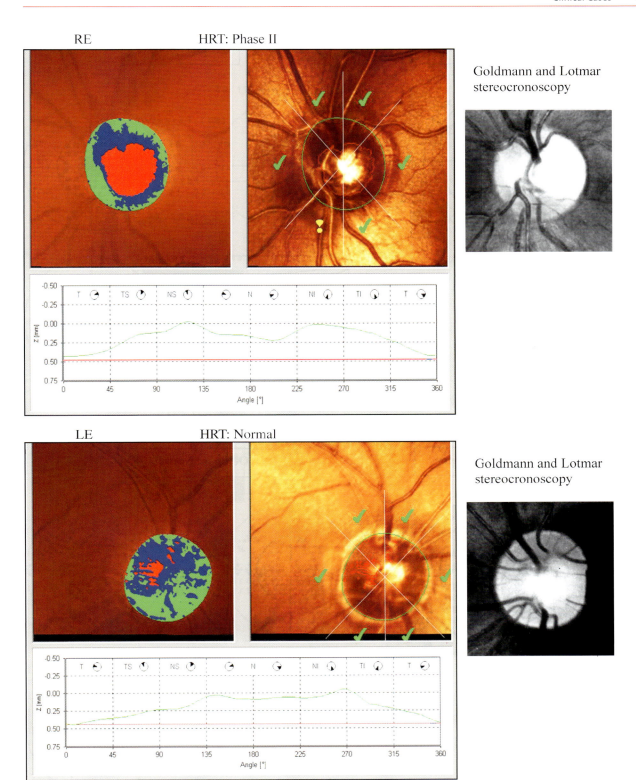

Fig. 17.53 HRT right and left eye, phase II in Goldmann stereochronoscopy

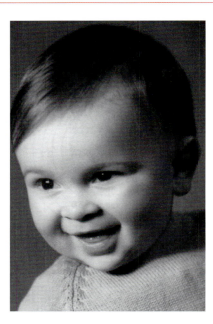

Fig. 17.57 A picture of the patient as a baby

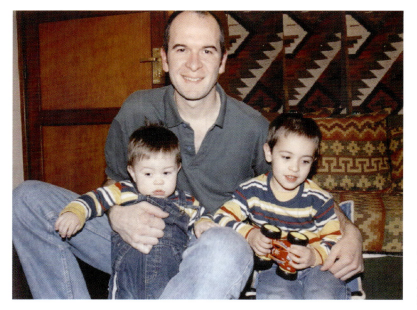

Fig. 17.58 The same patient 35 years later with his two normal children. The patient has become an engineer in computer systems

RE   HRT: Phase II

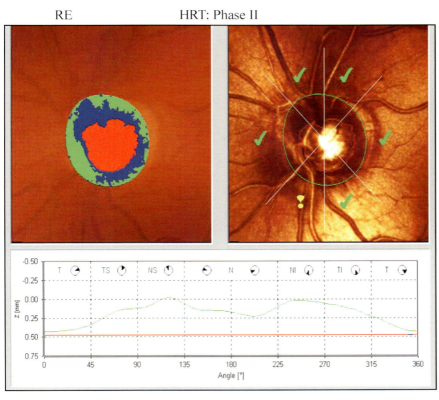

Goldmann and Lotmar
stereocronoscopy

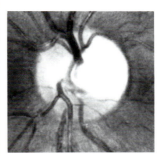

LE   HRT: Normal

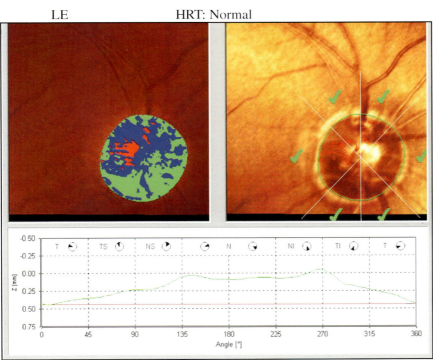

Goldmann and Lotmar
stereocronoscopy

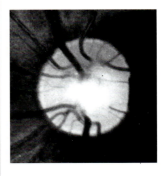

Fig. 17.53 HRT right and left eye, phase II in Goldmann stereochronoscopy

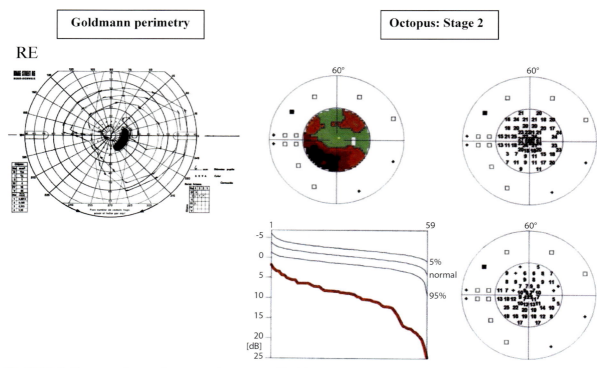

Fig. 17.54 Goldmann perimetry. Octopus perimetry, stage II, right eye

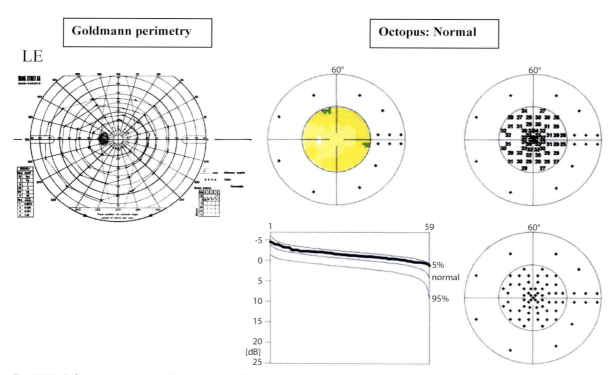

Fig. 17.55 Golmann perimetry in Octopus, normal, left eye

FDT: 09/14/2006:   RE: Stage 3

LE: Normal

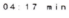

04:17 min

Umbral (dB)

```
    20   18  | 18   13
 16   24   24 | 19   24
 ---------23--------
    0   12   21 | 22   18
       0    4 | 14    5
```

Desviación total

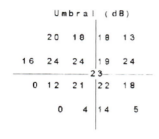

30°

Desviación del modelo

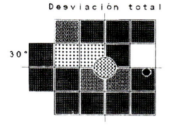

30°

```
  ▮    -11,36 dB  P  <  0,5%
 ·EP   +9,61 dB   P  <  1%

ERR. DE FIJACION:    0/6
ERR. POS. FALSOS:    0/8
ERR. NEG. FALSOS:    1/5
```

04:32 min

Umbral (dB)

```
    23   30  |28   23
 30   31  |28   28   22
 ---------29--------
 30   31  |24   24   22
 29   31  |31   30
```

Desviación total

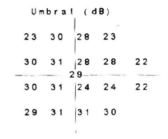

30°

Desviación del modelo

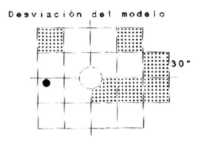

30°

```
 ▮M    -1,97 dB
 ;EP   +4,12 dB

ERR. DE FIJACION:    0/6
ERR. POS. FALSOS:    0/8
ERR. NEG. FALSOS:    0/5
```

Símbolos de probabilidad
```
  □       P  >=  5%
  ▦       P  <  5%
  ▨       P  <  2%
  ▩       P  <  1%
  ■       P  <  0,5%
```

Fig. 17.56 Double-frequency perimetry, right eye, stage III; left eye normal

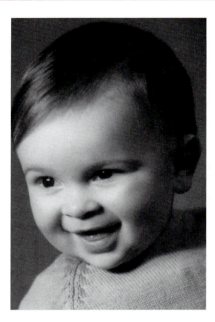

Fig. 17.57 A picture of the patient as a baby

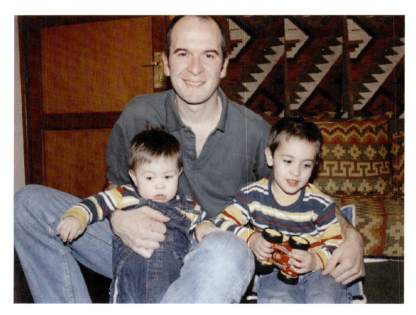

Fig. 17.58 The same patient 35 years later with his two normal children. The patient has become an engineer in computer systems

Case 3:
Congenital glaucoma Type I (Unilateral)
35 years of follow up

Family history: This female child, aged 8 months, was treated until 5 months of age for conjunctivitis. At 2 weeks, the left eye was seen to be much larger. She was examined under general anesthesia (by an another colleague) and not operated. Surgery was done at the age of 8 months. She was followed up for 25 years (Figs. 17.59, 17.60).

This case is very useful because it shows several things:

1. That one frequent error of the pediatrician is to treat a glaucoma as conjunctivitis.
2. One error of the ophthalmologist is to make an examination with general anesthetic and think that it is a case of normal child, because they do not know the normal values of ocular pressure and axial length.
3. Congenital glaucoma is like acute glaucoma. As Schaeffer said, when it is diagnosed under general anaesthetic for the exam, it should be operated immediately.
4. The 6-month delay produces a small lesion in the optic nerve that translates into a visual acuity of 0.9 20/60 in the operated eye vs 1.0 20/20 in the normal eye.
5. Normal frequency doubling perimetry and even more the Pulsar reveal a Bjerrum scotoma in the operated eye (Fig. 17.60).

	Right eye	Left eye
IOP	8 mmHg	**20 mmHg**
Axial length	20.32 mm	**22.61 mm**
Normal length	20 mm	20 mm
Chamber angle	Normal	**Type I**
Corneal diameter	11.75 mm	**12.75 mm**
Surgery (04/82)	–	**Trabeculotomy**
IOP	8 mmHg	8 mmHg
		Squint, left eye, amblyopia treatment
Visual acuity (1988)	20/25	20/60
Visual acuity (1989)	20/25	20/30 sph: −1.25, cil: −0.50 0°
Visual acuity (2001)	20/20	20/40 sph: −1.75, cil: −0.75 0°
Visual acuity (2007)	20/20	20/25 sph: −1.50, cil: −0.50 160°
Optic nerve (1996)		Lotmar and Goldman stereochronoscopy

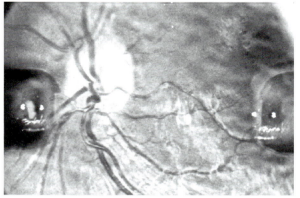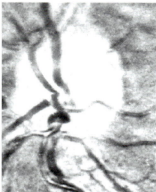

Fig. 17.59 Lotmar and Goldmann stereochronoscopy

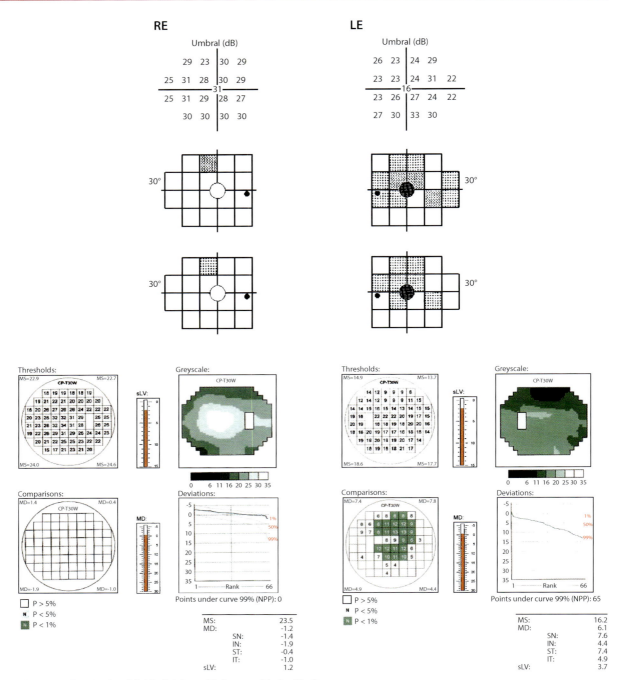

Fig. 17.60 Case 3, visual field of right and left eyes with double-frequency

Case 4:
Congenital Glaucoma Type I (Bilateral)
Follow up of 36 years

This female child was 2 months, 20 days old at consultation. When she was 8 days old, the mother noticed that the right eye was larger than the left eye. The next day, the right eye had edema. Two months later at a routine follow-up anesthesia, the intraocular pressure in the right eye was 10 mmHg and in the left eye 28 mmHg.

This patient is now a prima ballerina in the Colón Theater in Buenos Aires (Figs. 17.61, 17.62, 17.63).

	Right eye	Left eye
IOP (06/71)	30 mmHg	10 mmHg
Axial length	23 mm	19 mm
Chamber angle	Type I	–
Corneal diameter	12.5 mm	12 mm
Surgery (06/71)	Trabeculotomy	
IOP (16/08/71)	10 mmHg	28 mmHg
Axial length	23 mm	23 mm
Surgery		Trabeculotomy
IOP (1983)	12 mmHg	12 mmHg
Echometry	23.37 mm	23.37 mm
Optic nerve stereochronoscopy (Lotmar and Goldmann)		
IOP (2007)	14 mmHg	13 mmHg
Echometry	22.49 mm	22.86 mm
Visual acuity	20/20	20/20
Optic nerve	Normal	Normal

RE HRT 2007

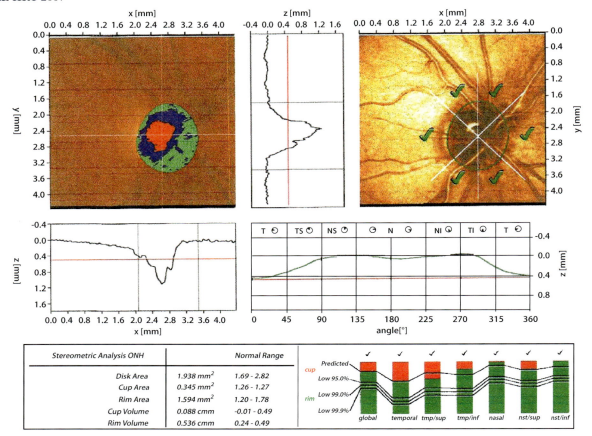

Stereometric Analysis ONH		Normal Range
Disk Area	1.938 mm²	1.69 - 2.82
Cup Area	0.345 mm²	1.26 - 1.27
Rim Area	1.594 mm²	1.20 - 1.78
Cup Volume	0.088 cmm	-0.01 - 0.49
Rim Volume	0.536 cmm	0.24 - 0.49

a

Fig. 17.61 a Right eye, HRT (*b see next page*)

LE HRT 2007

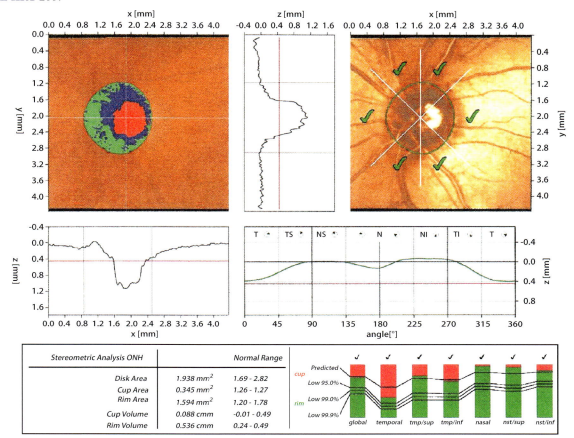

Stereometric Analysis ONH		Normal Range
Disk Area	1.938 mm²	1.69 - 2.82
Cup Area	0.345 mm²	1.26 - 1.27
Rim Area	1.594 mm²	1.20 - 1.78
Cup Volume	0.088 cmm	-0.01 - 0.49
Rim Volume	0.536 cmm	0.24 - 0.49

b

Fig. 17.61 (*continued*) **b** left eye, HRT 36 years after surgery

RE Octopus   Double Frequency

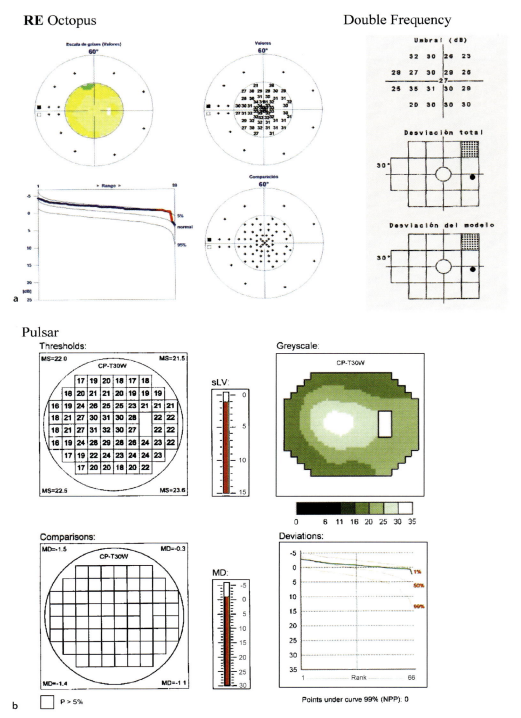

Fig. 17.62 a Right eye Octopus, **b** right eye Pulsar (*c,d see next page*)

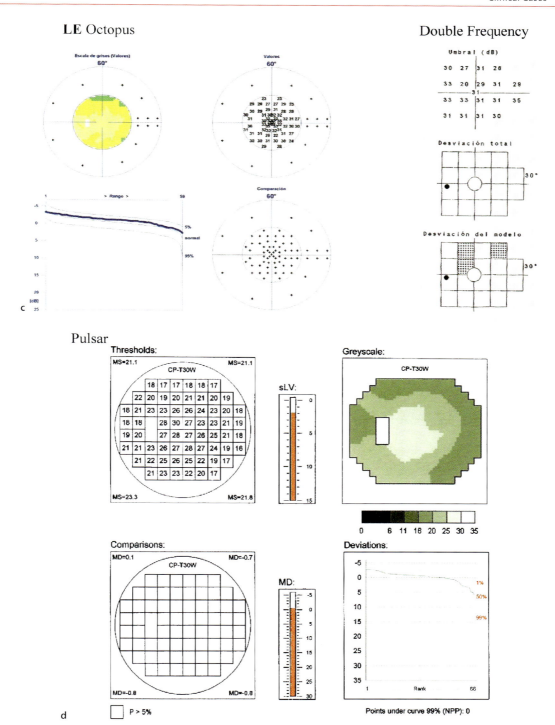

Fig. 17.62 (*continued*) **c** left eye Octopus, **d** left eye Pulsar

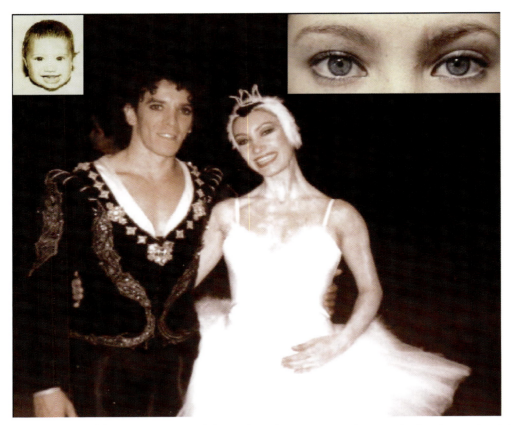

Fig. 17.63 In the *left* corner, patient as a baby. In the *right* corner, patient's eyes in 2007 and as a prima ballerina in the Colon Theater

Case 5:
Congenital Glaucoma Type I (Bilateral)
27 years of follow up

This is the second case of all the congenital glaucomas I have seen that also presented congenital glaucoma first in the left eye, while the right eye had a normal echometry and no symptoms. The left eye had three Haab lines just around the pupil. The chamber angle in the left eye was type I and trabeculotomy was performed. At the first postsurgical examination at 4 months of age, the echometry in the left eye decreased from 21.15 mm to 20.53 mm (due to surgery), while the right eye had an intraocular pressure of 10 mmHg, the echometry had increased from 20.19 to 21.79 mm.

When the patient was 7 months old, the echometry in the left eye remained 20.19 mm, whereas in the right eye was 22.20 mm and the intraocular pressure was 26 mmHg. Trabeculotomy was performed in the right eye as well.

The patient was followed up for 27 years. His visual acuity in the right eye is 20/20 and in the left eye is 20/30 (the lower visual acuity is due to the Haab lines in the cornea). The visual fields and the confocal tomographies are normal in both eyes, with binocular vision.

He is now a medical doctor specialized in neurology (Figs. 17.64, 17.65, 17.66, 17.67).

	Right eye	Left eye
1978		
Axial length	20 mm	21mm
IOP	10 mmHg	19 mmHg
Corneal diameter	12 mm	12.5 mm
Chamber angle	Normal	Type I
Surgery		Trabeculotomy at 3 months
Axial length	4 months: 21.44	20.53
	7 months: 22.20	20.29
IOP	26 mmHg	20 mmHg
Diagnosis	Congenital glaucoma begins at 7 months of age	
Surgery	Trabeculotomy at 7 months	
2005		
Axial length	22.97mm	22.20mm
Visual acuity	Sph −1.25, cil −1.25 5° = 20/20	Sph +1, cil −1.25 125° = 20/25
IOP	14 mmHg	15 mmHg
DPC	Normal	Normal
Optic nerve (HRT)	Normal	Normal
Visual field		
Octopus 101G2	Normal	Stage I
FDT	Normal	Stage I

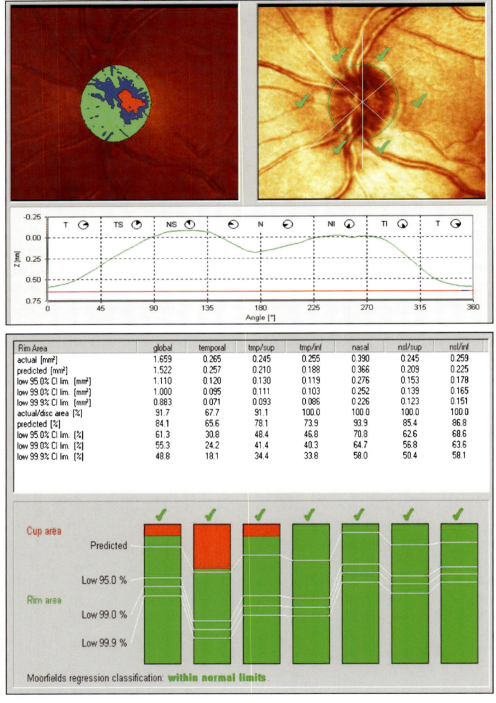

Rim Area	global	temporal	tmp/sup	tmp/inf	nasal	nsl/sup	nsl/inf
actual [mm²]	1.659	0.265	0.245	0.255	0.390	0.245	0.259
predicted [mm²]	1.522	0.257	0.210	0.188	0.366	0.209	0.225
low 95.0% CI lim. [mm²]	1.110	0.120	0.130	0.119	0.276	0.153	0.178
low 99.0% CI lim. [mm²]	1.000	0.095	0.111	0.103	0.252	0.139	0.165
low 99.9% CI lim. [mm²]	0.883	0.071	0.093	0.086	0.226	0.123	0.151
actual/disc area [%]	91.7	67.7	91.1	100.0	100.0	100.0	100.0
predicted [%]	84.1	65.6	78.1	73.9	93.9	85.4	86.8
low 95.0% CI lim. [%]	61.3	30.8	48.4	46.8	70.8	62.6	68.6
low 99.0% CI lim. [%]	55.3	24.2	41.4	40.3	64.7	56.8	63.6
low 99.9% CI lim. [%]	48.8	18.1	34.4	33.8	58.0	50.4	58.1

Moorfields regression classification: **within normal limits**.

Fig. 17.64 HRT, right eye

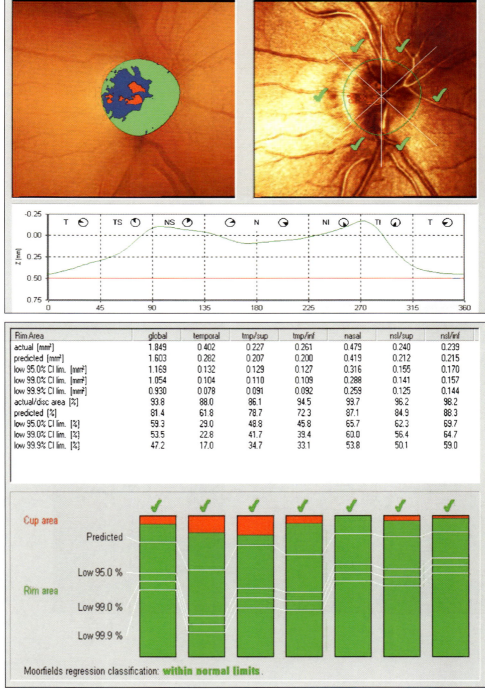

Rim Area	global	temporal	tmp/sup	tmp/inf	nasal	nsl/sup	nsl/inf
actual [mm²]	1.849	0.402	0.227	0.261	0.479	0.240	0.239
predicted [mm²]	1.603	0.282	0.207	0.200	0.419	0.212	0.215
low 95.0% CI lim. [mm²]	1.169	0.132	0.129	0.127	0.316	0.155	0.170
low 99.0% CI lim. [mm²]	1.054	0.104	0.110	0.109	0.288	0.141	0.157
low 99.9% CI lim. [mm²]	0.930	0.078	0.091	0.092	0.259	0.125	0.144
actual/disc area [%]	93.8	88.0	86.1	94.5	99.7	96.2	98.2
predicted [%]	81.4	61.8	78.7	72.3	87.1	84.9	88.3
low 95.0% CI lim. [%]	59.3	29.0	48.8	45.8	65.7	62.3	69.7
low 99.0% CI lim. [%]	53.5	22.8	41.7	39.4	60.0	56.4	64.7
low 99.9% CI lim. [%]	47.2	17.0	34.7	33.1	53.8	50.1	59.0

Moorfields regression classification: **within normal limits**.

Fig. 17.65 HRT, left eye

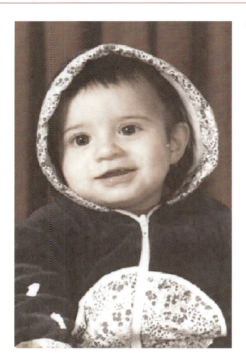

Fig. 17.66 The patient as a baby

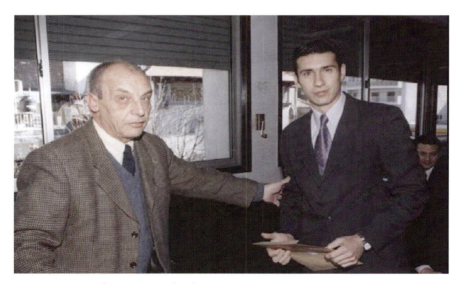

Fig. 17.67 25 years later, receiving his doctorate

Case 6:
Refractory Bilateral Congenital Glaucoma
Follow up of 29 years

This male child was first seen at the age of 6 months and followed up for 29 years. In 1977, at the age of 4 months, the pediatrician treated him for conjunctivitis and at 5 months the mother noticed photophobia and tearing.

This is an example of refractory congenital glaucoma for which combined surgery was used from the start: trabeculotomy + trabeculectomy in the same operation, as soon as diagnosed. The patient remains with normal axial length, 20/20 vision in both eyes, normal optic nerves and visual field. He is currently 28 years of age, working in Interpol, as an agent of the Argentine Federal police where he deals with the maintenance of networks and equipment. He also plays the piano and is still studying music (Figs. 17.68, 17.69, 17.70, 17.71, 17.72).

However, the most important aspect of this case is that the patient came in with an echometry of approximately 24 mm in both eyes, but corneas 15 mm in diameter. Today, at age 28, the eyes are still normal in size and the corneas 15 mm in diameter. This is a patient presenting refractory congenital glaucoma and a pure bilateral megalocornea that is unrelated to the glaucoma.

	Right eye	Left eye
1977		
Axial length	23.45	24.37
IOP	30 mmHg	23 mmHg
Corneal diameter	15 mm	15 mm
Chamber angle	Type II	Type II
Diagnosis	Refractory glaucoma	Refractory glaucoma
Surgery (1977)	Combined surgery: Trabeculotomy and trabeculectomy in the same section	
2006 Follow-up		
Axial length	23.59	24.33 (same in 1977)
IOP	13 mmHg	13 mmHg
Visual acuity	20/20	20/20
Optic disc (HRT)	Normal	Normal
Visual field		
Conventional perimetry	Normal	Normal
Nonconventional perimetry	Normal	Normal

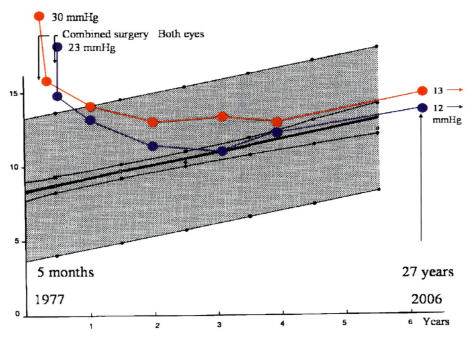

Fig. 17.68 Chart of intraocular pressure in children. Intraocular pressure of case no. 5. *Red dots*, right eye, *blue dots*, left eye. This shows how the IOP went into the normal range

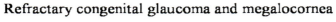

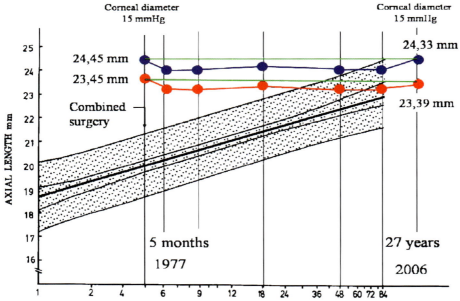

Fig. 17.69 Chart of the axial length of case no. 6

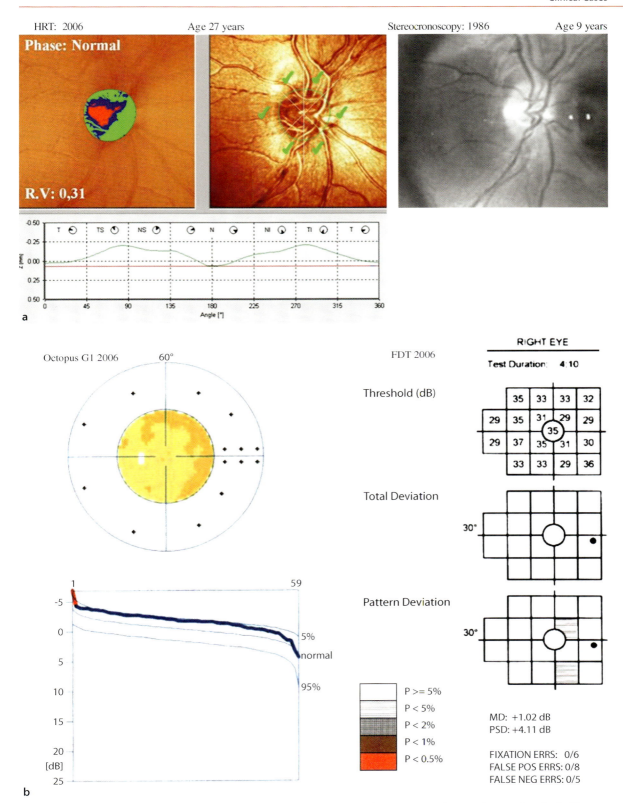

Fig. 17.70 **a** HRT 27 years after surgery of the right eye. On the right, stereochronoscopy at the age of 9 years (method of Lotmar and Goldmann). **b** Visual field with Octopus G1, right eye, with double-frequency technology

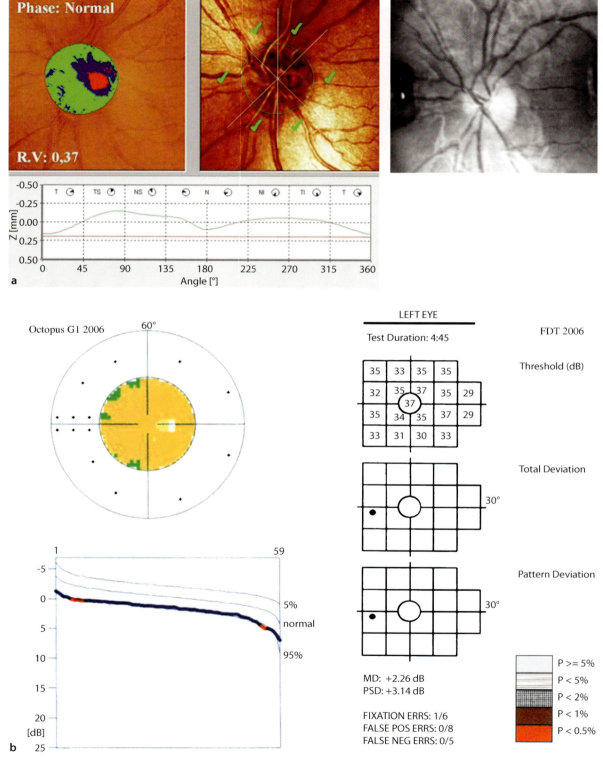

Fig. 17.71 a HRT 27 years after surgery of the left eye. On the right, stereochronoscopy at the age of 9 years (method of Lotmar and Goldmann). **b** Visual field with Octopus G1, left eye, with double-frequency technology

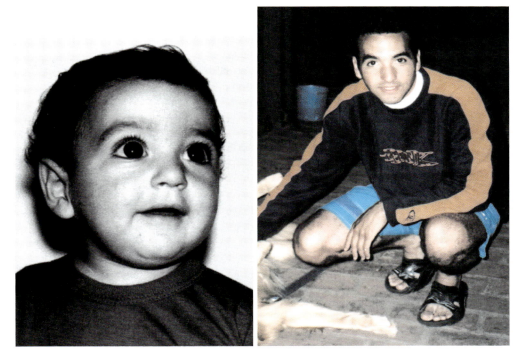

Fig. 17.72 The patient as a baby, case no. 7. On the right, at the age of 27 years

Case 7:
Refractory Bilateral Congenital Glaucoma

This is a 5-month-old boy whose mother noted his right eye was larger beginning at the age of 3 months, and whose first diagnosis was occlusion of the lacrimal ducts. The diagnosis we reached was refractory congenital glaucoma (type II chamber angle, apparent high insertion of the iris).

This case shows how the surgeon must always re-operate when presented with an increase in the axial length after the first operation. In this case, the clinical history shows that it was necessary to operate both eyes three times, and that the right eye had to be operated even a fourth and fifth time. The echometries were then normalized, but both eyes were left with a large axial length and myopia. Numerous check-ups have been made, with the latest in 2006, 9 years after; see Figs. 17.73, 17.74, 17.75, 17.76, 17.77, 17.78 for parameters.

In conclusion, the surgeon should not be discouraged by surgical failures. We operated this patient's right eye three times and left eye five times, achieving a grade III visual field in the right eye and grade II in the left eye, with vision of 20/60 in the right eye and 20/30 in the left despite high myopia.

	Right eye	Left eye
Axial length	26.03 mm	24.53 mm
IOP	36 mm	22 mm
Corneal diameter	14 mm	13.5 mm
Chamber angle	Type II (refractory congenital glaucoma)	Type II (refractory congenital glaucoma)
Surgery (1997, 1999)	(three surgeries) (Fig. 17.74)	(five surgeries) (Fig. 17.74)

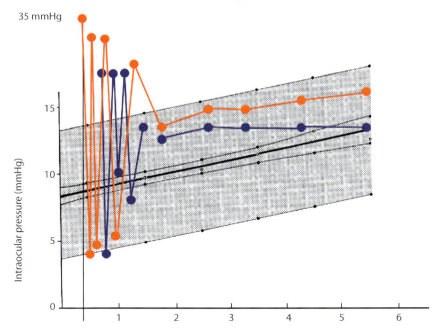

Fig. 17.73 Intraocular pressure values of case no. 6

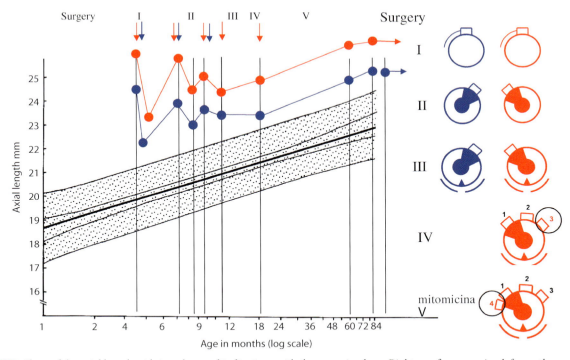

Fig. 17.74 Chart of the axial length with its values and indications with the surgeries done. Right eye, five surgeries, left eye, three surgeries

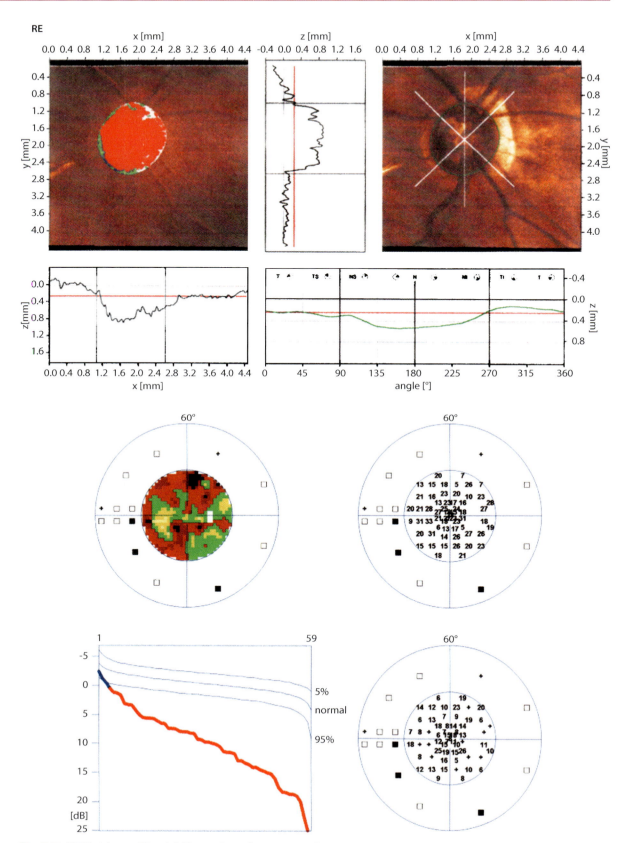

Fig. 17.75 HRT, right eye. Visual field stage III with conventional perimetry

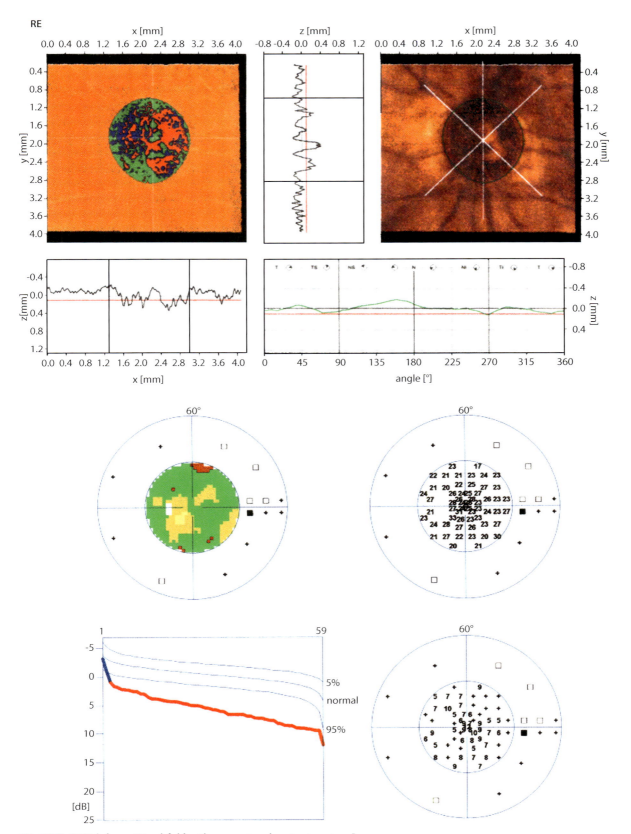

Fig. 17.76 HRT, left eye. Visual field with conventional perimetry, stage I

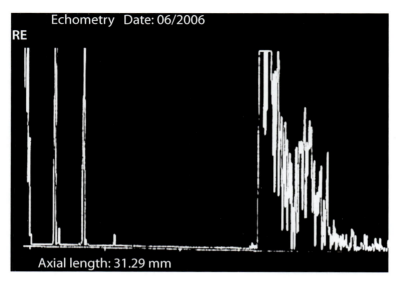

Fig. 17.77 Echometry of the right eye

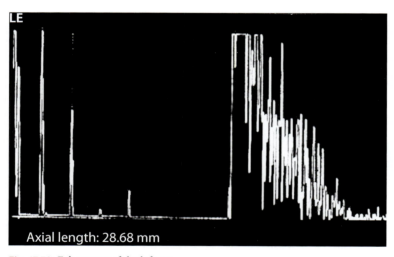

Fig. 17.78 Echometry of the left eye

Case 8:
Bilateral Refractory Congenital Glaucoma
18 years of follow up

At the age of 1 month, this male child presented lacrimation, photophobia, and corneal edema. The child was attended and operated in his city of birth. The mother and the aunt had keratoconus (Figs. 17.79, 17.80, 17.81, 17.82, 17.83, 17.84, 17.85).

In conclusion, we repeat that the ophthalmologist should not be discouraged by failure in surgeries and severe complications. The first two surgeries performed (goniotomies) were not successful in this child. The second surgery done in his right eye (trabeculo-

tomy) also failed. At 7 months, he was sent to us and we performed a combined surgery in the right eye (trabeculotomy and trabeculectomy) and trabeculotomy in the left eye. This third surgery in the right eye and the second in the left eye have regulated the pressure to date. Since the right eye had a tear in the Descemet membrane passing trough the pupil, we made a perforating corneal graft, because amblyopia and strabismus were starting. The first corneal graft was complicated by an abscess. We performed a second perforating corneal graft and then a refractive surgery. Today he is an outstanding 18-year-old student with no strabismus and a good bilateral visual field.

	Right eye	Left eye
IOP	30 mmHg	32 mmHg
Surgery 1	Goniotomy	Goniotomy (6 months)
IOP	20 mmHg	10 mmHg
Surgery 2	Trabeculotomy temporal	
1991: surgeon who operated the child earlier sent him to me for treatment		
Axial length	23.49 mm	23.70 mm
IOP	30 mmHg	22 mmHg
Corneal diameter	14 mm	13.5 mm
Chamber angle	Invisible because of corneal edema. Congential glaucoma type I, Haabs lines	
Surgery 3	Combined surgery Trabeculotomy + Trabeculectomy (6 o'clock)	Trabeculotomy (12 o'clock)
IOP (8 months)	15 mmHg	10 mmHg
	Divergent squint	*Divergent squint*
Surgery 4 (9.5 months)	First corneal graft	
Bronchitis (11 months)	Pneumococcus, corneal abscess	
Surgery 5 (16 months)	Second corneal graft	
Surgery 6 (astigmatism)	Incisional refractive surgery	

	Right eye	Left eye
	Squint disappears with occlusion and orthoptic exercises	
IOP (2 years)	14 mmHg	11 mmHg
DPC (10 years)	Normal	Normal
Axial length (15 years)	23.49 mm	23.79 mm
Refraction	Sph −8, cil −3 180°	Sph −0.50, cil −2.75 10°
Visual acuity	20/200	20/30
Optic nerve	Megalopapilla (disc area: 3.404 m³)	Normal
Visual field		
Conventional perimetry	Stage III	Normal
Nonconventional perimetry	Stage III	Normal

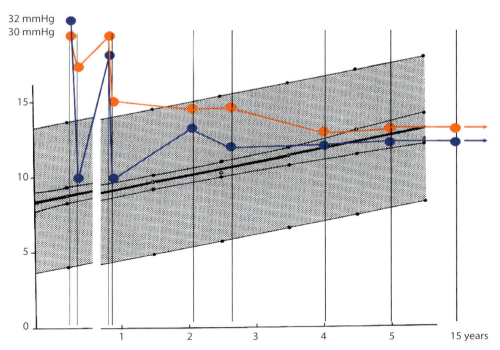

Fig. 17.79 Chart of intraocular pressure with the different intraocular pressures with *red dots*, right eye, with *blue dots*, left eye over 15 years

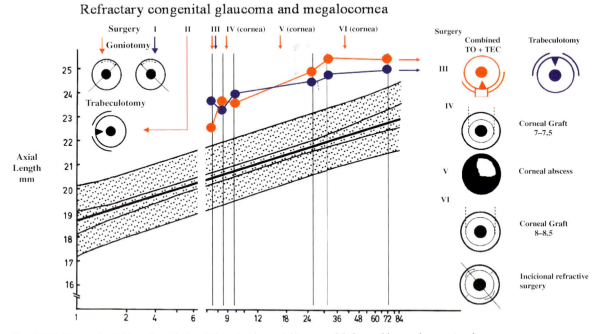

Fig. 17.80 Chart of axial length with the different values; right eye, *red*, left eye, *blue*, and surgeries done

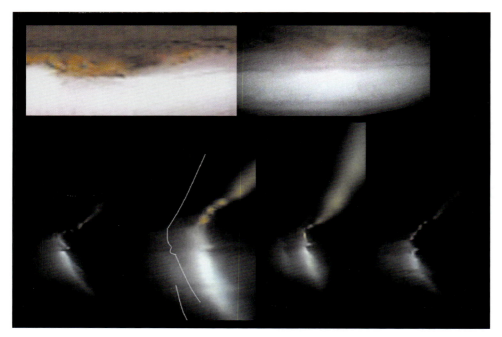

Fig. 17.81 Goniophotograph of the left eye after trabeculotomy

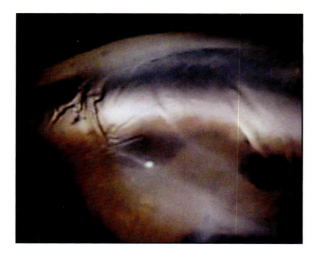

Fig. 17.82 Right eye ruptures in the Descemet membrane (Haab´lines) and two iridectomiess

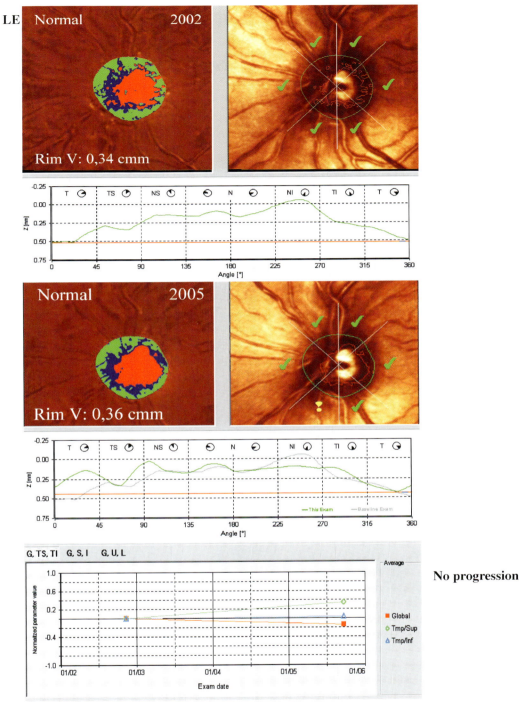

Fig. 17.83 HRT in right and left eyes, which shows that there is no progression

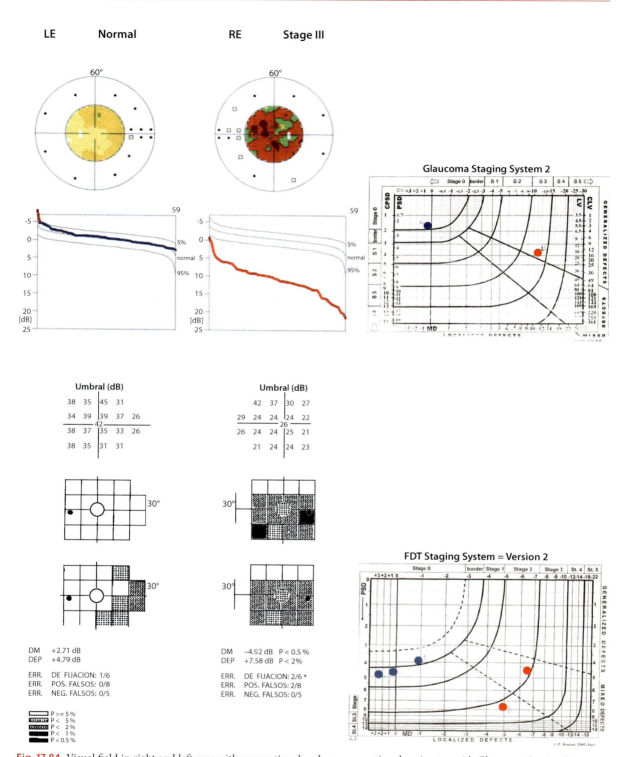

Fig. 17.84 Visual field in right and left eyes with conventional and nonconventional perimetry with Glaucoma Staging System

RE after the second perforating corneal graft   LE

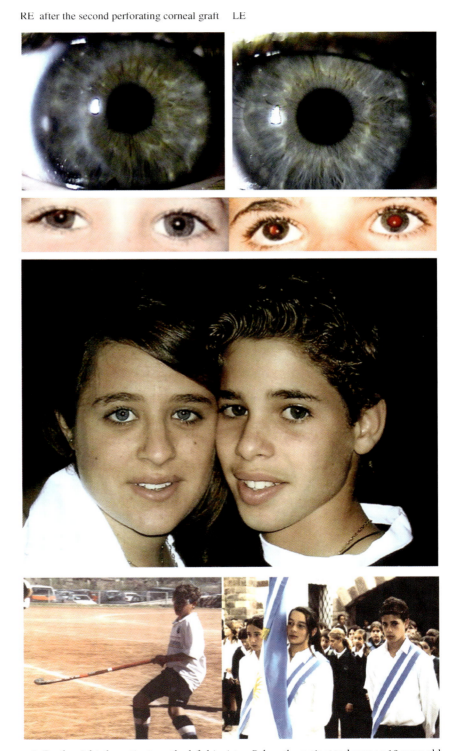

Fig. 17.85 Right and left eye of case no. 8. On the *right*, the patient, on the *left*, his sister. *Below*, the patient today as an 18-year-old student and playing hockey

Case 9:
Late Congenital Glaucoma or Juvenile Glaucoma (Goniodysgenesis)

This male child was 7 years old and presented with late congenital glaucoma (goniodysgenesis). Trabeculotomy had been performed in both eyes at 6 years of age.

As can be seen in the evolution diagram (Fig. 17.86), the right eye was regulated at between 18 and 20 mmHg, and the left eye was always around 10 mmHg, i.e., ap-

	Right eye	Left eye
Axial length	23.35 mm (normal for the age)	24.12 mm (normal for the age)
IOP	36 mmHg	11 mmHg
Corneal diameter	11 mm	11 mm
Chamber angle	Goniodysgenesis	Goniodysgenesis
Visual acuity	20/20	20/20
Surgery (1981)	Trabeculotomy	Trabeculotomy
IOP (check-up, 1985–1993)	18 mmHg	18 mmHg
Daily pressure curve	Pathological	Pathological
Optic nerve (1994, HRT)	Phase III	Normal
Visual field	Norma	Norma
Visual acuity	20/20	20/20

parently both eyes were regulated, but a deeper study showed that for the right eye, pressures of around 18–20 mmHg were not the target pressure needed. As the patient lived in another city, the ophthalmologist who followed him up started to make daily pressure curves at the age of 10 years, and told us that the pressures at 6 a.m. in bed were 25, 28, 28, 30, 27, and 33 mmHg.

As can be seen in Fig. 17.87, the action over the years of the ocular pressure (peaks at 6 a.m.) gradually wore down the optic nerve in the right eye. At the center, the HRT shows a pathological rim volume. In the retinofluoresceinography in Fig. 17.85c, corresponding to the right eye, there are no more capillaries in the capillary border of the disc. In Fig. 17.85f, corresponding to the left eye, the capillaries are normal in this zone. In Fig. 17.85b, e, the HRT image corresponds to what was said above.

In Fig. 17.88, the HRT corresponds to both eyes shows the pathology of the right eye. Since the intraocular pressure went down with medication and the diurnal pressure curve regulated (Figs. 17.89, 17.90), it seems for the moment to have stopped the progress of the optic nerve lesion of right eye. Figure 17.87 of the right eye shows with the ophthalmoscope, a pathological excavation. With HRT the optic nerve is very damaged. Interestingly, the photograph on the right (fluorescein) shows absence of the capillaries in the periphery of the optic nerve and vascular hooks. The figure below shows a normal optic disc with capillaries and no hooks.

The visual fields with conventional and nonconventional perimetry are normal in both eyes.

Fig. 17.86 Progression diagram of the intraocular pressure of right and left eyes of case no. 9

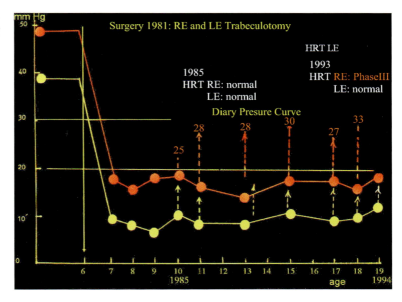

RE

LE

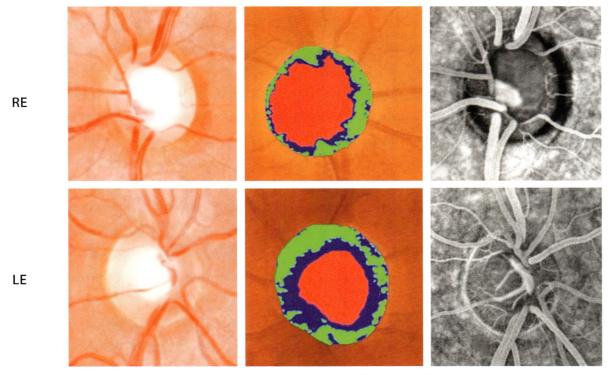

Fig. 17.87 Optic nerve right and left eye. On the *left*, photograph of the papilla in the *middle* HRT and on the *right* retinofluoresceinoangiography of case no. 9

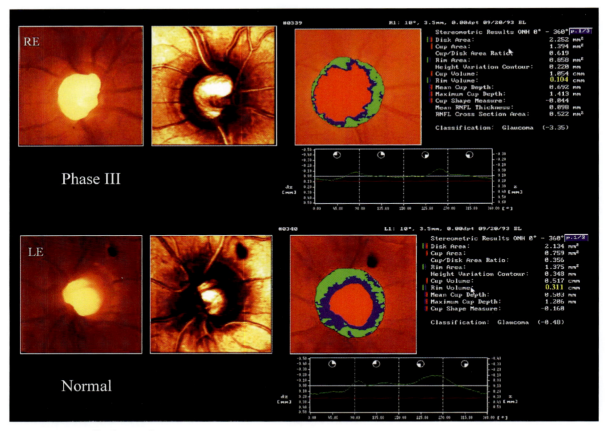

Fig. 17.88 HRT of both eyes of patient, case no. 9

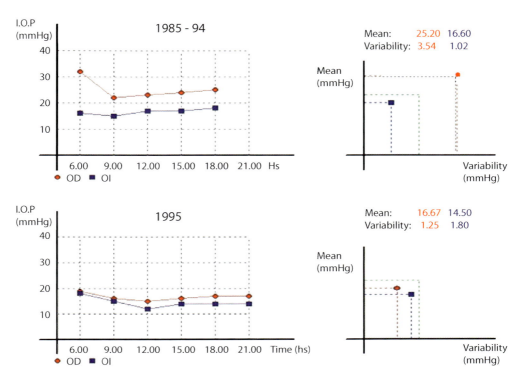

Fig. 17.89 Daily pressure curve from 1985 to 1995

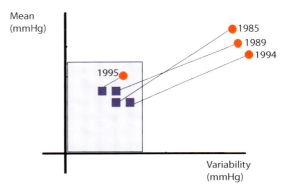

Fig. 17.90 Variability of the daily pressure curve, which was regulated with medical treatment

The daily pressure curve was regulated with medical treatment.

References

1. Helmholtz HV (1950) Beschreibung eines Augen-Spiegels zur Untersuchung der Netzhaut im lebenden Auge. In: Engelking D (ed) Dokumente zur Erfindung des Augenspiegels durch Herrmann von Helmholtz im Jahr 1850. Bergmann, Munich, pp 14–55

2. Varma R, Spaeth G (1993) The optic nerve in glaucoma. Lippincott, Philadelphia

3. Leydhecker W, Krieglstein GK, Colloni EV (1979) Observer variation in applanation tonometry and estimation of the cup disc ratio. In: Krieglstein GK, Leydhecker W (eds) Glaucoma update: International Glauacoma Symposium, Nara, Japan, 1978. Springer, Berlin Heidelberg New York, pp 101–117

4. Lichter PR (1976) Variability of expert observers in evaluating the optic disc. Trans Am Ophthalmol Soc 74:532–572

5. Varma R, Steinmann WC, Scott IU (1992) Expert agreement in evaluating the optic disc for glaucoma. Ophthalmology 99:215–221

6. Takamoto T, Schwartz B (1985) Reproducibility of photogrammetric optic disc cup measurements. Invest Ophthalmol Vis Sci 26:814–817

7. Airaksinen PJ, Drance SM, Douglas GR, Schulzer M (1985) Neuroretinal rim areas and visual field indices in glaucoma. Am J Ophthalmol 99:107–110

8. Goldmann H, Lotmar W (1977) Rapid detection of changes in the optic disc. Esterochronoscopy. Graefes arch Clin Exp Ophthalmol 202:87–90

9. Littmann H (1982) Zur Bestimmung der wahren Probe eines Objektes auf dem Hintergrund des lebenden Auges. Klin Mbl Augenheilk 180:286–289

10. Burk R, Konig J, Rohrschneider K, Noack H, Volcker HE, Zinser G (1990) Analysis of three-dimensional optic disk topography by laser scanning tomography. Parameter definition and evaluation of parameter inter-dependence. In: Nasemann J, Burk ROW (eds) Scanning laser ophthalmoscopy and tomography. Quintessenz, Munich, pp 161–176

11. Sampaolesi R, Sampaolesi JR (1999) Confocal tomography of the retina and the optic nerve head. City-Druck, Heidelberg

12. Sampaolesi JR, Sampaolesi R (1995) Lecture: Study of normality in the optic nerve head with H.R.T., in Curso y Simposio Argentino de Glaucoma, July 1995, Buenos Aires, Argentina

13. Vihanninjoki K, Teesalu P, Burk ROW, Läärä E, Tuulonen A, Airaksinen PJ (2000) Search for an optimal combination of structural and functional parameters for the diagnosis of glaucoma. Multivariate analysis of confocal scanning laser tomograph, blue-on-yellow visual field and retinal nerve fiber layer data. Graefes Arch Clin Exp Ophthalmol 238:477–481

14. Franceschetti A, Bock R (1950) Megalopapilla: a new congenital anomaly. Am J Ophthalmol 33:227–235

15. Brodsky CM (1994) Congenital optic disk anomalies. Sur Ophthalmol 39:89–112

16. Goldhammer Y (1975) Optic nerve anomalies: a basal encephalocele. Arch Ophthalmol 2:115–118

17. Theossiadis GP, Kollia AK, Theodossiadis PG (1992) Cilioretinal arteries in conjuction with a pit of the optic disc. Ophthalmologica 204:115–121

18. Caprioli J (1989) Basal encephalocele and Morning Glory syndrome. Br J Ophthalmol 107:145–150

19. Sampaolesi R, Sampaolesi JR (1998) Etude du nerf optique dans le glaucome congénital par la tomographie confocale au laser. Ophtalmologíe 12:205–213

20. Grimson BS, Perry DD (1984) Enlargement of the optic disk in childhood optic nerve tumors. Am J Ophthalmol 97:627–631

21. Collier M (1965) Megalopapilla and central pulverulent cataract. Bull Soc Fr Ophtalmol 9:719–724

22. Hirokane K, Kimura T, Kimura W, Savwada T, Ohte A, Kobayashi M (1995) Megalopapilla in four children. Folia Ophthalmol Jpn 46:731–735

23. Jonas JB, Zäch FM, Gusek GC, Naumann GOH (1989) Pseudoglaucomatous physiologic large cups. Am J Ophthalmol 107:137–144

24. Maisel JM, Pearlstein CS, Adams WH, Heotis PM (1989) Large optic discs in the Marshallese population. Am J Ophthalmol 107:145–150

25. Saruhan A, Orgül S, Kosak I, Prünte C, Flammer J (1998) Descriptive information on topographic parameters computed at optic nerve head with Heidelberg Retina Tonograph. J Glaucoma 7:420–429

26. Burk ROW, Rohrsneider K, Noack H, Völcker HF (1992) Are large optic nerve head susceptible to glaucomatous damage at normal intraocular pressure? Graefes Arch Ophthalmol 230:552–560

27. Sampaolesi R, Sampaolesi JR (1995) Tomografia confocal del nervio óptico y la retina. Arch Oftalmol B Aires 70:1–566

28. Sampaolesi R (1994) Congenital glaucoma. The importance of echometry in its diagnosis, treatment and functional outcome. In: Cennamo G, Rosa N (eds) Ultrasonography in ophthalmology XV, Procceding of the 15 SIDUO Congres, Cortina Italy, 1994. Kluwer, Dordrecht, pp 1–47

29. Orellana J, Friedman AH (1993) Chapters 24–40. In: Clinico-pathological atlas of congenital fundus disorders. In: Orellan J (ed) Springer, Berlin Heidelberg New York, pp 119–142

30. Apple DJ, Rabb MF, Walsh PM (1982) Congenital anomalies of the optic disc. Surv Ophthalmol 27:3–41

31. Brodsky MC (1994) Congenital optic disk anomalies. Surv Ophthalmol 39:89–112

32. Jonas JB, Koviszewski G, Naumann GO (1989) "Morning glory syndrome" and "Handmann's anomaly" in congenital macropapilla. Extreme variants of confluent optic pits. Klin Mbl Augenheilk 195:371–374

33. Hotchkiss ML, Green WR (1979) Optic nerve aplasia and hypoplasia of the optic nerve. J Pediatr Ophthalmol Strabismus 16:225–240

34. Mosier MA, Lieberman MF, Green WR, Knox DL (1978) Hypoplasia of the optic nerve. Arch Ophthalmol 96:1437–1442

35. Arslanian SA, Rothfus WE, Foley TO, Becker DJ (1984) Hormonal, metabolic and neuroradiologic abnormalities associated with septo-optic dysplasia. Acta Endocrin 139:249–254

36. Izenberg N, Rosenblum M, Parks JS (1984) The endocrine spectrum of septo-optic dysplasia. Clin Pediatr 23:632–636

37. Margalith D, Tze WJ, Jan JE (1985) Congenital optic nerve hypoplasia with hypothalamic-pituitary dysplasia. Am J Dis Child 139:361–366

38. Nelson M, Lessell S, Sadun AA (1986) Optic nerve hypoplasia and maternal diabetes mellitus. Arch Neurol 43:20–25

39. Hoyt WF, Kaplan SL, Grumback MM, Glaser JS (1970) Septo-optic dysplasia and pituitary dwarfism. Lancet 2:893–894

40. Brodsky MC (1991) Septo-optic dysplasia: a reappraisal. Semin Ophthalmol 6:227–232

41. Brodsky MC, Glasier CM (1993) Optic nerve hypoplasia: clinical significance of associated centra nervous system abnormalities on magnetic resonance imaging. Arch Ophthalmol 111:66–74

42. Novakovic P, Taylor DSI, Hoyt WF (1988) Localizing patterns of optic nerve hypoplasia-retina to occipital lobe. Br J Ophthalmol 72:176–182

43. Graether JM (1963) Transient amaurosis in one eye with simultaneous dilatation of retinal veins. Arch Ophthalmol 70:342–345

44. Kindler P (1970) Morning glory syndrome: unusual congenital optic disk anomaly. Am J Ophthalmol 69:376–384

45. Beyer WB, Quencer RM, Osher RH (1982) Morning glory syndrome: a functional analysis includuing gluorescein angiography, ultrasonography, and computerized tomography. Ophthalmology 89:1362–1364

46. Pollock JA (1987) The morning glory disc anomaly: contractile movement, classification and embryogenesis. Doc Ophthalmol 91:1638–1647

47. Haik BG, Greenstein SH, Smith ME et al (1984) Retinal detachment in the morning glory syndrome. Ophthalmology 91:1638–1647

48. Takida A Hida T, Kimura C et al (1984) A case of bilateral morning glory syndrome with total retinal detachment. Folia Ophthalmol 32:1177–1182

49. Irvine A.R, Crawford JB, Sullivan JH (1986) The pathogenesis of retinal detachment with morning glory disc and optic pit. Retina 6:146–150

50. Bonamour G, Bregeat P, Bonnet M, Juge P (1968) La papille optique, Masson, Paris, pp 63–68

51. Ebner R (1994) Application of confocal laser tomography in neuro-ophthalmology, Ch. 15. In: Sampaolesi R, Sampaolesi JR (eds) Confocal tomography of the retina and the optic nerve head. http://www.onjoph.com/global/heidelberg/300dpi/00.pdf. Cited 22 August 2008

52. Alezzandrini AA (1993) Sindrome de "Morning Glory". Arch Oftalmol B Aires 58:46–49

53. Chestler RJ, France TD (1988) Ocular finding in the CHARGE syndrome. Opthalmology 95:1613–1619

54. Russell-Eggitt IM, Blake KD, Taylor DSI, Wyse RKH (1990) The eye in the CHARGE association. Br J Opthalmol 74:421–426

55. Pagon RA (1981) Ocular coloboma. Surv Ophthalmol 25:223–236

56. Carney SH, Brodsky MC, Good WV et al (1993) Aicardi Syndrome: more than meets the eye. Surv Ophthalmol 37:419–424

57. Hoyt CS, Billson F, Ouvrier F et al (1978) Ocular features of Aicardi's syndrome. Arch Ophthalmol 96:291–295

58. Taylor D (1990) Optic nerve. In: Taylor D (ed) Pediatric ophthalmology. Cambridge MA, Blackwell, Cambridge MA, pp 441–466

59. Calhoun FP (1930) Bilateral coloboma of the optic nerve associated with holes in the disc and cyst of the optic nerve sheath. Arch Ophthalmol 3:71–79

60. Singh D, Verma A (1978) Bilateral peripapillary staphyloma (ectasia). Indian J Ophtahalmol 25:50–51

61. Jonas JB, Zach FM, Gusek GC, Naumann GOH (1989) Pseudoglaucomatous physiologic optic cups. Am J Ophthalmol 107:137–144

62. Franceschetti A, Bock R (1950) Megalopapilla: a new congenital anomaly. Am J Ophthalmol 33:227–235

63. Theodossiadis GP, Kollia AK, Theodossiadis PG (1992) Cilio-retinal arteries in conjunction with a pit of the optic disc. Ophthalmologica 204:115–121

64. Bonnet M (1991) Serous macular detachment associated with optic nerve pits. Arch Clin Exp Ophthalmol 229:526–532

65. Brown GC, Shields JA, Goldberg RE (1980) Congenital pits of the optic nerve head. II. Clinical studies in humans. Ophthalmology 87:51–65

66. Lincoff H, Lopez R, Kreissing I et al (1988) Retinoschisis associated with optic nerve pits. Arch Ophthalmol 106:61–67

67. Brown G, Tasman W (1983) Congenital anomalies of the optic disc. Grune and Stratton, New York, pp 31–215

68. Ferry AP (1963) Macular detachment associated with congenital pit of the optic nerve head. Arch Ophthalmol 70:106–117

69. Young SE, Walsh FB, Knox DL (1976) The tilted disc syndrome. Am J Ophthalmolo 82:16–23

70. Riise D (1975) The nasal fundus ectasia. Acta Ophthalmologica Suppl 126:3–128

71. Argento C, Mayorga E (1980) Frecuency in ophthalmological findings in the fundus nasal ectasia .Arch Oftalmol B Aires 55:153–164

72. Brusini P, Cabazza S, Della Mea G (1982) Duplicazione della papilla ottica e seudo duplicazione: problemi di diagnostica differenziale. Boll Ocul 61:609–618

Contents

In 1979, Robin et al. [1] and in 1980, Morin and Bryars [2] published perimetry studies in children operated for congenital glaucoma using the Goldmann perimeter. In 1989, Tejeiro and Domínguez [3] performed the first visual fields in children operated for congenital glaucoma with computed perimetry, using the Octopus 500 and the 2000, program G1. The children studied were aged between 6 and 17 years. They found a generalized depression: MD = 62 dB. Fifty-eight percent had truly pathological values of MD greater than or equal to 4 dB. They had 15.2% loss of visual field, which, as the authors comment, is certainly small. They say that this good result stems from:

1. The children being operated within 3 days of diagnosis.
2. After surgery, every eye that had an ocular pressure greater than 16 mmHg was reoperated.
3. Repeated correction of the refraction and prevention of amblyopia.

This work is extraordinary if we think that it was written 16 years ago and shows the authors' profound knowledge of congenital glaucoma disease.

Sampaolesi and Casiraghi´s [4] study titled "Computerized visual fields in pediatric glaucoma" had findings similar to Domínguez's study [3], i.e., a limited diffuse loss of sensitivity in children with pure congenital glaucoma. This good result stems from good early surgical treatment and frequent monitoring of the refraction, i.e., the three criteria described by Dominguez are respected. In refractory congenital glaucoma and in late congenital glaucoma, we found diffuse loss of sensitivity and scotomas. In these cases, the visual defects were greater and in some cases were at very advanced stages.

Material

In our 1990 study, we examined 46 eyes of 25 patients from three pediatric glaucoma groups, ranging from 6 to 21 years of age (Table 18.1). We divided the patients into three groups:

– Group 1: Pure congenital glaucomas;
– Group 2: Refractory congenital glaucomas;
– Group 3: Late congenital glaucoma (goniodysgenesis).

Table 18.1 Three pediatric glaucoma groups

Group	No. of eyes	Males	Females	Bilateral	Unilateral	Visual fields performed at age
1 (pure congenital glaucoma)	19	12	7	14	5	6–18 Years
2 (refractory glaucoma)	11	9	2		7	10–21 Years
3 (late congenital glaucoma)	16	4	12	16		8–17 Years
Total [a]	46	25	21	34	12	6–21 Years

[a] Mean 11.9

Method

The visual fields were examined with the Octopus 2000 perimeter, using both phases of the program G1 [5, 6] and analyzed with Octosmart including the Bebie curve [7]. In order to minimize learning effects, the number of visual fields performed was between two and five per eye [8].

Analysis of variance including the following elements was performed with both parametric and nonparametric tests: best corrected visual acuity in the 20/20 scale, refraction, corneal diameter, axial length, mean defect (MD), and corrected loss variance (CLV), and a reliability factor lower than 10. The visual fields were analyzed with Bebie cumulative frequency curve and classified as diffuse, scotomatous, or combined (diffuse plus scotomatous) loss.

To evaluate the normal threshold in the 10- to 20-year-old age group [9], we carried out both phases of the G1 program on ten young normal subjects with a visual acuity of 1.0 20/20 and axial length between 23.50 and 24.50, with a normal daily pressure curve and no ocular or associated systemic pathology.

Results

Group 1: Pure Congenital Glaucoma

The prognosis in these cases is very good when surgery normalizes intraocular pressure. The eyes stop enlarging, the optic disc is normal, the visual acuity is good, and the visual field is normal or nearly normal (Fig. 18.1).

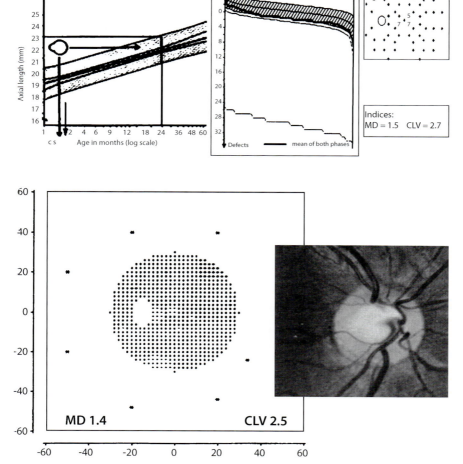

Fig. 18.1 Group 1. Pure congenital glaucoma

Group 2: Refractory Congenital Glaucoma

In many cases, the eyes were operated twice. The optic disc was pathological and the visual fields had diffused defects and scotomatous defects. In some eyes, the defects were larger and more advanced.

After the introduction of combined surgery for refractory glaucoma, only one surgery was necessary and the anatomical and functional results were very good (Fig. 18.2).

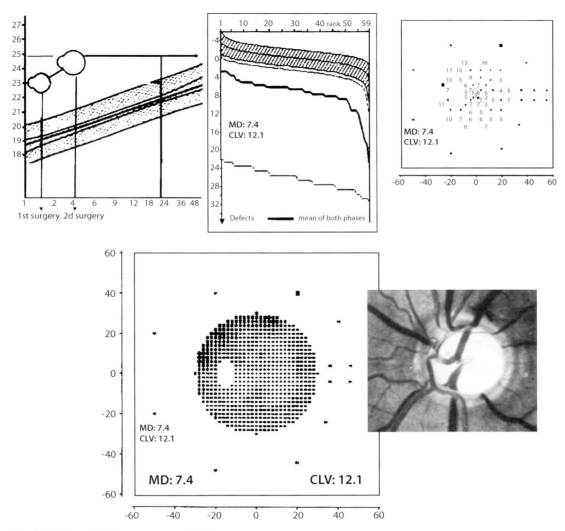

Fig. 18.2 Group 2. Refractory congenital glaucoma

Group 3: Late Congenital Glaucoma

In Fig. 18.3 corresponding to the right eye, it can be seen that the optic nerve (ON) is in phase IV, the conventional visual field is normal, and the nonconventional visual field is in phase III. For the ophthalmologists who think that glaucoma is an alteration of the optic nerve (ON) and of the visual field and who work with conventional perimetry, the diagnosis in this case is ocular hypertension. For those who work with nonconventional perimetry, the diagnosis is glaucoma, since the ON lesion corresponds topographically to the visual field (VF) lesion made with nonconventional frequency-doubling perimetry. Since in this patient the maximum medication, prostaglandins – carbon anhydrase inhibitors and beta blockers – did not regulate the pressure, we performed surgery: deep nonpenetrating sclerectomy and goniopuncture with Yag laser. The pressure regulated at 12 mmHg and the daily pressure curve was normal. We would stress here that this patient was on medication for 17 years while her ON and VF were deteriorating. We believe that she will not have the same fate as her glaucomatous predecessors.

The ON and the VF are generally the same as in group 2, but the defects are much greater.

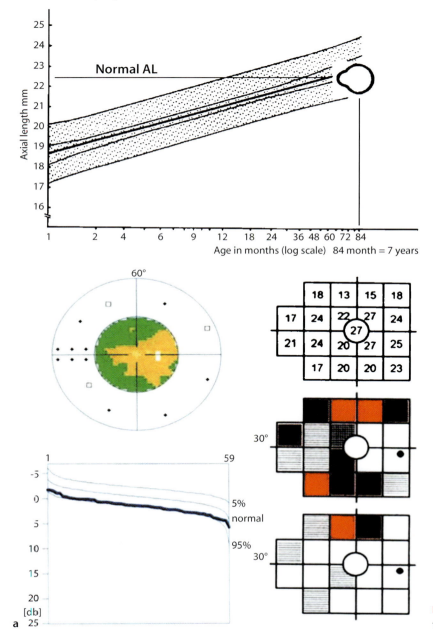

Fig. 18.3a,b Group 3. Late congenital glaucoma

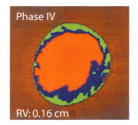
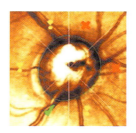

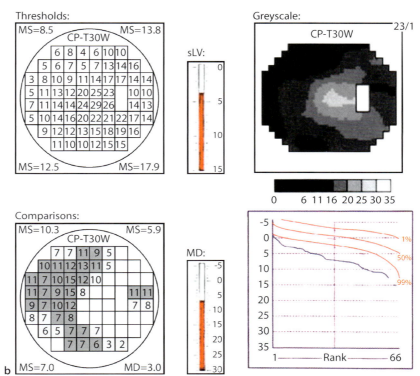

Fig. 18.3a,b *(continued)* **b**

High-Pass-Resolution Perimetry in Normal Children in Congenital Glaucoma

In 1983 [10], we conducted a comparative study between differential light sensitivity perimetry and high-pass-resolution perimetry in congenital glaucoma. The population of congenital glaucoma patients was studied by performing visual field examinations with the Octopus 1-2-3 and high-pass-resolution perimetry and confocal tomography with the Heidelberg Retina Tomograph, which was used to assess optic disc parameters. The population was divided into three groups:

G1   Pure congenital glaucomas;
G2   Refractory glaucomas;
G3   Late congenital glaucoma (goniodysgenesis).

Introduction

Differential light sensitivity (DLS) perimetry and high-pass-resolution perimetry (HRP) in adults have been compared by several researchers [11–14], but their relationship has not been studied in children with congenital glaucoma.

Material

See Table 18.2 for a description of the material.

Table 18.2. Patient material

	No.	Age (years)	Male	Female
Group 1	19	12–28	13	6
Group 2	12	7–22	10	2
Group 3	29	11–23	15	14
Total	60	7–24	38	22

Methods

Visual field examinations were performed with Octopus 1-2-3 (Interzeag, the G1 program, 59 locations within 30° of the visual field) and the Ophthimus high-pass-resolution perimetry (High-Tech Vision, Malmö, Sweden; version 2.0) (50 locations were measured within the central 30°s of the visual field).

In this study, Pearson's correlation coefficient was calculated between MD (mean defect) and NC (neural capacity), MD and GD (global deviation), and CLV (corrected loss variance) and LO (local deviation) in three groups. NC is an index estimating the total number of functioning retinal ganglion cells.

Results

The relationship between mean defect (MD) and global deviation (GD) showed in group 1 MD and GD correlated significantly: $r = 0.80$, $p < 0.0001$ (Fig. 18.4). In groups 2 and 3, the correlation was not significant.

The relationship between corrected loss variance (CLV) and local deviation (LD) was as follows. In group 1, CLV and LD correlated significantly, $r = 0.78$, $p < 0.0001$ (Fig. 18.5). In group 2, it was not significant. Group 3 had a fairly significant correlation: $r = 0.45$, $p < 0.01$.

The relationship between MD and neural capacity NC showed that in group 1, there was a significant correlation: $r = 0.78$, $p < 0.0001$ (Fig. 18.6). Group 2 was not significant. Group 3 had a fairly significant correlation, $r = 0.42$, $p < 0.02$.

However, when we tried to correlate the three groups together, we found two groups of cases: one located far from the zero line and the other surrounding zero. The correlation is not represented by a straight line but rather by a curve. This means that in many cases the MD is normal but the NC is pathological. The correlation between these two indices is far from perfect (Fig.18.7). In our opinion, these different methods of psychophysical tests measure different aspects of the visual field system.

Both at the 1990 IPS Meeting held in Malmö, Sweden, and now, we believe we were the first to study the visual field in children with differential light sensitivity perimetry (Octopus 2000 and 1-2-3 perimeters) and with high-pass-resolution perimetry. With both perimeters, it is possible to obtain reliable results in children between 5 and 10 years of age. To be sure of the accuracy of our results, we used a reliability factor not higher than 10.

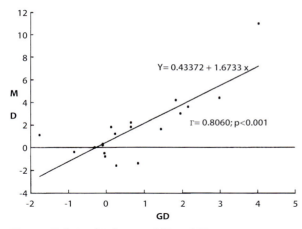

Fig 18.4 Relationship between MD and GD in group 1

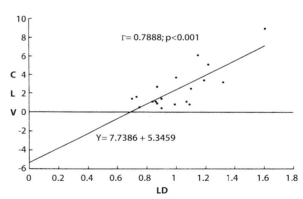

Fig 18.5 Relationship between CLV and LD in group 1

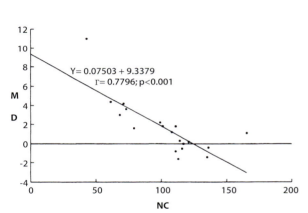

Fig. 18.6 Relationship between MD and NC in group 1

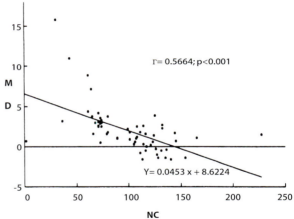

Fig. 18.7 Two groups of cases can be found: one located far from the zero line and the other surrounding it. The correlation is not represented by a straight line but rather by a curve. This means that in many cases, the MD is normal but the NC is pathological

Nonconventional Contrast Perimetry in Congenital Glaucoma

Nowadays, nonconventional perimetry is performed using the following perimeters: frequency doubling technology (FDT) (Carl Zeiss Meditec, Jena, Germany and Zeiss, Wellch Allyn, Skaneateles Falls, NY, USA), Matrix (Zeiss), and Pulsar (Haag-Streit, Wedel, Germany).

Throughout this book, we have presented perimetries taken in children with congenital glaucoma using conventional and nonconventional perimetry. We will give a short explanation why. The method is explained in full detail and the results correlate with lesions of the optic nerve (HRT). In 2003, we showed that in 50% of glaucoma patients with a normal visual field for conventional perimetry, there are defects marked with frequency doubling and that these are topographically perfectly correlated with the damage found in the optic nerve with confocal tomography (HRT). We will show an example here. The complete model and its results are presented in Volume II.

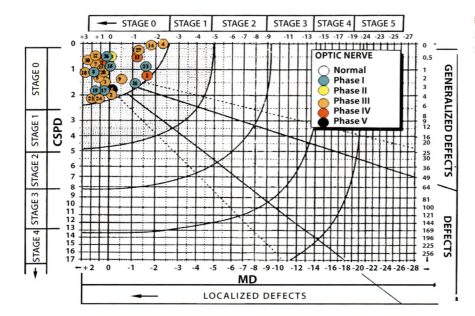

Fig. 18.8 Conventional perimetry (Octopus), all eyes have normal visual field

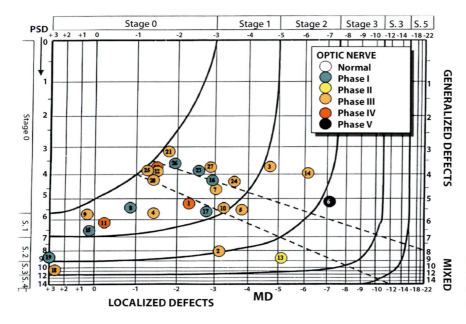

Fig. 18.9 Nonconventional perimetry (FDT), Group 3, all eyes have pathological visual field

With conventional perimetry (Octopus) all eyes had a normal visual field (Fig. 18.8). With nonconventional perimetry (FDT), in group 3, all eyes had a pathological visual field. Figures 18.8 and 18.9 show the Brusini Staging System for classifying the degree of development of the perimetry lesion, firstly for conventional perimetry (Octopus), and in the second for nonconventional perimetry (FDT). The upper part shows the developmental phase. Each numbered round dot represents an eye, and the color corresponds to the developmental phase of the ON for confocal tomog-

raphy (HRT), as can be seen in this group. Those performing only conventional perimetry will diagnose hypertension, and those who perform frequency doubling will diagnose glaucoma. In conclusion, Chap. 20 (see Figs. 20.11 and 20.13) presents a typical case of goniodysgenesis, or late congenital glaucoma, which is seen to be normal with conventional perimetry, although with nonconventional perimetry in the same field it shows ON lesions that correspond topographically to visual field lesions.

Fig. 18.10 Glaucoma staging system 2

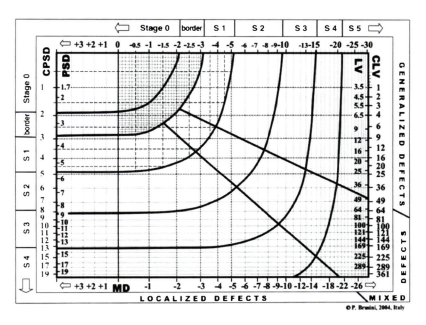

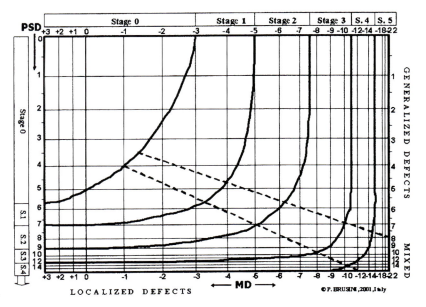

Fig. 18.11 FTD staging system

There are two very interesting studies on the application of the frequency doubling technique in pediatrics by Nesher et al. [16] and by Blumenthal et al. [17]. The authors show that the method is very useful in young patients beginning at 6 years of age, the reliability of the results increases as age increases, children are not frightened by it because the lights in the room can be switched on, because there is no dome, and finally because the stimulus is not static but moving, which attracts the child's attention.

We believe the Brusini Glaucoma Staging System 2 to be the best method to study the progression of the visual field for conventional perimetry (Fig. 18.10) and the FDT Staging System from the same author for non-conventional perimetry (Fig. 18.11) [18, 19, 20].

References

1. Robin AL, Quigley HA, Pollack IP et al (1979) An analysis of visual fields and disk cupping in childhood glaucoma. Am J Ophthalmol 88:847–858
2. Morin JD, Bryars JH (1990) Causes of loss of vision in congenital glaucoma. Arch Ophthalmol 98:1575–1576
3. Tejeiro A, Dominguez A (1990) Perimetría computarizada en el glaucoma congénito Arch Soc Esp Oftalmol LVIII:631–634
4. Sampaolesi R, Casiraghi JF (1991) Computerized visual fields in pediatric glaucoma. In: Mills RP, Heijl A (eds) Perimetry update 1990/1991.Kugler & Ghedini, Amsterdam, pp 455–464
5. Flammer J (1987) The Octopus glaucoma GI program. Glaucoma 9:67–72
6. Flammer J (1986) The concept of visual field indices. Graefes Arch Ophthalmol 224:389–392
7. Bebie H, Flammer J, Bebie T (1989) The cumulative defect curve: separation of local and diffuse components of visual field damage. Graefes Arch Ophthalmol 226:9–12
8. Wild JM, Dengler-Harles M, Searle AET, O'Neill EE, Crews SJ (1989) The influence of the learning effect on automated perimetry in patients with suspected Glaucoma. Acta Ophthalmol 67:537–545
9. Haas A, Flammer J, Schneider U (1986) Influence of age on visual fields of normal subjects. Am J Ophthalmol 101:199–203
10. Sampaolesi R (1983) Ocular echometry and the diagnosis of congenital glaucoma and its evaluation. In: Glaucoma update II, Springer, Berlin Heidelberg New York, pp 175–184
11. Wanger P, Persson HE (1987) Pattern-reversal electroretinogramms and high-pass resolution perimetryin suspected or early glaucoma. Ophthalmology 94:1098–1103
12. Dannheim F, Abramo F, Verlohr D (1989) Comparison of automated conventional and spatial resolution perimetry in glaucoma. In: Heijl A (ed) Perimetry update 1988/1989. Kugler & Ghedini, Amsterdam, pp 383–392
13. Lachenmayr BJ, Drance SM, Douglas GR, Mikelberg FS (1991) Light-sense, flicker and resolution perimetry in glaucoma: a comparative study. Graefe's Arch Ophthalmol 229:246–251
14. Kono Y, Maeda M, Yamamoto T, Kitazawa Y (1993) A comparative study between high-pass resolution perimetry and differential light sensitivity perimetry in glaucoma patients. In: Mills R (ed) Perimetry update 1992/1993. Kugler, Amsterdam, pp 409–413
15. Sampaolesi R, Brusini P, Sampaolesi JR (2003) Korrelation zwischen der konfokalen Tomographie des Nervus Opticus (HRT) und der perimetrischen Frequenzverdoppelugstechnik (FDT) Klin Monatsbl Augenheilkd 220:754–766
16. Nesher R, Norman G, Stem Y, Gorck L, Epstein E, Raz Y, Assia E (2004) Frequency doubling technology threshold testing in the pediatric age group. J Glaucoma 13:278–282
17. Blumenthal EZ, Haddad A. Horani A, Anteby I (2004) The reliability of frequency-doubling perimetry in young children. Ophthalmology 111:435–439
18. Brusini P, Filacorda S (2006) Enhanced Glaucoma Staging System (GSS 2) for classifying functional damage in glaucoma. J Glaucoma 15:40–46
19. Brusini P (2006) Frequency doubling technology staging system 2. J Glaucoma 15:315–320
20. Brusini P, Johnson CA (2007) Staging functional damage in glaucoma: review of different classification methods. Surv Ophthalmol 52:156–178

Contents

Nasolacrimal Duct Obstruction

Epiphora and blepharospasm are signs of this disease, but never photophobia. However, many cases have reached us 7 months or more after the onset of symptoms because the family consulted a neonatologist or pediatrician who mistook the diagnosis. We always give courses in the hospital neonatology and pediatrics departments to alert them to this possibility. If there is any doubt, a permeability test of the lachrymal ducts can always be made with fluorescein or probing at the lachrymal point and passing a drip. It should be remembered that in a congenital glaucoma case, there is always photophobia, tearing, blepharospasm [1, 2], increased axial length, and reversible optic nerve cupping.

Megalocornea

Megalocornea may simulate congenital glaucoma and lead to confusion in the diagnosis. In general, the corneal diameter is greater than 14 mm, which leads to the anterior chamber being deeper, and to iridodonesis, but it does not present ocular hypertension, increased axial length, or reversible ON cupping. The chamber angle is normal. There are rare cases of families in which some members have glaucoma and others megalocornea.

Rubeola

This inflammatory disease in mothers may cause a chamber angle anomaly identical to that in congenital glaucoma with ocular hypertension, which responds to antiglaucoma operations. However, these cases are differentiated by cataract, deafness, cardiac anomalies, and mental retardation. Nevertheless, there are cases, generally occurring when the rubeola virus infection occurs in the first 3 months of pregnancy, where these alterations are not present and the risk of confusion is greater.

Obstetric Trauma

Often when the child is extracted with forceps, there is a breakage of the endothelium and the Descemet membrane (Haab's striae). These striae are generally unilateral.

Myopia

In general, it is very difficult to differentiate myopia from congenital glaucoma [3]. Echometry can help, since in glaucoma the anterior chamber, the length of the vitreous, and axial length are noticeably increased, but the lens is less thick, which does not occur in myopia. It should also be remembered that in myopia there is no hypertension.

Corticoids and Ocular Pressure

History

The first case of glaucoma described was provoked by the use of cortisone in patients who had been treated for long periods as a result of a uveitis or spring conjunctivitis [4].

Lijó-Pavía [5] described the first case in Argentina. Similar situations were presented by Dejean et al. [6]. In 1953, Stern [7] reported acute glaucoma produced by the application of cortisone administered locally. In 1954, Covell [8] published a paper on glaucoma produced by systemic corticosteroid therapy. In 1954, François published a study on cortisone and ocular pressure, and in 1962, Goldmann et al. [9] reported the characteristics of the disease in six patients and called it cortisone glaucoma.

Becker [10] and Armaly [11, 12] classified the population by their response to cortisone as high, medium, or low, and concluded that this response was hereditary. This interpretation is not currently accepted, because of identical twin studies conducted by Schwartz et al. [13, 14], and because the response to corticoids can be produced only in the group that reacts with high pressure [15].

Glaucoma has also been described as provoked by corticoids when they are applied internally: MacLean [16], Woods [17], Laval and Collier [18]. These authors reported that corticoids used internally can provoke or worsen glaucoma.

Discussing a study by Bárany on the exit of aqueous humor, Chandler [19] said that cortisone treatment given internally can hamper the control of simple chronic glaucoma. Berstein and Schwartz [20] found a statistically significant slight increase in ocular pressure in 48 patients who, for various reasons, were submitted to long-term corticoid treatments.

Glaucomas have also been described that originated from endogenous corticoids. Bayer [21] and Bayer and Neuner [22] showed glaucoma in patients with subtotal adrenalectomie in suprarenal glands, and Haas and Nootens in a case of Cushing's syndrome [23].

Physiopathology

Bárany [24] showed that locally applied hyaluronidase acts on the hyaluronic acid of the trabecular meshwork, depolymerizing it and increasing the exit of aqueous humor from the anterior chamber. Corticoids have an antihyaluronidase action and thus act on the trabecular meshwork, reducing the ease of the outflow of aqueous humor.

In cortisone glaucoma, aqueous humor exit is reduced because of an alteration of the trabecular meshwork. The amount of already existing polymerized glycosaminoglycans (hyaluronic acid) in the trabecular meshwork increases, because degradation (depolymerization) fails. This alteration occurs because of the inhibition of the release of enzymes contained in the lys-

osomes in the cellular cytoplasm that are responsible for depolymerization. The inhibition of enzyme release is produced by the stabilization of the lysosome membrane provoked by corticoids (the stabilizing action of the membrane has been demonstrated experimentally). Another theory in 1975 suggested that the corticoids block phagocytosis of the trabecular meshwork by the endothelial cells (this is their normal function, called self-cleaning).

The third theory was developed by Yun et al. [25], who suggest that the increase in elastin observed in human trabecular meshwork cells, cultivated intra- and extracellularly after being treated with dexamethasone, could be related to a possible obstructive mechanism in the drainage system of the aqueous humor. Quaranta and Serafini [26] showed that, in this type of glaucoma, intraocular pressure increases because in tonography the value of C is reduced.

Clinical Picture

Describing his first six cases, Goldmann [9] listed the characteristics as an open-angle glaucoma, with generally high ocular hypertension, in white eyes, with optic disc pallor but without cupping, and uncharacteristic lesions of the visual field.

In cortisone glaucomas, there are no symptoms. It is like open-angle glaucoma, with the diagnosis generally made fortuitously when measuring ocular pressure. These patients have often been treated for months or years for conjunctivitis, blepharitis, uveitis, or intolerance to contact lenses. Weekers et al. [27] also studied it from this point of view.

Development

Almost all the cases improved after 2–4 weeks, simply by interrupting corticoid use. In others, however, this improvement did not occur and in these patients, chronic irreversible glaucoma was established.

In many cases in which removing the corticoid led to normalization of ocular pressure, the visual field defects persist irreversibly. It should be remembered that today these patients are confused with normal-pressure or low-tension glaucoma and become part of the great arsenal of these diagnoses that we described in Chap. 1 as glaucomas that are inactive as a result of local medication.

Treatment

Treatment can be reversible:
1. Corticoid suppression;
2. Antiglaucoma medical therapy;
3. Subconjunctival hyaluronidase.

Or irreversible:
4. Surgical therapy.

Any fistulizing surgical therapy can be chosen, but it should be stressed that Bietti and Quaranta [28] used goniotomy in eight cases of irreversible corticoid glaucoma, seven of which obtained perfect regulation of ocular pressure and thus could continue using corticoids. We currently prefer trabeculotomy and, if necessary, trabeculectomy.

Prophylaxis

Any local application of corticoids must be accompanied by precise indications and strict monitoring of ocular pressure. Careless self-medication in cases of contact lenses, conjunctivitis, etc., which is common today, and even treatment indicated by general clinicians, should be avoided (Table 19.1).

In extreme cases, the use of FML (fluorometholone) has a greater anti-inflammatory effect and does not cause ocular hypertension. Flurbiprofen (Tolerane, Plos NR), which is a corticoid and analgesic anti-inflammatory, is in our opinion the best medication today.

Table 19.1 Side effects of corticoids

General	Ocular	
	Oral	Local
Pseudo-Cushing's syndrome	Cataracts	Glaucoma
Activation of peptic ulcer	Optic disc edema	Keratitis
Aggravation of diabetes		
Sodium retention		
Acute pancreatitis		
Susceptibility to infections		
Iatrogenic suprarenal insufficiency		
Reactivation of tubercular foci		

Clinical History No. 1

The following clinical history is an example of corti-sone glaucoma.

This 16-year-old female, had a history of toxoplas-mosis (bilateral peripheral uveitis). She received gen-eral and local corticoids for 4 years. The left eye pre-sented a slight dysgenesis in the chamber angle, with pathological mesodermal tissue up to the spur, an anomaly not present in the right eye, with visual acuity 200/200, ocular pressure 14 mmHg, and normal daily pressure curve. The left eye has the following features, as well as the gonioscopic elements mentioned above, corresponding to the first examination at the time the patient was referred to us in 1974.

	Left eye
IOP	42 mmHg with maximum medication 1 g. of acetazolamide per day
Visual acuity	−1 at 0°: 20/80
Anterior chamber	3.5 mm
Optic disc	Cupping 4/6
Visual field (Goldmann)	Only exclusion of blind spot

Faced with irreductible levels of tension and a reduction of visual acuity, I made a trabeculectomy. From then on, ocular pressure was regulated around 16 mmHg with the diurnal pressure curve at normal values and visual acuity reached 20/60.

The pathological anatomy of the trabeculectomy piece can be seen in Fig. 19.1.

In 1988, after missing check-ups for 3 years, she re-turned at age 30 because of reduced vision in the left eye. Visual acuity had fallen to less than 20/200 because of a cortisone posterior subcapsular cataract. In 1989, I inserted an intraocular lens, achieving visual acuity of 20/40, and she has maintained ocular pressure within normal limits to date, 2008.

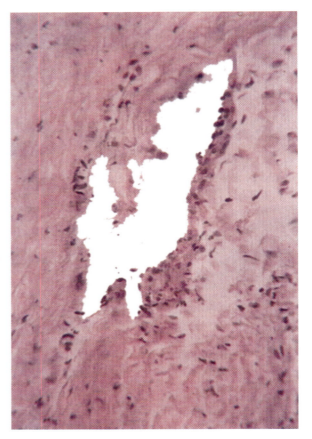

Fig. 19.1 Pathological anatomy

Pseudocongenital Cortisone Glaucoma

Cortisone glaucoma in the newborn child in the first 2 years of age is relatively frequent.

Congenital obstruction of the lacrimal ducts, which is generally resolved with a needle to inject physiological solution in the upper and lower tear points and, more rarely, probing the tear duct with a Bangerter probe, does not require corticoids. Unfortunately, clinicians, family doctors, and pediatricians prescribe cortisone abundantly, with dexamethasone eye drops several times a day for months, and unleash an iatrogenic glaucoma known as pseudocongenital cortisone glaucoma. The same happens with other newborn children with uveitis, conjunctivitis, blepharitis, dacryocystitis, with equally disastrous results. It should be added that in some cases they coincide with a congenital glaucoma, with lacrimal duct obstruction and, in this case, the ophthalmologist must resolve both pathologies. Therefore, it is essential that any clinician or pediatrician treating a newborn with tearing or photophobia should immediately refer them to an ophthalmologist.

Symptoms

Signs and symptoms similar to those of congenital glaucoma appear at once: increased ocular pressure, increased axial length, deeper anterior chamber, and thinner crystalline lens. Sometimes there is an increase in corneal diameters in advanced cases with long-term treatment of 8 months or more and breakages of the Descemet membrane and endothelium. Glaucoma cupping of the optic disc can also be seen as in congenital glaucomas. This cortisone glaucoma is distinguished from pure congenital glaucoma by the chamber angle, which is absolutely normal.

The clinical picture is sometimes solved by suspending the corticoids, but this is rare. Generally it is necessary to operate, and this condition responds remarkably well to trabeculotomy.

If the chamber angle presents the elements of congenital glaucoma (type 1 or type 2 angle) with pathological mesodermal remnants, this is not a case of pseudocongenital cortisone glaucoma but of a congenital glaucoma in which corticoids have contributed to bringing it out or have worsened it. François published a comment on a 1973 study by Bietti questioning whether it was possible for one of the cases described by the latter to develop pseudocongenital cortisone glaucoma with an increase in axial length. We are inclined to favor Bietti's description, because in our clinical experience we have seen that the axial length continues increasing from birth to 4.5 years of age.

There are two fundamental studies on this topic in the literature: Gnad and Martenet's, of Zurich, in 1973 [29] and that of Calixto, presented in the 95th meeting of the French Society of Ophthalmology, in 1984. The literature also contains other interesting studies on this subject: Alfano [30], Bietti [31], Mascaro et al. [32], Calixto and Cronemberg [33], and Kass et al. [34].

The following clinical history is an example of pseudocongenital cortisone glaucoma:

Clinical History No. 2

A 6-month-old male presented with conjunctivitis with photophobia and epiphora in the left eye at the age of 6 days. The pediatrician, without consulting the ophthalmologist, gave him hydrocortisone in eye drops, 0.5 g four times a day for 1 month and the following 3 months dexamethasone 0.1 g four times a day, also in eye drops. At 4 months, the mother noticed that the left eye was larger than the right eye and took him to the ophthalmologist, who referred him to the university hospital.

	Right eye	Left eye
Axial length	20.73 mm	22.52 mm
IOP	12 mmHg	26 mmHg
Corneal diameter	11.5 mm	11.5 mm
Chamber angle	Normal	Normal
Surgery		A trabeculotomy was performed

See Fig. 19.2 for echometry. Follow-up continued until the child reached 4 years of age. Ocular pressure was controlled at normal values and the echography showed good progress.

It is remarkable that in this case the examination of the fundus shows the optic disc with a cupping of 5/6 (Recas classification) in the left eye as opposed to the normal cup of the other eye of 1/6. The visual field cannot be determined yet, and acuity is 20/30 in the unoperated eye and 20/40 in the operated eye.

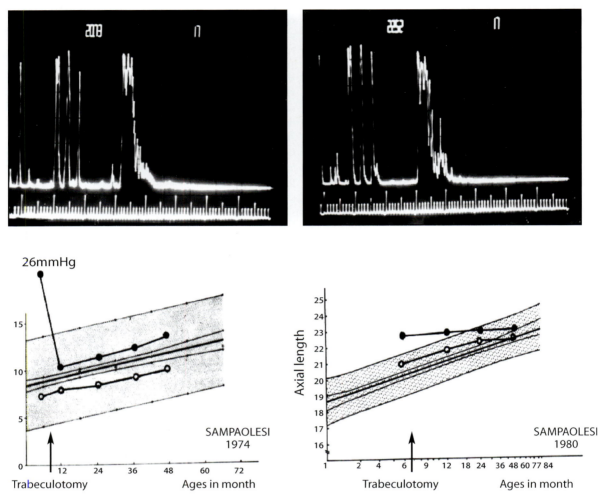

Fig. 19.2 Development of ocular pressure and axial length of both eyes

Clinical History No. 3

A 6-month-old male presented with pseudocongenital cortisone glaucoma with a completely normal chamber angle. Trabeculotomy was done in the left eye.

For echometry results, see Fig. 19.3.

	Right eye (normal)	Left eye (pseudocongenital cortisone glaucoma)
IOP	10 mmHg	20 mmHg
Chamber angle	Normal	Normal
Axial length	22.42	24.67
Cornea	0.56	0.77
Anterior chamber	2.21	3.02
Thickness of lens	4.39	3.87

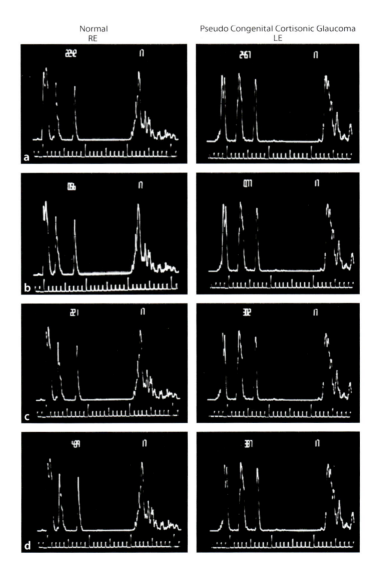

Fig. 19.3a–d Morphological alteration of the dimensions of the eye is identical to that in pure congenital glaucoma, as it has increased its axial length (a), the cornea is thicker because of the edema (b), the anterior chamber is deeper (c) and the lens is thinner (d)

Clinical History No. 4

A 16-month-old male was treated for conjunctivitis and dacryocystitis of the newborn at the age of 10 months with cortisone drops, three or more times per day, and then for 6 months, once a day. The ophthalmologist performed a lacrimal probe. Photophobia and tearing persisted.

	Right eye	Left eye
IOP	30 mmHg	28 mmHg
Corneal diameter	12 mm	12 mm
Descemet membrane and endothelium	Normal	Haab striae
Chamber angle	Normal	Normal
Surgery	Trabeculotomy	Trabeculotomy

The child recovered in 1 week, the symptoms disappeared, and ocular pressure was regulated between 10 and 14 mmHg. Since age 7, a diurnal pressure curve has been made annually, which always shows normal values both in the mean and in the variability. The progression of the axial length since surgery is shown in Fig. 19.4a.

At age 11 (1991), the condition of the optic nerve can be seen in Fig. 19.4b and 19.4c. Remember that the right eye was slightly larger than the left eye and had suffered more, as it presented tears in the paracentral endothelium and Descemet membrane. This led to a different surgical therapy since, while in the right eye only trabeculotomy was performed, in the left eye combined surgery was undertaken: trabeculotomy and trabeculectomy, despite the good visual acuity in both eyes (right eye, visual acuity, 20/200 with cylinder −0.50 at 10° and left eye, 20/200 with cyl. −0.50 at 170°). The optic disc cupping is asymmetric, barely 1/3 in the right eye and slightly more than 4/6 in the left eye.

In addition, the good acuity with ocular dimensions at 11 years of age, above normal, indicates the emmetropization that takes place in eyes with glaucoma, which distends the ocular globe in the first months of life.

In summary, it is remarkable that with an almost equal mean defect in both eyes, the optic disc of the left eye, which is longer, showed much more cupping than the right eye's disc, the axial length was greater and had tears in the Descemet membrane, i.e., the visual field in this case is not an index to know which eye is the most damaged, whereas the optic disc, the Descemet tears, and the axial length can provide this indication. It should also be emphasized that both eyes with a myopia below 1 diopter (D) had emmetropization.

In Fig. 19.5, the visual fields made with Octopus 2000 in 1991, show a greater mean defect (MD) in the left eye (4 dB).

The pathological anatomy also confirmed the diagnosis (Fig. 19.6).

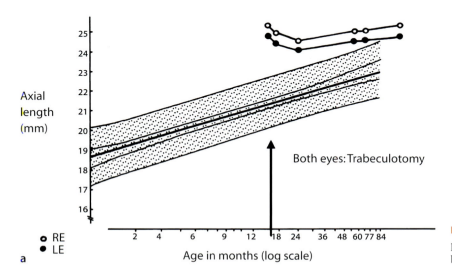

a

○ RE
● LE

Both eyes: Trabeculotomy

Axial length (mm)

Age in months (log scale)

Fig. 19.4a–c Clinical history no. 5, progression of the axial length can be followed in this graph

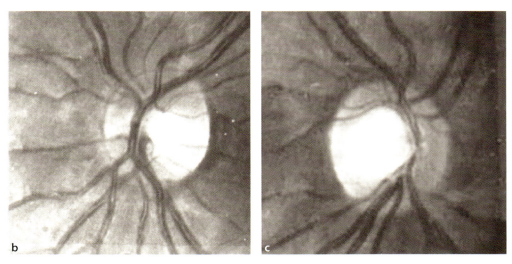

Fig. 19.4a–c (*continued*)

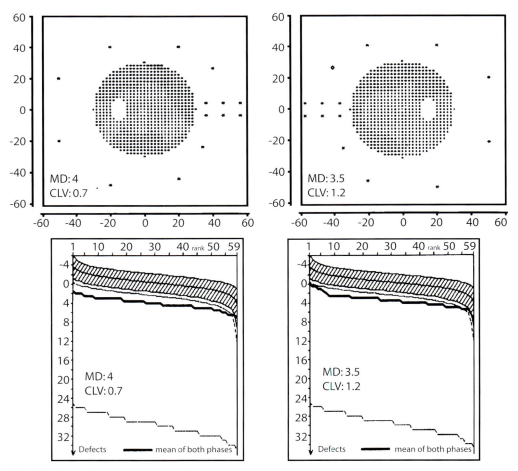

Fig. 19.5 Clinical history no. 5, visual fields

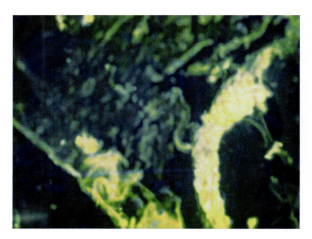

Fig. 19.6 Clinical history no. 5, pathological anatomy. Material placed in dry ice (30'), later inclusion in Tissue-tek, placed in cryostat. Semi-serial 3- to 6-μm sections. Staining with hematoxylin and eosin and incubation at 5°C (15 h) with C3, IgG, IgA, and IgM, conjugated with fluorescein isothiocyanate. Microscopy: partial piece of sinusectomy that includes scleral flap, the Schlemm canal, and trabecular meshwork, lax in parts and with sectors partially homogenized. With immunofluorescence techniques, a strong, dense granular deposit of C3 can be seen at trabecular level. There are scant deposits of IgG at trabecular level. IgA and IgM are negative

References

1. Becker B, Shaffer RN (1965) Diagnosis and therapy of congenital glaucoma. Mosby, St. Louis

2. Kolker AE, Hetherington J (1976) Diagnosis and therapy of glaucoma. Mosby, St. Louis, pp 276–321

3. Sampaolesi R, Caruso R (1982) Ocular echometry in the diagnosis of congenital glaucoma. Arch Ophthalmol 100:574–577

4. François J (1954) Cortisone et tension oculaire. Ann Ocul 187:805

5. Lijo-Pavia 1 (1952) Cortisona y tensión ocular. Rev Oto-Neurooftal B Aires 27:14

6. Dejean C, Viallefont H, Champion J, Vidal L (1952) De l'action aggravante de l'acth et de la cortisone sur l'hypertension oculaire. Montpellier Med 41:38

7. Stern J (1953) 1. Acute glaucoma during cortisone therapy. Am J Ophthalmol 36:389–390

8. Covell LL (1958) Glaucoma induced by systemic steroid therapy. Am J Ophthalmol 45:108–109

9. Goldmann H (1962) Cortisone glaucoma. Arch Ophthal 68:621

10. Becker B (1965) Intraocular pressure response to topical corticosteroids. Invest Ophthalmol 4:198–220

11. Armaly MF (1966) The heritable nature of dexamethasone induced ocular hypertension. Arch Ophthalmol 75:32–35

12. Armaly MF (1967) Inheritance of dexamethasone hypertension and glaucoma. Arch Ophthalmol 77:747–752

13. Schwartz JT, Reuling FH, Feinleib M et al (1973) Twin study on ocular pressure after topical dexamethasone. 1. Frequency distribution of pressure response. Am J Ophthalmol 76:126–136

14. Schwartz JT, Reuling FH, Feinleib M et al (1973) Twin study on ocular pressure following topically applied dexamethasone. II. Inheritance of variations in pressure responses. Arch Ophthalmol 90:281–286

15. Palmberg PF, Mandell A, Wilensky JT et al (1975) The reproducibility of the intraocular pressure response to dexamethasone. Am J Ophthalmol 80:844–856

16. McLean IM (1950) Discussion of the communication of AC Woods. Trans Am Ophthalmol Soc 48:259–296

17. Woods AC (1951) The present status of the ACTH and cortisone in clinical ophthalmology. Am J Ophthalmol 34:945–960

18. Laval J, Collier R Jr (1955) Elevation of intraocular pressure due to hormonal steroid therapy in uveitis. Am J Ophthalmol 39:175–182

19. Chandler P (1955) In glaucoma. Josiah Macy Jr Foundation, New York

20. Bernstein HN, Schwartz B (1962) Effects of long term systemic steroids on ocular pressure and tonographic values. Arch Ophthalmol 68:742–753

21. Bayer JM (1959) Ergebnisse und Beurteilung der subtotalen Adrenalektomie beim hyperfunktions-Cushing, Langenbecks Arch Klin Chir 291:531

22. Bayer JM, Neuner NP (1967) Cushing-Syndrom und erhöhter Augeninnendruck. Dtsch Med Wochenschr 92:1971

23. Haas JSY, Nootens RH (1974) Glaucoma secondary to benign adrenal adenoma. Am J Ophthalmol 78:497–500

24. Barany EH (1955) Glaucoma. The physiology and pathology of the filtering angle. Masson, Paris, pp 91–102

25. Yun AJ, Murphy CG, Polansky JR, Newsome DA, Alvarado JA (1989) Proteins secreted by human trabecular cells. Invest Ophthal 30:2012–2022

26. Quaranta CA, Serafini S (1963) Indagini tonografiche in corso di stati ipertensivi oculari da terapia cortisonica locale. Atti Soc Oftalmol Ital 21:294

27. Weekers R, Grieten J, Watillon M, Prijot E (1964) Les formes cliniques des glaucomes dus à la cortisone. Ophthalmologica 148:81–90

28. Bietti GB, Quaranta CA (1966) Considerazioni sulla terapia di particolari forme di "glaucoma de cortisone" con speciale riguardo a quella chirurgica mediante goniotomia. Doc Ophthalmol 20:25–271

29. Gnad HD, Martenet AC (1973) Kongenitales Glaukom und Cortison. Klin Mbl Augenheilk 162:86–90

30. Alfano JE, Plait D (1966) Steroid (ACTH)-induced glaucoma simulating congenital glaucoma. Am J Ophthalmol 61:911–912

31. Bieiti GB, Quaranta CA, Bucci MG, Roll A (1973) Contribution au tableau clinique du glaucome cortisonique et à son traitement. Bull Mem Soc Ophthalmol Fr 86:167–173

32. Mascaro F Quintana M, Zamora M (1980) Glaucoma congenital iatrogenique. Bull Mem Soc Ophthalmol Fr 92:215–217

33. Calixto NE, Cronemberger Sobrinho A (1981) Glaucoma cortisonico; Etudo de 15 casos. Rev Bras Oftalmol 40:19–42

34. Kass MA, Kolker AE, Becker B (1972) Chronic topical corticosteroid use simulating congenital glaucoma. J Pediatr 81:1175–1177

Contents

Late Congenital Glaucoma: Goniodysgenesis

The diagnosis of late congenital glaucoma is basically made through the chamber angle. These are children over 6 years of age, young people, or adults up to 45 years of age, presenting persistence of pathologic mesodermal tissue reaching at least to the spur, the trabecular meshwork, the height of the Schlemm canal, or even further up to the Schwalbe line. The most outstanding sign in gonioscopy is the absence of the ciliary body band, which may be total or partial. This is a fetal alteration of the development of the iridocorneal angle called goniodysgenesis and it is accompanied by a halt in the development of the superficial mesodermal layer of the iris that enables the radial vascular and avascular columns of the deep iris to be seen, and at the avascular columns, the black triangles can be seen corresponding to the posterior pigmentary epithelium of the iris. In general, peripheral atrophy of the superficial layer of the iris is visible.

At other times, there is mesodermal tissue, but its appearance is modified: it looks like a grayish white band. This led Busacca to name this metaplasia of the mesodermal tissue. Even though he includes it in child congenital glaucoma, we have rarely seen it there. Moreover, Busacca and Carvalho [1] describe metaplasia of the mesodermal tissue in 28 cases, 22 of whom were adults and only six were children.

Heredity is dominant in late congenital glaucomas, contrary to what occurs in pure congenital cases in newborns. The most important difference with pure congenital cases in newborns is that in these cases the axial length is increased, and in late congenital glaucomas the axial length of the eye is normal.

Clinical experience shows that in addition to the cases we have described, in which the dimensions of the anterior segment are normal with an open angle, there are others that also have late onset but present enlargement of the cornea and at times of the eye as a whole. Heredity is dominant in these as well, but hypertension must surely have been present since childhood without giving rise to noticeable signs, because functionally the eye compensates in part for the defect [2]. Patients come late to consultation, with a transparent cornea, good vision, very high ocular pressure, and a highly damaged visual field.

Kniestedt et al.'s article [3] is useful to consult. We also advise reading the book *Goniodysgenesis* by Jerndal et al. [4], which is the most complete work on this topic, as well as the work of Boles Carenini [5].

It is very important to be able to recognize this clinical form of glaucoma, since, if the ocular pressure is not regulated, as occurs in some cases, surgery will be necessary, and special care will have to be taken in the location of the incision and in the transillumination (the Minsky maneuver), to avoid severe complications that are a consequence of the malformation of the chamber angle (Table 20.1).

Table 20.1 Goniodysgenesis

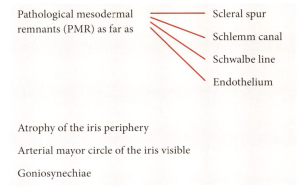

Pathological mesodermal remnants (PMR) as far as — Scleral spur / Schlemm canal / Schwalbe line / Endothelium

Atrophy of the iris periphery

Arterial mayor circle of the iris visible

Goniosynechiae

Gloor's team [3] found goniodysgenesis in 48%–77% of adults, in open angle glaucoma.

Figure 20.1a illustrates the chamber angle, where a new element, the pathological mesodermal remnants (1), appears, located between the outer and inner wall of the angle, in the recess of the angle, which are chestnut or brown in color.

In Fig. 20.1b, a goniophotograph of the angle shows (1) pathological mesodermal remnants, (2) the last circular fold of the iris, and (3) the Schlemm canal. It is quite clear that the mesodermal remnants completely hide the ciliary body band; therefore, goniodysgenesis is defined as a lack of visibility of the ciliary body band.

Figure 20.2a shows a diagram and 20.2b a goniophotograph of a normal angle. The iris processes can be seen, reaching the spur and leaving the ciliary body band perfectly visible behind in a bluish color. Figure 20.2c illustrates goniodysgenesis: the pathological mesodermal remnants can be seen hiding the entire ciliary body band.

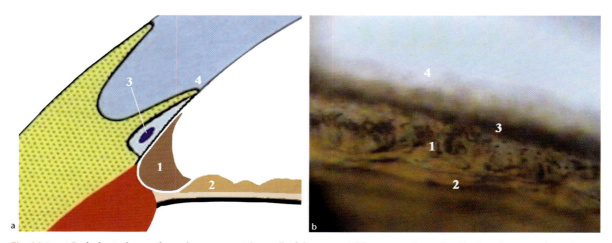

Fig. 20.1 a *1* Pathological mesodermal remnants; *2* last roll of the iris; *3* Schlemm canal; *4* Schwalbe line. **b** *1* Mesodermal remnants; *2* last roll of the iris; *3* Schlemm canal

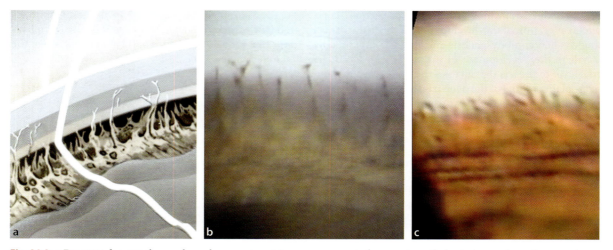

Fig. 20.2 a Diagram; **b** normal mesodermal remnants; **c** iris processes, goniodysgenesis, pathological mesodermal remnants

The iris root is inserted, as can be seen in the upper part of Fig. 20.3, always in the internal face of the ciliary body, in hyperopic patients in the anterior part of the face, in emmetropic patients in the middle, and in myopics in the rear part, but always in the internal face of the ciliary body. The pathological congenital remnants occupy the recess of the angle in front of the iris root.

Even in type II congenital glaucomas, mistakenly called high iris insertion, which should be called apparent high insertion of the iris, since, as can be seen in Fig. 20.3b, the root adheres to the lower wall of the angle, and when it is seen with the gonioscope, it seems to insert itself at the level of the Schwalbe line.

Kluyskens [6] wrote: *"Most writers, even the most careful ones, observing the angle in cases of congenital glaucoma, have the impression that the iris is inserted higher than normal, but in fact it is not a case of an insertion abnormally high from the base of the iris, which is always in its normal position, but of the presence in the recess of the angle of an abnormal tissue that gives this false appearance."*

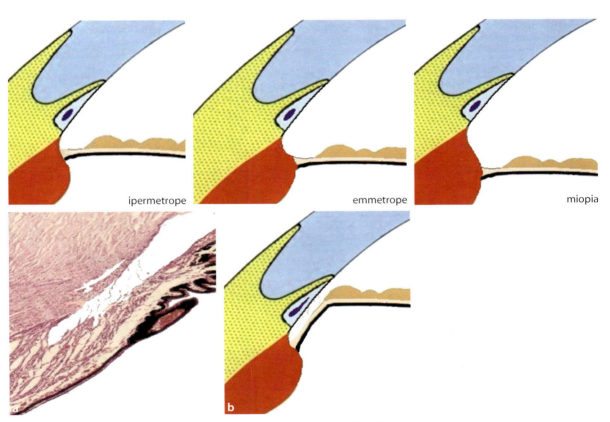

Fig. 20.3a,b In the *upper part, left*, iris insertion in the internal face of the ciliary muscle in hypermetropia. In the *center* in emmetropia and on the *right* in myopia. **a** At the *bottom*, histology of an apparent high insertion of the iris. **b** Diagram of this histological preparation

Purscher, in correspondence to Busacca, presented a personal study on this matter in which he shows that the iris insertion is always on the internal face of the ciliary body, showing this histologically. Figure 20.4 shows the goniophotograph of a case of goniodysgenesis with a great atrophy of the iris and an apparent insertion of the iris at the level of the scleral spur.

Figure 20.5 shows a goniophotograph of pigmentary glaucoma (late congenital glaucoma, or goniodysgenesis) and apparent high insertion of the iris at the spur.

In 2000, Prof. Balder Gloor's team [3] wrote a very important paper on dysgenetic chamber alterations in patients with glaucoma or suspect glaucoma before 40 years of age. They used 200 eyes of 104 patients who had been examined but were now reexamined and photographed with Roussell and Fankhauser's CGA-1 gonioscopic lens. In 24 of these 200 eyes (12%), slight goniodysgenesis was found, in 81 eyes (40.5%) intermediate goniodysgenesis, and in 49 eyes (24.5%) severe goniodysgenesis. On reexamination, the number

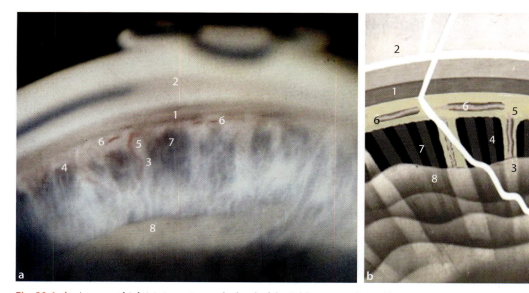

Fig. 20.4a,b Apparent high iris insertion at the level of the Schlemm canal. *1* Schlemm canal, *2* Schwalbe line, *3* vascular pillars, *4* avascular pillars, *5* vessel in vascular pillars, *6* major arterial circle of the visible iris, *7* black triangles (pigment epithelium of the posterior face of the iris), *8* last roll of the iris, *SP* scleral spur

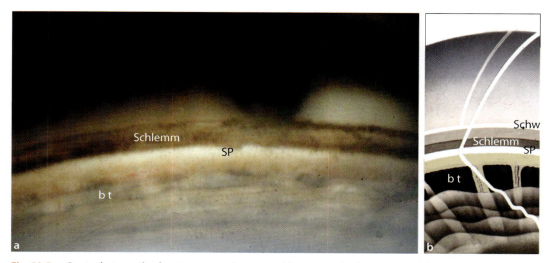

Fig. 20.5 **a** Goniophotograph of a pigmentary glaucoma with apparent high insertion of the iris at the scleral. This is similar to type I congenital glaucoma. **b** Diagram of the same

of dysgeneses increased from 48% to 78%. They concluded that the high frequency of dysgenetic changes in the chamber angle of glaucoma patients affected under the age of 40 suggests that in this age group developmental glaucoma is predominant and has to be separated as a special entity from POAG. Two questions arise: (1) were these dysgenetic changes overlooked most of the time in the newer genetic studies of patients with GLC1A? (2) If not, do patients suspected of having glaucoma and patients with open-angle glaucoma before the age of 40 with and without dysgenetic changes belong to groups with different glaucoma genes, those with dysgenetic changes belonging to genes IRID1 and IRID2 and those without belonging to genes GLC1A to GLC1F?

The following figures, reproduced with the permission of Prof. Gloor, show great similarity with those that we reproduced on the pages above (Figs. 20.6, 20.7, 20.8).

When the diagnosis is goniodysgenesis, however slight it may be, it is important to investigate the presence of glaucoma thoroughly using all the corresponding studies. The presence of this phenotype in the angle suggests the existence of a glaucomatous genotype.

We studied 27 cases up to 1994 (the second edition of Sampaolesi 1994) and the most interesting will be presented here. We wish to emphasize that six of the 27 patients had pigmentary glaucoma. Of 46 cases, only 20 patients were 6–25 years of age; the others were adults.

We present two very interesting clinical cases: one is a 7-year-old child with late congenital glaucoma in whom I operated both eyes at the same time (see Chap. 17, clinical history no. 37). The second is a 45-year-old female, clinical history no. 5 below.

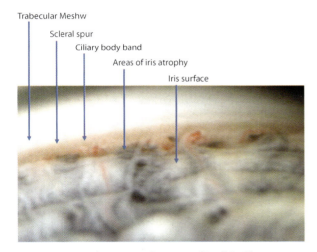

Fig. 20.6 Goniodysgenesis. Courtesy of Prof. B. Gloor

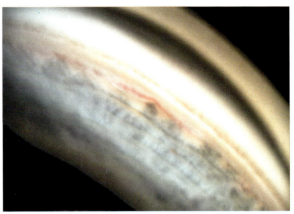

Fig. 20.7 Goniodysgenesis. Courtesy of Prof. B. Gloor

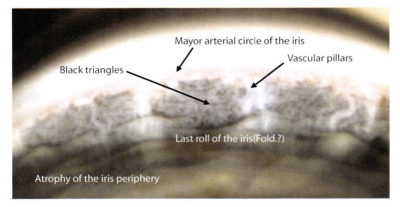

Fig. 20.8 Goniodysgenesis. Courtesy of Prof. B. Gloor

Clinical Cases

Late Congenital Glaucomas in Young People

Clinical history No. 1 was a 21-year-old female sent to us from the Clinical Medicine department to study her visual field, with a diagnosis of Turner syndrome; pterygium colli, amenorrhea, menstrual period presenting only after medical treatment at age 15, and remaining only if the treatment was not interrupted. The patient presented harmonious dwarfism, gonadal dysgenesis, infantilism (womb, labia minora, lack of hair in the pubis and armpits), as well as reddish chestnut color marks on the face and arms. The karyotype was XO.

	Right eye	Left eye
Visual acuity	Sph. +0.50 = 20/20	Sph. +0.50 = 20/20
IOP	19 mmHg	24 mmHg
Anisocoria	Pupil 4 mm	Pupil 5.5 mm
Corneal diameter	11 mm	12 mm
Diffuse limbus		In the upper temporal and lower nasal quadrants
Tonography C1.3~7	0.13	0.09
Visual field	Normal	Exclusion of the blind spot and Bjerrum scotoma
Funduscopy	Normal	Disc excavation 5/6 Nasal border < 1/3
Chamber angle	Normal	Severe goniodysgenesis

Late Congenital Glaucomas in Adults

Clinical history No. 2 was a 49-year-old female who presented glaucoma in the right eye, diagnosed 3 years before as chronic congestive glaucoma. She was operated three times by other colleagues abroad. The first operation was an Elliot operation at 12 o'clock with iridectomy in the sector. The second operation was an Elliot operation with lower basal iridectomy, and the third was a cyclodiathermy.

At the time of examination, the patient's IOP had remained under control for 3 years, with a daily pressure curve in the right eye at a mean 15 mmHg, variability, 3 mmHg, and in the left eye at a mean 14 mmHg, variability, 0.5 mmHg. Tonographic values were normal.

	Right eye	Left eye
Visual acuity	20/25	20/20
IOP	60 mmHg	16 mmHg
Tonography C1.3~7	0.02	0.15
Visual field	Loss of the upper half of the visual field maintaining the macula, with exclusion of the optic disk	Normal
Funduscopy	Glaucomatous excavation 5/6. Temporal border 0.5/3	Normal
Chamber angle	Alterations in chamber angle development in lower nasal sector with depression of the iris, severe goniodysgenesis, and atrophy at the periphery of the iris	Normal
Surgery	Trabeculectomy	

Clinical history No. 3 was a 42-year-old female presented glaucoma in the left eye with lower nasal coloboma of the iris and posterior embryotoxon.

	Right eye	Left eye
Patient		
IOP		50 mmHg
Funduscopy		Excavation of optic disc 5/6, great loss of visual field
Patient's sister		
IOP	35 mmHg	28 mmHg
Chamber angle	Severe goniodysgenesis	Severe goniodysgenesis
Visual field	Loss of visual field: Seidel's scotoma	Loss of visual field: Bjerrum scotoma
Surgery	Trabeculectomy	Trabeculectomy

Her 30-year-old sister accompanied the patient. Knowing the importance of the hereditary factor we examined her. She showed in both eyes a severe goniodysgenesis and an IOP of 35 mmHg and 28 mmHg, loss of visual field and it was necessary to perform Trabeculectomy in both eyes.

Clinical history No. 4 was another 42-year-old female. The patient presented a pigmentary retinopathy, albinism, and bilateral glaucoma.

	Right eye	Left eye
Visual acuity	Sph. +1 = 20/200	Finger counting
IOP	24 mmHg	60 mmHg
Funduscopy	Characteristic of a pigmentary retinopathy in albino	Characteristic of a pigmentary retinopathy in albino
Visual field	Typical of a pigmentary retinopathy	Typical of a pigmentary retinopathy
Chamber angle	Severe goniodysgenesis Deformation of the frill of the iris in the lower nasal zone	Severe goniodysgenesis Deformation of the frill of the iris in the lower nasal zone

As we have just seen in the clinical histories presented, in many of the gonioscopies in the lower nasal zone, there was a peripheral depression of the iris with displacement of its root in the form of a hollow or depression. At other times, there were colobomas of the superficial layer of the iris or a change in iris color in the same place. These observations led us to investigate this sign, and that we call late congenital glaucoma with lower nasal malformation.

Clinical history No. 5 was a 45-year-old woman. This patient consulted at age 28 to see if she had glaucoma, because of the considerable family background she had (Fig. 20.9). Her grandfather was operated for glaucoma in both eyes and was left blind.

	Right eye	Left eye
IOP	24 mmHg with medication	24 mmHg with medication
Visual acuity	Finger counting	Finger counting
Refraction	Esf. −3.50, Cil. −1 to 176°: 20/25	Esf. −3, Cil −2 to 1.5°: 20/25
ON (HRT)	Phase IV	Phase III
Conventional visual field	Normal	Borderline
Unconventional visual field	Stage III	Stage II
Gonioscopy	Goniodysgenesis 360°	Goniodysgenesis 360° (Fig.20.10)

Figure 20.11, corresponding to the right eye, shows that the ON is in phase IV, the conventional visual field is normal, and the nonconventional visual field is in phase III. For ophthalmologists who think that glaucoma is an alteration of the ON and the visual field and who work with conventional perimetry, the diagnosis in this case is ocular hypertension. For those who work with nonconventional perimetry, the diagnosis is glaucoma, since the ON lesion topographically corresponds to the VF lesion made with nonconventional frequency doubling perimetry. Since this patient was on the maximum medication – prostaglandins, carbon anhydrase inhibitors, and beta blockers did not regulate IOP – we performed surgery: deep nonpenetrating sclerectomy and goniopuncture with Yag laser. The pressure regulated at 12 mmHg and the DTC was normal following surgery.

We stress here that this patient was on medication for 17 years while her ON and her VF were deteriorating. We believe that she will not have the same fate as her glaucomatous forebears.

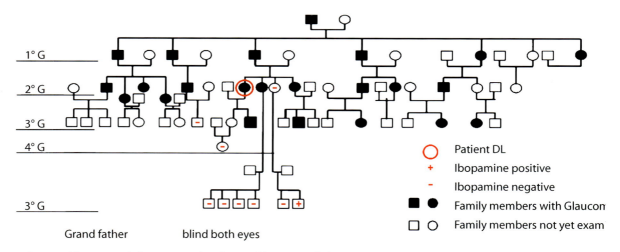

4 sons with operated glaucoma, 2 daughters with operated glaucoma, 1 normal daughter
14 grand children, 4 male with glaucoma, 10 females, 7 with glaucoma, 3 normal
27 grand grand children, 21 males, 2 with glaucoma, 6 females, 3 with glaucoma

Fig. 20.9 Family tree of the patient in Clinical History No. 5

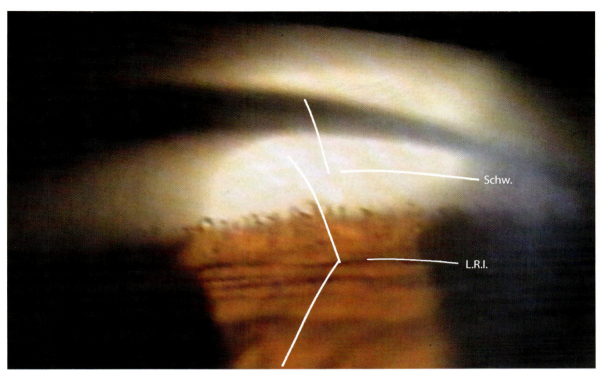

Fig. 20.10 Goniodysgenesis 360º. *Schw* Schwalbe line. *LRI* last roll of the iris. It is a dysgenesis in which the pathological meso-dermal tissue extends from the last circular fold of the iris as far as the coneoscleral trabeculum. The mesodermal remnants cover completely the scleral spur

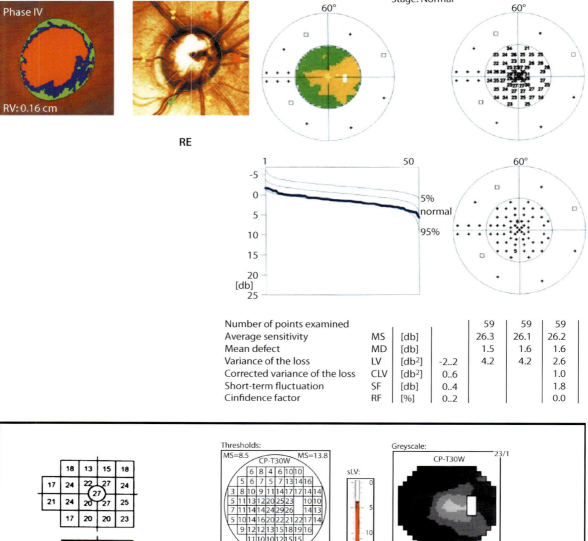

Number of points examined				59	59	59
Average sensitivity	MS	[db]		26.3	26.1	26.2
Mean defect	MD	[db]		1.5	1.6	1.6
Variance of the loss	LV	[db²]	-2..2	4.2	4.2	2.6
Corrected variance of the loss	CLV	[db²]	0..6			1.0
Short-term fluctuation	SF	[db]	0..4			1.8
Cinfidence factor	RF	[%]	0..2			0.0

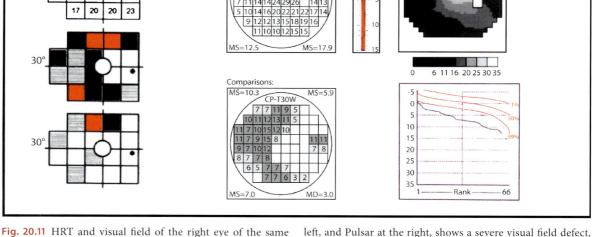

Fig. 20.11 HRT and visual field of the right eye of the same patient. In the upper right part, the visual field with conventional perimetry Octopus is normal, meanwhile, in the lower part the non conventional perimetry double frequency at the left, and Pulsar at the right, shows a severe visual field defect, topographicaly corresponding to the big lesion of the optic nerve show by the HRT

Figure 20.12, corresponds to the chamber angle of the left eye. Figure 20.13 shows that the ON of the left eye is in phase III, the conventional visual field is normal, and the nonconventional visual field is in phase III. For ophthalmologists who think that glaucoma is an alteration of the ON and of the visual field and who work with the conventional perimetry, the diagnosis in this case is ocular hypertension. For those who work with nonconventional perimetry, the diagnosis is glaucoma, since the ON lesion topographically corresponds to the VF lesion made with nonconventional frequency doubling perimetry. Since this patient on the maximum medication – prostaglandins, carbon anhydrase (FDT and pulsar showed defects topographically corresponding to the lesion of the ON), inhibitors, and beta blockers did not regulate pressure – we performed surgery, as in the other eye, deep nonpenetrating sclerectomy and goniopuncture with Yag laser. The pressure regulated at 12 mmHg and the DTC was normal.

As with the other eye, this patient was on medication for 17 years while her ON and her VF were deteriorating.

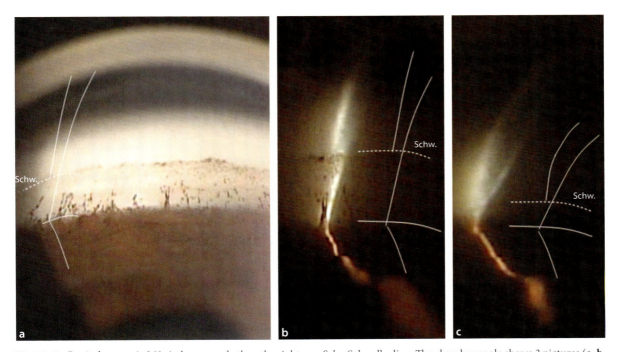

Fig. 20.12 Goniodysgenesis 360° in lesser grade then the right eye. *Schw* Schwalbe line. The chamber angle shows 3 pictures (**a**, **b**, and **c**)

In **a**: the Right Eye of the same patient, the ciliary body band ist not visible because it is covered by the pathological mesodermal tissue

In **b**: enlargement of the same

In **c**: in one part of the chamber angle the mesodermal remnants reach the Schwalbe line. Prolongations of this pathological tissue reach Schlemm canal

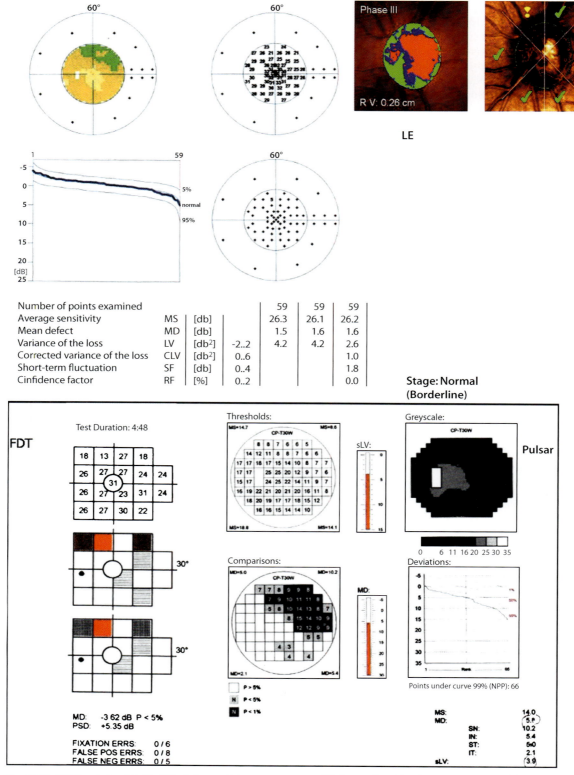

Stage: Normal (Borderline)

Number of points examined				59	59	59
Average sensitivity	MS	[db]		26.3	26.1	26.2
Mean defect	MD	[db]		1.5	1.6	1.6
Variance of the loss	LV	[db²]	-2..2	4.2	4.2	2.6
Corrected variance of the loss	CLV	[db²]	0..6			1.0
Short-term fluctuation	SF	[db]	0..4			1.8
Cinfidence factor	RF	[%]	0..2			0.0

Fig. 20.13 HRT and visual field of the left eye of the same patient. In the *upper left part*, the visual field with conventional perimetry Octopus is normal, meanwhile, in the *lower part* the non conventional perimetry double frequency at the *left*, and Pulsar at the *right*, shows a severe visual field defect, topographicaly corresponding to the big lesion of the optic nerve show by the HRT

Late Congenital Glaucoma with Lower Nasal Malformation

In our experience with glaucomas, we find cases that, despite presenting clinically as simple glaucomas, were actually late-onset congenital glaucomas. These were glaucomas whose etiology stemmed from an anomalous development of the chamber angle. We should classify them as true late congenital glaucomas. Studying the angle of the anterior chamber, particularly in all its circumference, a malformation involving both the iris wall and the scleral wall can be found by Sampaolesi (1962, 1968) [7, 8].

Topographically, this anomaly appears in the low nasal quadrant of the chamber angle. This constant location led us to relate this malformation to the fissure of the optic vesicle, as its closure occurs in this area. At this level, the iris shows a retrocession of its root, a surface depression, and an increase in the depth of the anterior chamber. This sign in itself already demonstrates goniodysgenesis and is accompanied by the features we described in slight or intermediate goniodysgenesis (Fig. 20.14).

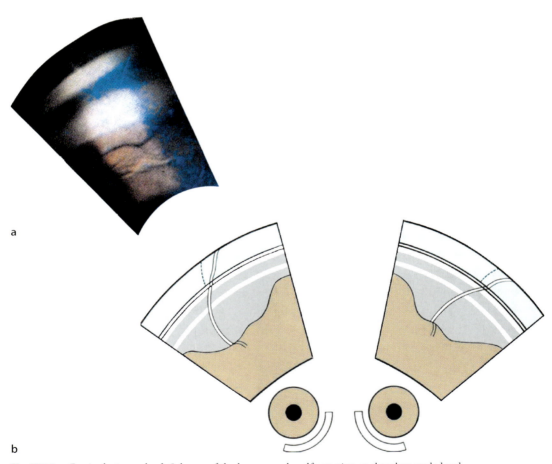

a

b

Fig. 20.14 **a** Goniophotography. **b** Schema of the lower nasal malformation at chamber angle level

The lower part represents the iris and pupil and the affected part is marked. In the upper part, a schema of the malformation of the chamber angle from the Schwalbe line backward (Fig. 20.14).

In the scleral wall of the chamber angle remnants of dark pigment can be seen (Fig. 20.15) or a tissue that is different from the iris tissue, which fills the chamber angle, or ramified pathological mesodermal remnants (Fig. 20.16), or a prominent Schwalbe line, etc.,

but these variations are always limited to the lower nasal zone. This anomaly often appears together with a change in the iris pigmentation in that area, which sometimes reaches the pupil (Fig. 20.17). There are also eccentricities in the frill of the iris.

One feature of this anomaly is the presence of mesodermal pathological remnants (mesodermal tissue) in the lateral parts of the iris depression (Figs. 20.18, 20.19).

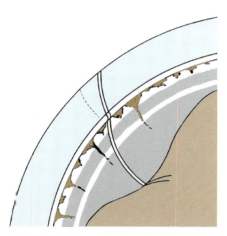

Fig. 20.15 Schema showing the lower nasal anomaly of the chamber angle with remnants of dark pigment at the level of Schwalbe's line

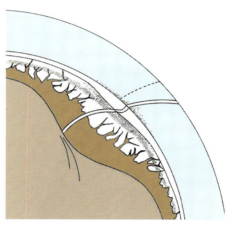

Fig. 20.16 In the zone of the lower nasal anomaly, ramified iris processes and greatly thickened Schwalbe line

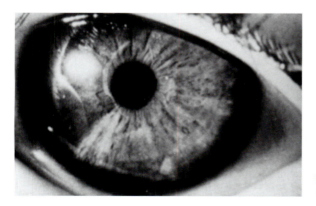

Fig. 20.17 Inferior nasal coloboma of the iris shaped like a white triangle

Fig. 20.18 Pathological mesodermal remnants in the lateral parts of the iris depression

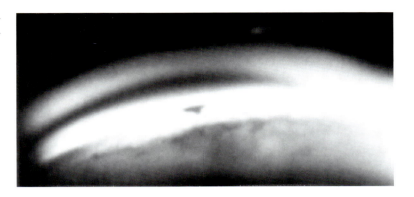

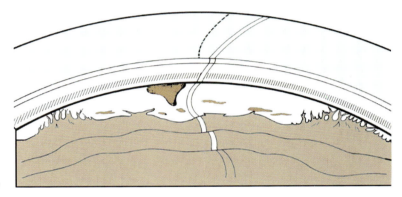

Fig. 20.19 Diagram of the same

Clinical history No. 6 is a 42-year-old man diagnosed with late congenital glaucoma, with lower nasal malformation and coloboma of the iris mesenchymal layers at 6 o'clock. He had been treated for the previous 2 years since the hypertension had been discovered accidentally during a routine check-up for refraction. The results were as follows:

	Right eye	Left eye
IOP	26 mmHg	26 mmHg
Visual acuity	20/20, (with sph. + 1)	20/20 (with sph. + 1)
Tonography C1.3-7	0.12 (pathological)	0.08 (pathological)
Chamber angle	Persistence of mesodermal remnants and lower nasal depression	Persistence of mesodermal remnants and lower nasal depression
Iris	Coloboma of the iris, mesenchymal layers, from 6 o'clock pupillary border, through the pigmentary layer of the iris can be seen (Fig: 20.20a)	In the pupillary zone, at 6 o'clock a very small coloboma can be see. Almost subclinical in the same shape as that of the RE (Fig: 20.20b)
Optic disc	Excavation 5/6	Excavation 5/6
Visual field	Stage II	Stage II
Gonioscopy	Goniodysgenesis 360º	Goniodysgenesis 360º (Fig. 20.10)

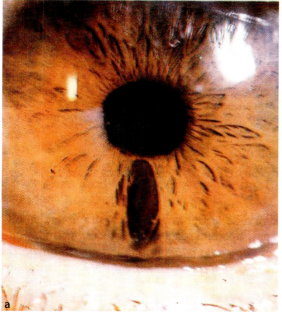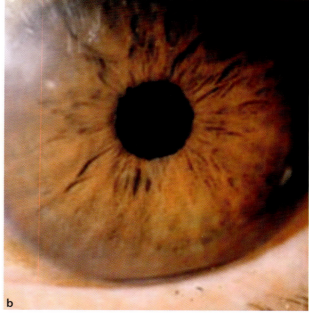

Fig. 20.20 **a** Partial coloboma of the iris, both mesenchymal layers were missing and the posterior ectodermic pigment could be seen at 6 o'clock. **b** The other eye of the same patient, with a subclinical coloboma

Apparently, this malformation is new in the literature. However, Busacca called our attention to work published by Arnold (1911) [11] and Streiff (1915) [12], which are closely related to our findings. Arnold's paper shows iris pigmentation anomalies at 6 o'clock and partial coloboma of the anterior mesodermal layer of the iris in the same way as these were described by Fuchs. Arnold says that these alterations in the iris surface run in families and are hereditary. They occur with alterations to the pigmentation and show varying degrees of insufficient development that may lead to a real anomaly.

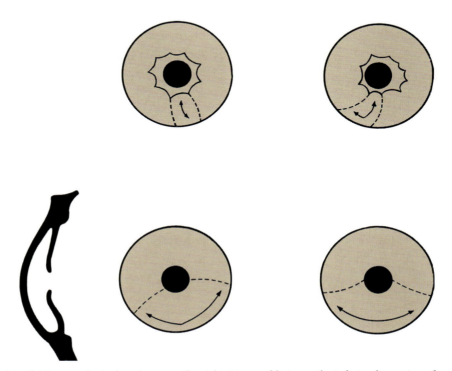

Fig. 20.21 Arnold and Streiff's design of this anomaly, in the schema on the right it is possible to see the inferior depression of the chamber angle

In Fig. 20.21 in Streiff's paper shows the lower nasal positioning, the eccentricity of the collarette, and the greater depth of the anterior chamber at this point.

In Fig. 15.50 of his book, Vogt [13] also describes a case of hypoplasia of the superficial mesodermal layer of the iris in the lower nasal quadrant and relates it to an optic vesicle fissure closure defect. At the end of his description of this figure, he says that the patient suffered from simple glaucoma and had optic disc excavation. This last remark in the clinical history is highly suggestive.

It should be remembered that in all these cases of late congenital glaucoma, heredity is highly dominant and it is necessary to examine all the members of the family.

Clinical history No. 7 involves a 17-year-old female whom we followed up from 2002 to 2008, diagnosing late congenital glaucoma, goniodysgenesis 360° (Figs. 20.22, 20.23, 20.24, 20.25).

This case shows that at 17 years of age glaucoma with high intraocular pressures, which is not regulated to normal target values with maximum medical treatment, the visual field defects are stage II and the optic nerve phase III in both eyes: surgery had to be done. The decision was not easy to make, but 6 years later, with no medical treatment, the patient's visual field improved, the optic nerve defect had not progressed, and the visual acuity was exactly the same as at the beginning.

	Right eye	Left eye
2002		
IOP	20 mmHg with prostaglandin and beta blockers	21 mmHg with prostaglandin and beta blockers
DPC	M: 21 mmHg V. 1.5 mmHg	M: 21 mm Hg. V. 1.3 mmHg
Pachimetry	541	544
Optic nerve (HRT)	Phase III	Phase III
Visual acuity	Sph. −2.50, cil. −1, 150° = 20/25	Sph. −3.50 = 20/25
Surgery	August 2002, combined surgery	August 2002, combined surgery
Visual field	Stage II	Stage II
2008		
IOP	12 mmH, without treatment	12 mmHg, without treatment
DPC	M: 13.8 mmHg, V. 1.6mmHg	M: 14.2 mm Hg V. 1.1 mmHg
Optic nerve (HRT)	Phase III (no progression)	Phase III (no progression)

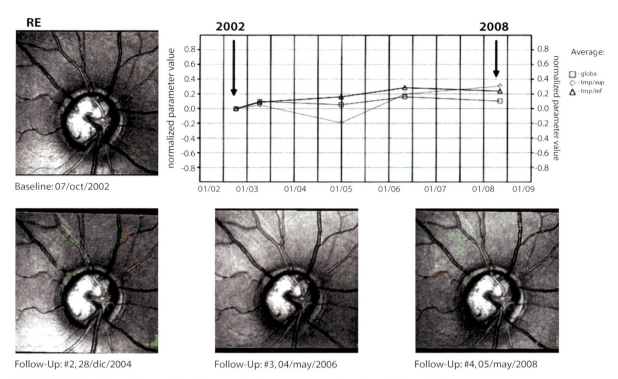

Fig. 20.22 HRT of the right eye with a diagram that shows no progression from 2002 to 2008

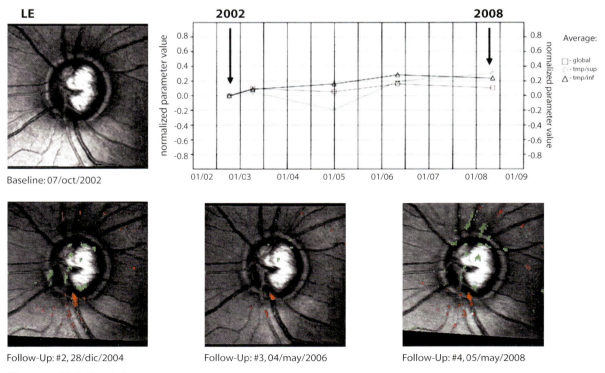

Fig. 20.23 HRT of the left eye

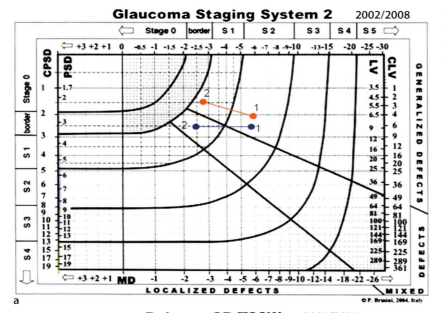

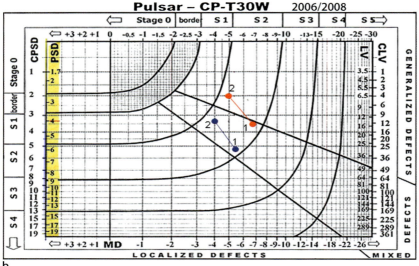

Fig. 20.24a,b Brusini glaucoma staging system. **a** Improvement in right and left eyes. **b** Brusini staging system for Pulsar-CP-T30W

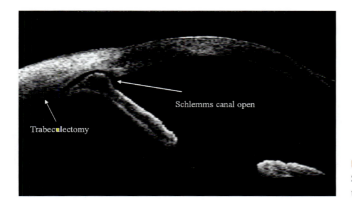

Fig. 20.25 SL-OCT of the right eye that shows the Schlemm canal open and in communication with the trabeculectomy

Pigmentary Glaucoma

In the first edition of Glaucoma, Sampaolesi 1974, we presented statistics of 27 cases of pigmentary glaucoma. In the second edition (Sampaolesi 1994) there were 107, and now in this book the number of patients has reached 180, with 5–36 years of follow-up. In most of the cases, we found anomalies of the chamber angle (goniodysgenesis).

The first clinical description of this condition was published in 1949 by Sugar and Barbour [14], and the association between pigmentary glaucoma and congenital glaucoma was described for the first time in 1957 by Malbrán [15]. Etienne [16], Etienne and Pommier [17], Weekers and Watillon [18], Di Tizio and Lepri [19], Nordmann [20], Jerndal et al. [4], Heinzen and Lueder [21] and Shaffer and Weiss [22] share this opinion.

Literature Review

We believe it is very useful to carefully review the literature relating to pigmentary glaucoma and its clinical manifestations.

Mauksch (1925) [23] refers to an observation made in 21-year-old twin brothers: "both have Krukenberg's spindle and an extraordinary disintegration of the pigment of the iris epithelial layer. The pigment is also deposited on the posterior face of the lens, at the bottom of the bag between the hyaloid membrane and the crystalloids. The irregular borders seen in this ring are probably produced by the insertion of the more posterior zonular fibres."

In a paper on the study of the Krukenberg's spindle, Cavara [24] describes several cases in which there is great pigment dispersion originated by the atrophy of the iris. He says that this, like Koby's work, supports the idea of the pigment line of the periphery of the lens as being acquired and relates it with the hemorrhages of the posterior chamber that are in the same place as the pigment.

Koby [25] describes the case of a 46-year-old woman and her daughter, 22, who have a pigment ring in the posterior face of the lens and also pigment at the arciform boundary. Toward the edge of the lens, the granulations separate from its posterior face to occupy the surface of a transparent substrate in the vitreous body. He describes the following kinds of pigment dispersion in the posterior face of the lens: disseminated, in bands, perihyaloid, inferior, and circular.

Focosy [26], in a paper titled "On the pigment deposits in the posterior crystalloid," describes the intense pigment dispersion that occurs in these cases and

remembers that in the exfoliative syndrome, as Baumgart described it, there is also great pigment dispersion, and mentions Streiff's observation on similar cases, with great aplasia of the iris pigment layer, and Collebati's case with subluxation of the lens and coloboma of the iris. To my knowledge, this is the first reference to pigment dispersion occurring in exfoliative syndrome, made describing the pigment deposits in the posterior capsule of the lens that are seen in pigmentary glaucoma. As we know, Sugar associated this ring in the posterior capsule of the lens with the condition of pigmentary glaucoma after its discovery. Since then, numerous authors have made the mistake of associating pigmentary glaucoma with exfoliative syndrome but these are actually two completely different disorders, clearly distinct, with their own characteristics, even though they may coincide in the same patient.

Focosy concludes, "Even though the cases of Koby (mother and daughter) and of Mauksch (twins) might suggest that it is a congenital lesion, in fact, my cases, like those of Cavara and Bietti, show that it is an acquired alteration, for two reasons: (1) Because of the great atrophy that is always seen in the pigment layer, (2) because in the cases which I have been able to follow up for a long time, the pigmentation steadily increases."

Bietti (1934) [27] gives us the most accurate description of this sign: "The pigment accumulates in the capsulohyaloid angle, i.e., in the place where the anterior surface of the vitreous body joins the posterior capsule of the lens. At this point a triangular shaped blind bottom forms. This ring is almost always bilateral, although at times it may be unilateral as in Koby's case and in one of mine. There are granules of pigment that can sometimes also be present in the vitreous body. This ring is due to the disintegration of the pigment layer of the iris and the pigment collects at the height of Wieger's capsulohyaloid ligament in the capsulohyaloid angle. This pigment is carried by the flow of the aqueous humor through the zonular fibres to the retrolental space that Reslob described. This ring is an acquired manifestation."

In her book on congenital defects of the eye, Mann [28] says, "In the 100 mm embryo, the vertex of the ciliary processes is found in contact with the periphery of the lens; in some animals this continues throughout life, and in birds the ciliary processes depress the lens. This contact of the ciliary processes with the lens would leave pigmentation on the posterior face."

Zentmayer (1938) [29] was the first writer in the United States to describe the association of the Krukenberg spindle with the pigment ring in the posterior face of the lens. He presents two drawings which illustrate zonular fibers with pigment in the lower part, and he thinks that this arrives there carried by the circulation of the aqueous humor.

Evans et al. [30] describe 202 cases of Krukenberg spindle in the United States, of which 14 present the pigment ring in the posterior face of the lens. They deduce from their study that it is an acquired malformation.

Cameron (1941) [31] states that the transillumination of the iris shows a well-advanced atrophy and that the ring of the posterior face of the lens is formed by rectangular masses of pigment.

Bellows [32] considers that the ring is formed as a consequence of depigmentation, resulting from degenerative changes in the iris and mentions Mann's study.

As for genetic differences, Becker et al. [33] conclude that pigmentary glaucoma in general is differentiated from open-angle glaucoma by a study with the antigen HLA-7, HLAB13, and HLAB12.

In examining the behavior of the pupil, Kaiser-Kupfer [34] divide the pigmentary syndromes into three groups: (1) pigmentary syndrome without glaucoma, (2) pigmentary syndrome with ocular hypertension, and (3) pigmentary syndrome with ocular hypertension and defects of the visual field. This author studied age, sex, iris, gonioscopy, tonography, color of the iris, transillumination, refraction, and pupilography, based on the pathological anatomy of the iris that showed hypertrophy of the dilator muscle. Using the pupilography with infrared rays, he studied the behavior of the pupil and found alterations correlating with the pathological anatomy.

In pigmentary syndrome and pigmentary glaucoma, Farrar et al. [35] analyzed 93 patients with pigmentary glaucoma and 18 with pigmentary syndrome, 75% of whom were men. The pigmentary glaucomas had greater myopia and a higher incidence of Krukenberg spindle. Fundamentally, the authors studied the risk factors that transform a pigmentary syndrome into a pigmentary glaucoma, such as myopia, family history, etc. More than half the patients with pigmentary syndrome developed pigmentary glaucoma over time. Of 111 patients, 61 (55%) developed pigmentary glaucoma.

Campbell [36] thought that the rubbing of the iris against the zonular fibers due to the trapezoidal shape of the anterior chamber is the factor responsible for the peripheral atrophy of the iris pigment layer.

Calixto [37] and Calixto and Cronemberg [38] conducted detailed studies of pigmentary glaucoma. The latter study refers to retinal detachment in pigmentary syndrome and they quote Cardozo's 1986 study in the bibliography, but make no mention of the first documented study that we know of, by Brachet and Cher-

met (1974) [39], or of our study published in *Archivos de Oftalmología de Buenos Aires* (1975) [40].

Richter et al. [41] share our opinion that it is a progressive glaucoma that worsens without treatment.

Richardson [42] divides the progress of pigmentary glaucoma into two stages, a first stage that he calls pigmentary dispersion, which is reversible if treated, and a second stage that is not reversible. In the first stage, there are transitory peaks of ocular pressure. The author advances a hypothesis about its pathogenesis based on the pathological anatomy: the endothelial cell is altered by phagocytosis of the pigment and separates from the connective tissue of the trabecula, leaving it bare.

All these bibliographical references (except Mann's study) show that the pigmentation on the posterior face of the lens is an acquired phenomenon.

Mauksch's observation in a set of twins and Koby's in the mother and daughter point to something hereditary and congenital; this is in accordance with the anomalies presenting in the chamber angle that we described earlier. Pigmentation is a phenomenon that develops gradually, accompanying the congenital component in the chamber angle and ocular hypertension. We suggest reading Rosen's papers [43], which are most useful for the biomicroscopy interpretation of this pigmentation that we have just described.

Epidemiology

Pigmentary glaucoma has a frequency of 1%–1.5% among the glaucomas, according to Scheie et al. [44] and Mapstone [45], cited by Campbell in the book by Ritch et al. [46]. In reality, this percentage cannot be so precise, because gonioscopy is not always performed, and this is the only method that enables a correct diagnosis of pigmentary glaucoma, as there can be Krukenberg spindle without pigmentary glaucoma. This is also true of the frequencies found in the literature on the amount of pigment dispersion (which is not pigmentary glaucoma) and pigmentary glaucoma; we have seen many patients classified as pigmentary dispersion, because the ophthalmologist took a single spot-check IOP during the day and did not carry out a DPC: daily pressure curve. This disorder affects young adult men between 20 and 45 years of age, with a deep anterior chamber and myopia. In women, it generally appears 10 years later.

Clinical Features: Diagnosis

We will examine the clinical manifestations of pigmentary glaucoma in the following order:

1. Intraocular pressure;
2. Anterior chamber;
3. Pigmentary syndrome;
4. Congenital anomalies of the chamber angle;
5. Refraction;
6. Heredity;
7. Possible associations with other ocular problems;
8. Pathological anatomy;
9. Pathogenesis;
10. Differential diagnosis.

Pigmentary glaucoma is a bilateral disease that occurs particularly in young men and women, generally under 50 years of age, at an average age of 48.3 (average age in men, 49; in women, 47.6). Of our 107 cases studied, 86 (80.4%) were men, and 21 (19.6%) were women.

The diagnosis of glaucoma is made as follows.

Intraocular Pressure

a. As in simple glaucoma, by accident, when measuring ocular pressure during a routine check-up.
b. Sometimes, because of a brusque increase in ocular pressure following medical dilatation of the pupil, due to a papillary block.
c. From symptoms of the congestive glaucoma type (the rarest ones). The patients have blurred vision, see colored rings around lights, etc.
d. It should be remembered that seeing colored rings is often not accompanied with hypertension in these patients and it is probably due, as Sugar says [48, 49], to the presence of a Krukenberg spindle in the cornea. Pressure varies between 21 and 50 mmHg; in rare cases it reaches 80 mmHg.

Since in all cases the initial ocular pressure gave pathological values, the daily pressure curve was taken not for diagnostic purposes, but only to check the effectiveness of medical or surgical therapy. In some borderline cases, it is necessary for the diagnosis of hypertension.

Anterior Chamber

The anterior chamber is characteristically deep and the iris assumes a concave configuration, most prominent in the mid-periphery. The shape of the anterior chamber is trapezoidal. This configuration results in rubbing the pigment epithelium against the zonular bundles, dislodging pigment granules [36].

Pigmentary Syndrome in the Anterior Segment and Chamber Angle

1. Atrophy of the pigment epithelial layer of the iris [50];
2. Krukenberg spindle [51];
3. Pigmentation on the surface of the lens, in the peripheral part of its posterior face, irregular in shape, half-ring, whole ring, or double ring;
4. Chamber angle: a dark pigment ring in the scleral trabecular meshwork at the height of the Schlemm canal and goniodysgenesis;
5. Pigment dispersion in the anterior face of the iris.

Atrophy of the Pigment Epithelial Layer of the Iris

This is visible only by means of transillumination. This is very easy if the retroillumination of the iris is made during the examination with the slit lamp, using the lens of the eye as a diffusing medium for the light. To do this, a slit 3 mm high and 2 mm wide is focused on the pupil zone, so that the beam does not touch the iris tissue (retroillumination in the red field).

The direction of the beam of light must be normal to the eye and coincide with the axis of the observation microscope, as occurs with an ophthalmoscope; in this way, the red image of the pupil and the red image corresponding to the atrophic region of the iris will be obtained. If pigmentary glaucoma is already well developed, irregular but rounded zones of atrophy will be seen, sometimes isolated, with others running together in the periphery of the iris (atrophy in rings) (Fig. 20.26).

If pigmentary glaucoma is of recent onset and has developed little, the atrophy always starts in the inferior nasal region of both eyes and this is where it should be looked for. When we discuss the congenital component later, we will present this topographical location of the atrophy of the iris pigment layer in pigmentary glaucoma at onset (Fig. 20.27).

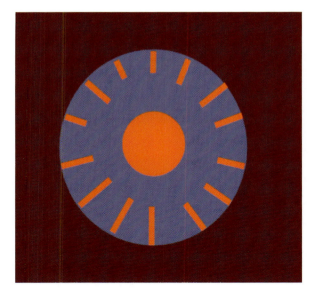

Fig. 20.26 Atrophy of the pigmentary layer of the iris in a well-developed pigmentary glaucoma

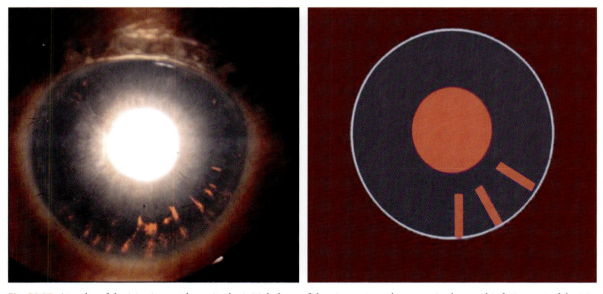

Fig. 20.27 Atrophy of the iris pigment layer, in the initial phase of the pigmentary glaucoma, in the nasal inferior part of the iris, at the place of closure of the optical vesicle (photo and diagram)

Krukenberg Spindle

This was described for the first time by Krukenberg in 1899 [51] in a mother and daughter. It is formed from the accumulation of pigment on the posterior face of the cornea. Its dimensions are approximately 6 mm in height by 3 mm in width. The pigment is phagocytosed by the endothelial cells covering the Descemet membrane.

We will not spend time studying the Krukenberg spindle since there are publications [30] that have investigated 202 cases in the United States. Hansen [52] shows a very good histological preparation of the Krukenberg spindle. Possibly the formation of the Krukenberg spindle is caused by the thermal flow that occurs in the anterior chamber. Of all our patients, 68.6% showed a Krukenberg spindle and 31.4% did not. However, these are pigmentary glaucomas (Fig. 20.28).

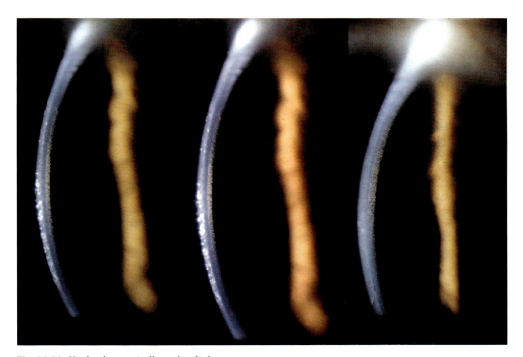

Fig. 20.28 Krukenberg spindle at the slit lamp

Pigmentation on the Surface of the Lens

In pigmentary glaucoma, we have also found pigment deposited on the lens, on the anterior and posterior capsule, in the zonular fibers, and in the anterior border of the vitreous body, anterior (zonular) hyaloids at the zonular fibers. The most important of these pigmentations is found on the posterior face of the lens, deposited toward the periphery on the capsule. This pigmentation on the peripheral surface of the lens is irregular in shape: a half-ring, ring, or double ring.

We believe this ring is almost constant in advanced pigmentary glaucoma (Fig. 20.29a,b). In the group of patients studied, 93.4% presented pigmented rings in the posterior face of the lens, 60.6% presented two pigmented rings, one of them sometimes more complete, 30.3% presented a pigmented ring, sometimes incomplete, and 9.1% presented a half-ring.

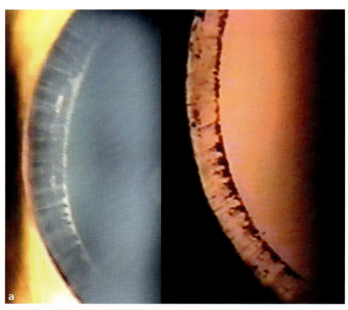

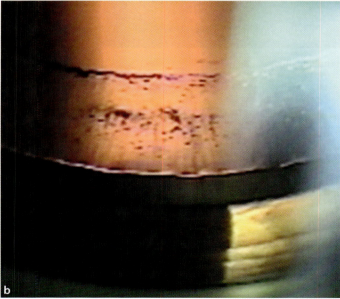

Fig. 20.29 a *Left*, insertion of the zonule in the equator of the lens with direct lighting; on the *right* with retroillumination. **b** Below the equator of the lens with two lines of pigment located at the level of the insertion of the zonular fibers

Pigmentary Ring in the Chamber Angle

This characteristic pigmentation is found in all our patients. It presents as a very clearly defined band, dark brown in color, almost black, homogeneous and thick in the region of the scleral trabecular meshwork corresponding to the Schlemm canal. In some eyes, this pigmentation extends to all the filtering trabecular meshwork and even beyond it in the form of fine granules, some passing the Schwalbe line and others on the surface of the iris.

When the pigment dispersion is extensive, the trabecular meshwork is also pigmented up to the Schwalbe line and sometimes the pigment passes over this line and deposits on the posterior face of the cornea in a random way. It can accumulate in the steepest part of the angle. This pigment ring in the chamber angle is the clearest, most constant sign that permits a diagnosis of pigmentary glaucoma, once ocular hypertension has been found. Gonioscopy has diagnostic value (Fig. 20.30).

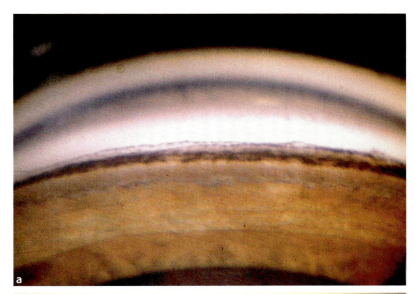

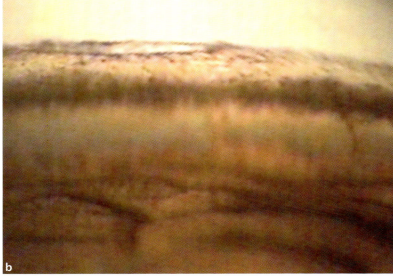

Fig. 20.30a,b Goniophotograph of a chamber angle in pigmentary glaucoma with the goniolens of Roussel Fankahause, **a** low magnification, **b** bigger magnification

Figure 20.31 sketches the biomicroscope study findings. Figure 20.31a, with maximum, almost limbic, pupil dilation, shows the lens equator and two concentric pigment rings. The inner one is thicker and is made up of rectangular pieces. The outer one is thinner, and, with great magnification, a structure can be seen made up of overlapping granules of pigment.

A careful study locates these two rings accurately. Figure 20.31b corresponds to a section of the anterior segment, in which the cornea, sclera, iris, ciliary body, periphery of the lens, zonular fibers, and anterior hyaloids can be seen. In Fig. 20.31c, Z indicates the insertion of the posterior zonular fibers and W marks where the anterior hyaloids meet the posterior face of the lens, a structure known anatomically as the Wieger capsulohyaloid ligament. The zonular fibers and the posterior capsule of the lens form an acute angle open toward the periphery. The anterior hyaloids and the posterior capsule of the lens form another acute angle open toward the periphery. The latter is called the capsulohyaloid angle. The section of both spaces is triangular in shape.

Following up patients over the years, we have been able to observe that, in general, the pigment stops first in the angle that the zonular fibers form with the lens and so constitutes the first pigment ring. The pigment then passes to the Petit perilenticular space (which is formed by the anterior and posterior zonular bundles), passing through the posterior zonular fibers to the Hannover space, which in these diseases is real, not virtual, and this reaches the capsulohyaloid angle, where it forms the second pigment ring, at the capsulolenticular ligament of Wieger. In normal persons, this Hannover space is commonly virtual, but it is real in cases of pigmentary glaucoma.

In Fig. 20.31b, a section of the lens can be seen, obtained by placing the slit horizontally and at an angle. The precise location can be seen of the accumulations of pigment that start the formation of the rings. Looking with greater magnification, it can be clearly observed that in the section the pigment has the same triangular shape corresponding to the capsulohyaloid angle and the zonular angle. As well as these rings, granules of pigment may be observed sticking to the zonular fibers, which are more numerous nearer their insertion, where they form macroscopically the first ring.

Having followed up these patients for years and observed how these rings slowly form, in addition to what has just been described, has convinced us that this sign is an acquired formation.

The pigment epithelial layer of the iris is destroyed and not in the region next to the pupil but in the peripheral part; the pigment, carried by the flow of the aqueous humor, enters through the anterior zonular fibers into the Petit perilenticular space, from there passes to the Hannover space and deposits on the posterior face of the lens. Moreover, the structure just described definitely does not represent a contact of the ciliary processes with the lens in the embryo stage that might leave pigment impressions. Sometimes the pigment reaches the ora serrata, and at other times passes it and deposits at those levels.

Chamber Angle in Pigmentary Glaucoma

As stated earlier, pigmentary glaucoma is a type of goniodysgenesis, a late congenital glaucoma. Figure 20.32a shows a scheme in which the most important point is the brown triangle (Fig. 20.32a, 1), showing the pathological tissue remnants that can, to a greater or lesser extent, reach the Schwalbe line, as in the congenital glaucomas. The notable pigmentation of the Schlemm canal (Fig. 20.32, 3) marks the diagnosis of pigmentary glaucoma.

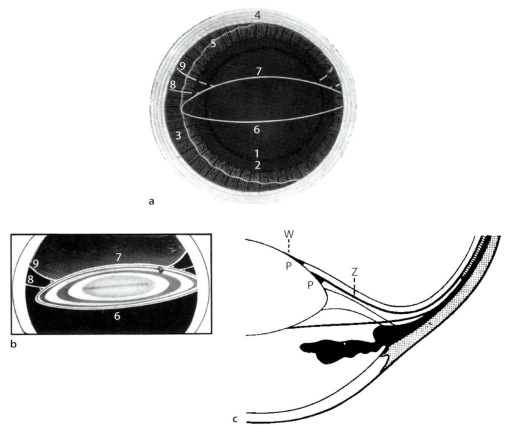

Fig. 20.31a–c Zones of pigment accumulation in pigmentary glaucoma. In **a**, *1* wide internal pigment ring; *2* thinner external pigment ring, corresponding to the insertion of the posterior zonular fibers; *3* posterior zonular fibers; *4* dilated iris; *5* lens equator. **b** Optical section with oblique horizontal slit: *6* profile line of the anterior face of the lens; *7* profile line of the posterior face of the lens; *8* profile line of the posterior zonular fibers; *9* profile line of the anterior hyaloids. **c** *Z* indicates the insertion of the posterior zonular fibers and *W* marks where the anterior hyaloids meet the posterior face of the lens, a structure known anatomically as the Wieger capsulohyaloid ligament. The two letters *P* mark the section of the pigment rings

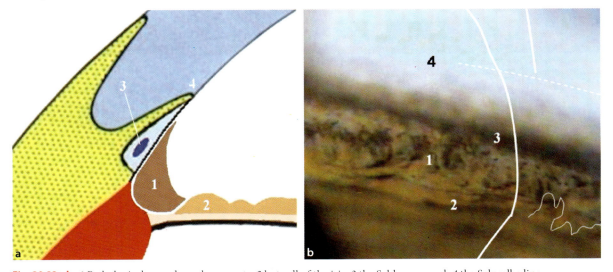

Fig. 20.32a,b *1* Pathological mesodermal remnants; *2* last roll of the iris; *3* the Schlemm canal; *4* the Schwalbe line

Figure 20.33 shows the goniophotograph of another pigmentary glaucoma; Fig. 20.33b is a diagram distinguishing the different elements of this pathology corresponding to another case. In Fig. 20.33a, the Schlemm canal can be seen as a thick, absolutely black line, which is what in most cases provides the diagnosis when performing gonioscopy. Here the zone should be noted that runs from the last roll of the iris to the following roll of the iris (vertical black line), because this zone presents iris atrophy, another feature of goniodysgenesis. Above the last fold of the iris, the strings forming the pathological mesodermal remnants can be clearly seen, and below they are blurred.

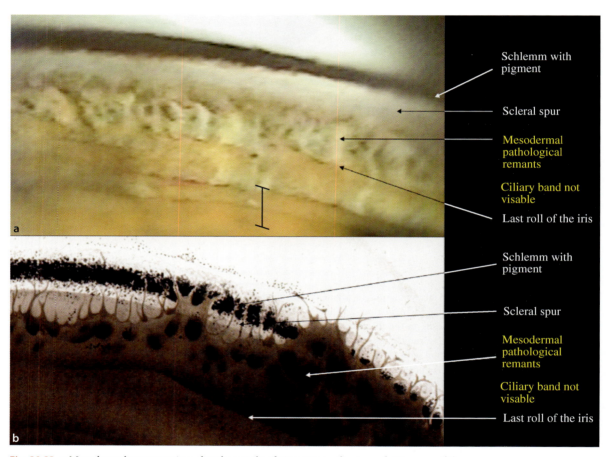

Fig. 20.33 **a** Mesodermal remnants in a chamber angle of pigmentary glaucoma. **b** Diagram of the same

Apparent High Insertion of the Iris in Pigmentary Glaucoma

Just as in a congenital glaucoma with type I and type II angles, the apparent high insertion of the iris can be at different levels: the ciliary body band, scleral spur, the Schlemm canal, the Schwalbe line or above it. In pigmentary glaucoma, the height of the apparent insertion of the iris can also vary. Figure 20.34 shows a pigmentary glaucoma with its apparently high insertion of the iris occurring at the level of the scleral spur. In Fig. 20.35, we have reproduced the angle of a refractory congenital glaucoma (type II) with an apparently high insertion of the iris at the level of the Schwalbe line, to compare it with the chamber angle of pigmentary glaucoma, which in some cases resembles the type II chamber angle. Figure 20.36 is another example of the same situation. Figure 20.37 is what we consider an extraordinary example of the angle of a pigmentary glaucoma, taken, like the other goniophotographs, with the Roussell and Fankhauser lens, which enables us to see the atrophy of iris tissue at the periphery and through it, the pathological mesodermal remnants, and the pigment accumulated among them.

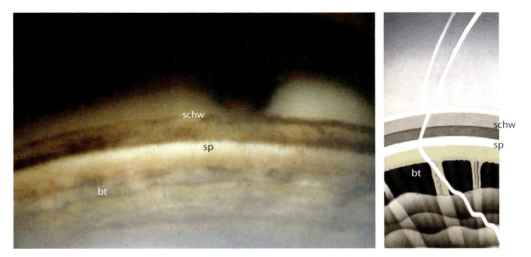

Fig. 20.34 Apparent high insertion of the iris at the level of the scleral spur. On the *right*, diagram of the same

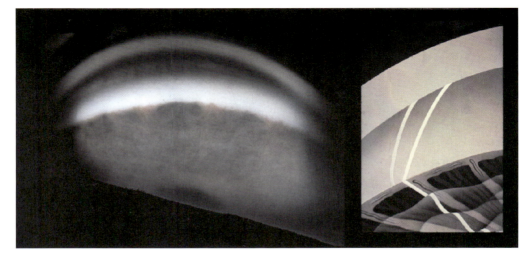

Fig. 20.35 Goniophotograph of a chamber angle of congenital glaucoma type II. On the *right*, diagram to compare with the figure

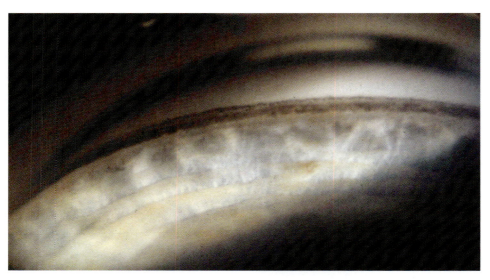

Fig. 20.36 Goniophotograph of a chamber angle of pigmentary glaucoma with great peripheral atrophy of the iris

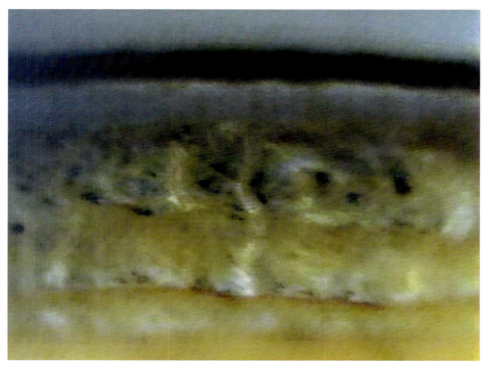

Fig. 20.37 Goniophotograph with large magnification of pigmentary glaucoma. The gonioscopy was made with the Roussel and Fankhauser lens

Congenital Anomalies of the Chamber Angle (Frequency)

Of the 107 cases studied in our statistics, 77% presented a congenital anomaly of the chamber angle and 23% did not. In the latter cases, then, these were pigment dispersion syndromes with ocular hypertension and, sometimes, visual field defects.

The pictures of those presenting chamber angle anomalies could be different types: in the first type, the three forms presented together (pathological mesodermal remnants, absence of the ciliary body band, and inferior nasal depression), and accounted for 43% of anomalies. A second type showed only two of the forms in combination, either pathological mesodermal remnants and absence of the ciliary body band, or pathological mesodermal remnants and inferior nasal depression: this accounted for 4%. The other presented any of three completely isolated forms: pathological mesodermal remnants (36.4%), absence of the ciliary body band (10.2%), and inferior nasal depression (6%) (Table 20.2).

Refraction

In the group in which we made the statistics, 73.5% presented myopia between sph. −1 and sph. −27 D distributed as follows: 25%, between −1 and −2.5 D; 18%, between −3 and −5 D; 21.9%, between −6 and −13 Ds; 7%, between −14 and −18 D and two eyes, one −25 D and the other −27 D. In total, 19.5% were emmetropic and 7% hypermetropic, between +1 and +6 diopters (Table 20.3).

Table 20.2 Congenital anomalies of the chamber angle, in pigmentary glaucoma (107 cases) (frequency)

Forms		
With congenital anomalies of the chamber angle (77%)	RMP, ABCC and DNI	43%
	RMP and ABCC	11.9%
	RMP and DNI	4%
	RMP	36.4%
	ABCC	10.2%
	DNI	6%
Without congenital anomalies of the chamber angle (23%)		

Cong congenital, *RMP* pathological mesodermal remnants, *ABCC* absence of the ciliary body band, *DNI* inferior nasal depression

Table 20.3 Refraction of myopia, emmetropia and hypermetropia

Reference disorder	Reference between	No. of eyes	%
Myopia (73%)	SPH. −1 and −2.5 D	32	25
	SPH. −3 and −5 D	23	18
	SPH. −6 and −13 D	28	21.9
	SPH. −14 and −18 D	9	7
	SPH. −25 D	1	0.8
	SPH. −27 D	1	0.8
Emmetropia		25	19.5
Hypermetropia	SPH. +1 and +6 D	9	7

REF refraction, *SPH* spherical, *D* diopters

Heredity

Congenital glaucoma has recessive heredity and late congenital glaucoma has dominant heredity, as does pigmentary glaucoma. The following paragraph from François [53] explains this clearly.

1. "The penetrance and expressivity of a gene may vary from 0 to 100%; it is known that gene penetrance of a gene expresses the frequency of its phenotypical manifestations, and the expressivity the degree of this manifestation."

2. "A gene in heterozygotic state always determines a less severe clinical manifestation than a gene in homozygotic state. This explains why a recessive disorder is often less severe than a dominant disorder. Considering these two facts, it is easy to imagine that there is no fundamental difference between recessive and dominant or intermediate heredity. If the penetrance and the expressivity are nil or very weak, the heredity will be recessive; if they are strong, dominant, and if they are average, intermediate. Dominance and recessivity do not indicate opposing forms of heredity but only, as Cuendeti and Streiff said: 'the opposite ends of the same unbroken chain, of variable modes of heredity but basically identical.'

In pigmentary glaucoma, one can also think of a phenomenon of gene linkage, i.e., a linking up of different genes in the same chromosome. In one chromosome, there may be a link between the glaucoma gene and the one that causes the pigment dispersion (Shaffer 1967 [54]).

Genetics

Anderson and Anderson et al. [55, 56] located the responsible gene in the telomeric extremity of the long arm of chromosome 7 (7q35-q369) and more recently found a second place in chromosome 18q.

Heredity: Clinical Cases

Family 1. A brother with typical pigmentary glaucoma, whose sister presented late-onset congenital glaucoma with all the signs in the chamber angle but without pigment. The mother was glaucomatous (Fig. 20.38).

Family 2. This family had of one generation of nine siblings, one of whom had died. We examined the remaining eight, calling them after diagnosing pigmentary glaucoma in patient no. 6 in the Table below, and we found pigmentary glaucoma also in a 42-year-old brother and late congenital glaucoma in a 49-year-old sister. The other five siblings were normal (Fig. 20.39). Of 15 descendants of the second generation, we checked only seven and found glaucoma in none of them, but we must point out that the eldest of them was only 25.

It is remarkable that in all the siblings the Schwalbe line was more prominent than normal. This prominence is not evident in the 360° of the angle but in particular zones.

Figure 20.39 and the table above show the various elements we studied in Family 2: refraction, depth of anterior chamber, shape of anterior chamber, ocular pressure, corneal diameter, transillumination, ring on the posterior face of the lens, chamber angle, and Krukenberg spindle. Pigmentary glaucomas occurred in two brothers; in one sister, there was late-onset congenital glaucoma. The three siblings with glaucoma are myopic, and the greater the myopia, the more severe the glaucoma; the rest of the siblings are emmetropic or hyperopic. The depth of the anterior chamber is significantly larger in the siblings with glaucoma. The three siblings with glaucoma have chamber angles typical of congenital glaucomas. The shape of the chamber is trapezoidal in the three siblings with glaucoma, planoconvex in four siblings, and concave-convex in the sister with the flattest chamber. We analyzed seven members of the second generation. From these it is interesting to point out that one of them, 9 years of age, has myopia of −6 D and a pressure of 18 mmHg in one measurement. Two brothers, one 25 and the other 13, have peripheral iris atrophy, which reveals the iris epithelial layer, as occurs in children, one of them with myopia of −3 D in both eyes.

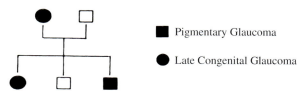

Fig. 20.38 Genealogic tree corresponding to the patient in Family 1

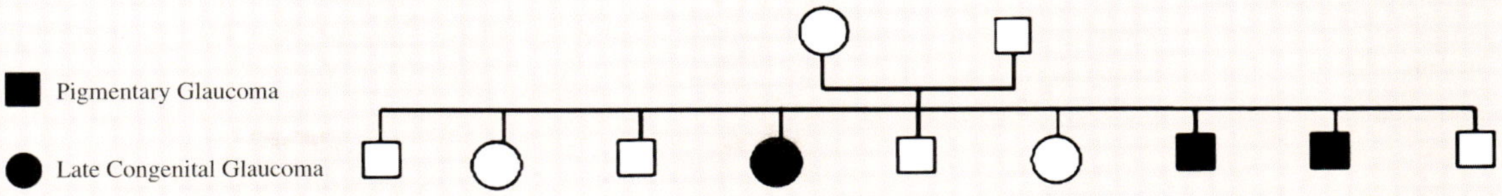

Clinical history no.	+	1	2	3	4	5	6	7	8
Age		53	51	49	47	46	43	42	40
Refraction		+1	E	−1.5	E	+1	−6	−4.5	E
		+1	E	−1.5	E	+1	−8	−4	E
Anterior chamber depth		1.88	2.24	2.9	2.4		2.97	2.78	2.62
		1.80	2.19	2.9	2.4		2.97	2.78	2.62
IOP		19	17	**19**	15	16	**40**	**22**	20
		19	17	**23**	15	16	**24**	**25**	19
Corneal diameter		11			11.8		12	11	12
		10.8			11.8		12	10.5	12
Transillumination		−	−	−	−	−	+	−	−
Ring on posterior face of lens		−	−	−	−	−	+	−	−
Chamber angle		Narrow	Open	l. p. Sch.	l. p.	Open	l. p. Sch.	l. p. Sch.	Open
			Normal			Narrow	DNI		
Krukenberg spindle		−	−	−	−	−	+	−	−

Fig. 20.39 Study of heredity in pigmentary glaucoma (Family 2). *E* Emmetropic, *l. p. Sch.* pathological mesodermal remains up to Schlemm canal. *IOP* intraocular pressure, *l. p* pathological mesodermal remains, *DNI* inferior nasal depression, *l. p.Schw.* Pathological mesodermal remains up to Schwalbe line

Family 3. The patient is a male who attended for consultation and pigmentary glaucoma was diagnosed. His brother, who accompanied him, had his ocular pressure taken "just in case" and was found to have 34 mmHg in the right eye and 27 mmHg in the left. A sister is normotensive. The mother has late congenital glaucoma (Fig. 12.40).

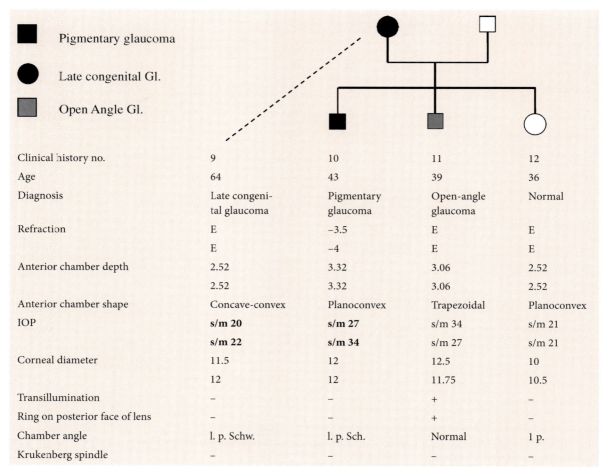

	Clinical history no.	9	10	11	12
	Age	64	43	39	36
	Diagnosis	Late congenital glaucoma	Pigmentary glaucoma	Open-angle glaucoma	Normal
	Refraction	E	−3.5	E	E
		E	−4	E	E
	Anterior chamber depth	2.52	3.32	3.06	2.52
		2.52	3.32	3.06	2.52
	Anterior chamber shape	Concave-convex	Planoconvex	Trapezoidal	Planoconvex
	IOP	**s/m 20**	**s/m 27**	s/m 34	s/m 21
		s/m 22	**s/m 34**	s/m 27	s/m 21
	Corneal diameter	11.5	12	12.5	10
		12	12	11.75	10.5
	Transillumination	–	–	+	–
	Ring on posterior face of lens	–	–	+	–
	Chamber angle	l. p. Schw.	l. p. Sch.	Normal	1 p.
	Krukenberg spindle	–	–	–	–

Fig. 20.40 Study of heredity in pigmentary glaucoma (Family 3). *E* Emmetropic, *l. p. Sch.* pathological mesodermal remains up to Schlemm canal, *IOP* intraocular pressure, *l. p.Schw.* Pathological mesodermal remains up to Schwalbe line, c/m with medication, *s/m*: without medication, *l. p.* pathological mesodermal remains

Family 4. A male patient attended for consultation and pigmentary glaucoma was diagnosed; his father was myopic and his 16-year-old son presented late-onset congenital glaucoma (Fig. 20.41).

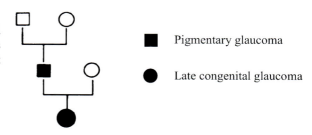

Fig. 20.41 Study of heredity in pigmentary glaucoma (Family 4)

Optic Nerve

The optic nerve was studied with direct ophthalmoscopy, retinography with double magnification and finally with HRT 1, 2, and 3, depending on the stage.

The study of normality and the five phases of glaucomatous alterations was made following our personal system (Chap. 18). There is always a good correlation between ocular pressure, optic nerve, and visual field. Because the majority of cases of pigmentary glaucoma have very high myopia, the evaluation is more difficult.

In some case it is possible to see an anomaly of the optic disc (dysversion of the disc). Figure 20.42 and 20.43 show a retinography with a congenital optic disc anomaly: dysversion of the optic disc, or situs inversus, a very pronounced glaucomatous excavation, papillary cone toward the inferior nasal region, partial albinism in the sector from the optic disc to the inferior nasal region (closing point of optic vesicle).

Fig. 20.42 Retinography with congenital dysversion of the optic disc

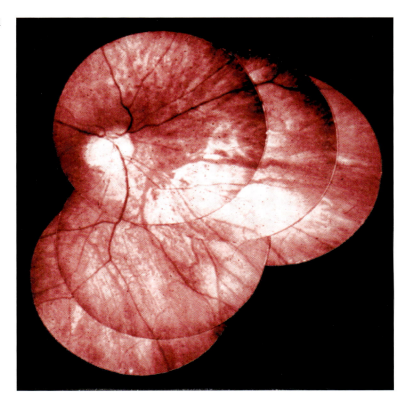

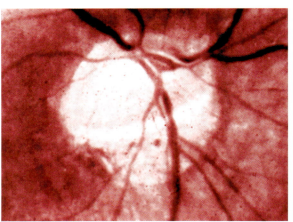

Fig. 20.43 Retinography with congenital dysversion of the optic disc with an inferior nasal coloboma

Visual Field

The staging of the visual field was made in accordance with the Brusini staging system, in six stages depending on the gravity. We should remember that the defects appear 4–5 years earlier with nonconventional perimetry (FDT) than with conventional perimetry (SAP).

Today we use the perimeter Octopus 101 program G2, the FDT, Matrix, and the Pulsar.

The defects prevail in a combination of diffuse defects and scotomatous effects.

We will provide examples later in the clinical histories.

Natural History

Pigmentary glaucoma is a progressive disease that requires medical or surgical management. In some cases, it becomes less severe and the pigment dispersion may regress and sometimes the intraocular pressure returns toward normal after treatment. This is why in some cases it is necessary to perform a differential diagnosis with low-tension glaucoma.

Robert Ritch [57] called the first (clinically irreversible) condition pigmentary glaucoma and the second pigment dispersion syndrome (clinically reversible).

Differential Diagnosis

Among the juvenile forms of glaucoma can be found congenital, late congenital, pigmentary, and simple glaucoma.

I. Congenital component of the chamber angle (peripheral depression of the iris at 6 o'clock, persistence of pathological mesodermal remnants over the trabecular meshwork, prominent Schwalbe line, peripheral atrophy of the iris, etc.);
II. Deep chamber and myopia.
III. Pigmentary syndrome (trabecular ring, Krukenberg spindle, pigment rings on the posterior face of the lens);

In general, pigmentary glaucoma shows components I, II, and III. In late congenital glaucoma, components I and II are found. In simple glaucoma, in the young person, these elements are absent. Pigmentary glaucoma seems to be a special form of late congenital glaucoma.

Capsular Pseudoexfoliation and Glaucoma

There are cases of this pathology with great pigmentary dispersion that develop from the posterior of the iris around the pupil where there is also atrophy. Pseudoexfoliation and pigmentary glaucoma can also be found together, as we have seen in several cases.

Severe Uveitis

These cases of uveitis are so severe that they have lost pigment from the posterior face of the iris but never have the characteristic signs of pigmentary glaucoma.

Cysts of the Ciliary Body Band or of the Iris Periphery

In these cases, though there is pigmentary dispersion, there is no Krukenberg spindle or deposit of pigment on the crystalline lens as in pigmentary glaucoma. Pigmentary dispersion may also be found in the melanomas of the ciliary body or in melanomas of the angle, but with a very different picture.

Pigmentary Glaucoma and Glaucoma for Pseudoexfoliation

It is rare, but both pigmentary glaucoma and glaucoma for pseudoexfoliation (PEX) can coexist in a single eye, as we have seen in our practice. Figure 20.44 shows the features differentiating the two pathologies. On the right can be seen the chamber angle (Fig. 20.44a); peripheral atrophy of the pigment layer of the iris in a well-developed case (Fig. 20.44b); with dilated pupil, pigment rings in the rear face of the len (Fig. 20.44c). On the left is illustrated a case of exfoliative syndrome and glaucoma is schematized (Fig. 20.44a): the chamber angle shows fine pigment in the form of waves that cross the Schwalbe line toward the rear face of the cornea (Fig. 20.44b); atrophy of the pigment layer of the iris, peripupillary (Fig. 20.44b); with dilated pupil, typical image in the anterior face of the lens (Fig. 20.44c). Figure 20.44d and Fig. 20.44e illustrate pigment distribution in pigmentary glaucoma and exfoliative syndrome. Figure 20.44e shows the location of pigment in exfoliative syndrome and Fig. 20.44f, the location of pigment in pigmentary glaucoma. In Fig. 20.44d, the pigment joins the exfoliative material and, since it forms a larger mixture, it cannot pass through all the trabecular meshwork and therefore remains at surface levels, not even reaching the juxtacanalicular tissue. In Fig. 20.44e, the granules of pigment come together in larger quantities opposite the Schlemm canal, but they can pass through the trabecular meshwork and settle inside the Schlemm canal and in the external collectors.

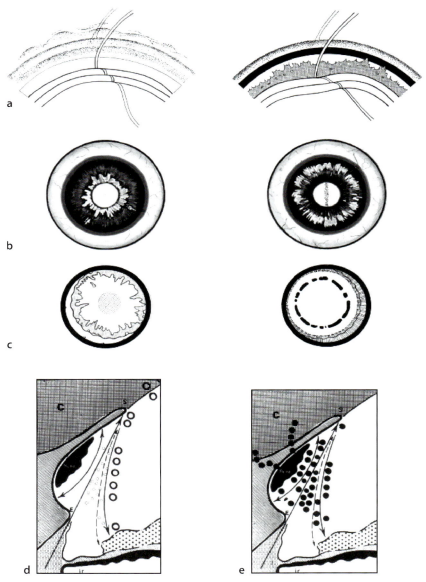

Fig. 20.44a–e On the *left*, glaucoma in pseudoexfoliation, and on the *right*, pigmentary glaucoma. **a**, Chamber angle with pigment that passes the Schwalbe line and deposits on the posterior face of the cornea in the form of waves (the Sampaolesi line). On the *right*, chamber angle in pigmentary glaucoma shows dark pigmentation in the Schlemm canal and pathological mesodermal remnants. **b** The pigmentation of the pigment layer of the iris: on the *left*, peripupillary, and on the *right*, peripheral. **c** With dilated pupil in pseudoexfoliation, the typical deposit on the anterior face of the lens in *two circles*. On the *right*, in the posterior surface of the lens, the deposit of pigment, in *two circles* at the place of the insertion of the posterior zonula. **d** The deposit of the exfoliative material of the pseudoexfoliation on the posterior face of the trabecular meshwork. **e** The deposit of pigment on the posterior face of the trabecular meshwork, inside the trabecular meshwork, inside the Schlemm canal and in the collector channels

Retinal Detachment and Pigmentary Glaucoma

In a series of statistics [58–61], we have steadily increased the number of cases of pigmentary glaucoma to 107 and we reached the conclusion that the incidence of retinal detachment in pigmentary glaucoma is 12.6%, while in the normal population it is 0.0001% [58–61]. Some months earlier in France, Brachet and Chermet [62] wrote an article on the association between pigmentary glaucoma and retinal detachment.

Pigmentary glaucoma is accompanied by myopia between sph −1 and −27 D in 73.5% of cases. A careful examination shows that not only is posterior hyaloid detachment very common, with its consequent posterior vitreous detachment, but the anterior hyaloid also detaches from the Wieger capsulohyaloid ligament up to the ora serrata. This posterior vitreous detachment and anterior vitreous detachment mean that it remains suspended only by its base (Fig. 20.45). Sometimes this base of the vitreous detaches, especially in the upper region, and the pigment of the posterior chamber passes through the ora serrata, over the retina. These changes, added to the peripheral degeneration of the retina, often lead to retinal detachment, in general,

bags with tears in their rounded (metacystic) ends (Fig. 20.46).

In pigmentary glaucomas, a careful study of its peripheral retina is always essential, and if lesions are found, they must be treated. For this reason also, miotics are contraindicated because, in these conditions, they provoke retinal detachment. This occurred in two patients in whom we provoked retinal detachment with pilocarpine.

The first manifestation of pigmentary glaucoma may be that of glaucoma or of retinal detachment. In the latter case, the diagnosis of pigmentary glaucoma is missed and the patient as well as the doctor may continue to be unaware of it. If the retinal detachment department makes a gonioscopic examination as a matter of routine, these cases are detected as pigmentary glaucoma. Even though the ocular pressure is very low at that time, if the retina attaches, the ocular pressure gradually increases and reaches pathological levels. If the medication is not sufficient to regulate the ocular pressure and there are progressive visual field defects, it is preferable to make a trabeculotomy instead of a trabeculectomy, since this regulates ocular pressure at rather higher levels between 20 and 24 mmHg, better for an eye that has suffered retinal detachment.

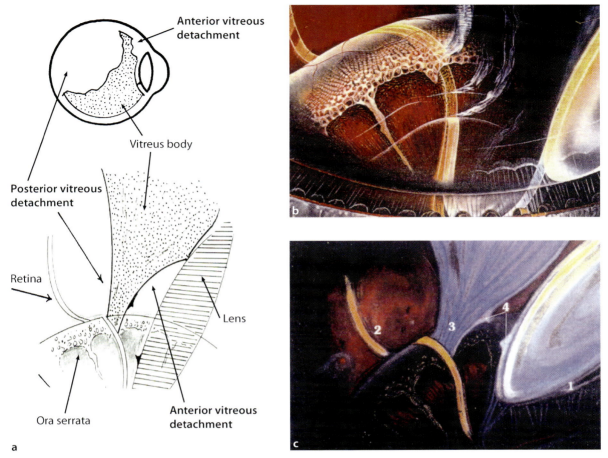

Fig. 20.45 a Drawing in the clinical chart of the first patient in which pigmentary glaucoma and retinal detachment were found. **b** Periphery of normal retina (from Eisner). **c** *1* lens, *2* retina, *3* vitreous body, *4* rupture of Wieger capsulohyaloid ligament found in pigmentary glaucoma

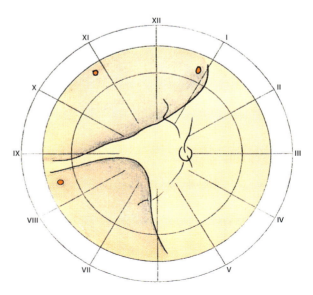

Fig 20.46 Retinal detachment, two bags with tears rounds (metacystic)

Case History No. 13

This patient was a 49-year-old female who had been operated for retinal detachment in the left eye 10 years earlier. During a check-up, the ocular pressure was found to be high.

	Right eye	Left eye
Visual acuity (c/c)	Sph. −7. Cyl. −0.50 to 165° = 20/25	Sph. −5 Cyl. 0.75 to 30° = 20/40
IOP	29 mmHg	23 mmHg
Chamber angle	Persistence of pathological mesodermal remnants, typical picture of pigmentary glaucoma	Persistence of pathological mesodermal remnants, typical picture of pigmentary glaucoma
Optic disc	5/6	5/6
Visual field	Stage III	Stage III
Surgery	Trabeculotomy (on the right part of the chamber angle)	
IOP	15 mm Hg	

The postsurgical gonioscopic picture is very interesting because the pigment disappeared in the zone of the trabeculotomy. This case is the opposite of the previous ones, because the retinal detachment presented first and then the pigmentary glaucoma became evident (Fig. 20.47).

Blockage of the Chamber Angle After a Pupillary Dilatation During Examination

In a young, 39-year old patient with typical pigmentary glaucoma with all the characteristics present, on dilating the pupil a pupillary block occurred in that eye, which raised the intraocular pressure to 55 mmHg. The UBM (Fig. 20.48) gave a typical picture of pupillary block. A UBM should always be done in cases of pigmentary glaucoma because it gives an idea of the morphology of the anterior chamber.

Medical Therapy

In the past, we have treated patients using adrenergic antagonists and agonists, beta blockers, etc. Today we treat them directly with prostaglandins from the start. If this does not regulate the IOP we add other drugs. In our experience, miotics should never be used, and even less the strong miotics, in this type of glaucoma. The high frequency of retinal detachment must not be forgotten. We have produced a retinal detachment by applying miotics.

Surgery

Campbell [63] proposed using peripheral iridectomy for pigmentary glaucoma. More than ten authors with long experience have communicated that peripheral iridectomy does not work. Jampel [64] published a paper titled "Lack of effect of peripheral iridectomy in pigmentary dispersion syndrome," just as Lehto did [65]. In our hands, the surgery that gives best results is trabeculectomy. In the series comprising 107 cases, the operation performed was trabeculectomy in most cases, and in eight patients, trabeculotomy: 79.1% of them without medication and 16.2% with medication regulated their pressure and stopped the development of their visual field defect. The daily pressure curve, visual field, and optic disc monitoring showed the defect to be regulated. In the cases in which the daily pressure curve was not regulated, the field continued to deteriorate. And when the IOP was not regulated with medication, they were reoperated.

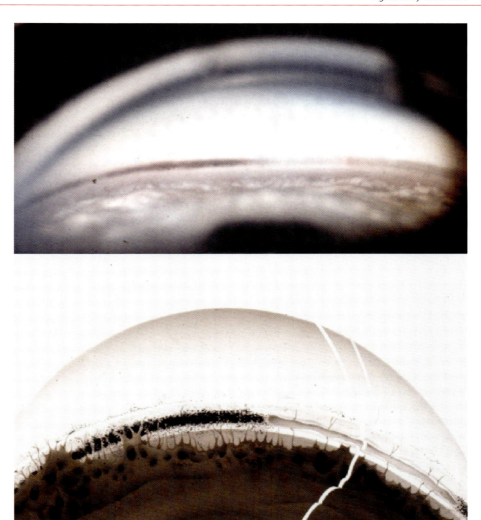

Fig. 20.47 Hemitrabeculotomy in a patient who had been operated 10 years before for retinal detachment, in whom pigmentary glaucoma was not diagnosed at that time

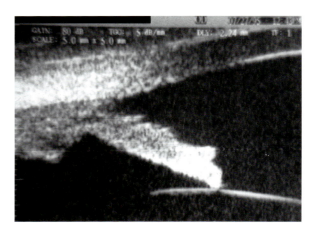

Fig. 20.48 Acute hypertension from pupillary block in pigmentary glaucoma. UBM made by Dr. Grigera

Pathological Anatomy in Pigmentary Glaucoma

Clinical History No. 14

A 33-year-old man came for consultation in 1974. He had worn glasses for myopia for 12 years, renewing them every 2 years. The ophthalmologists had never taken his ocular pressure. In 1971, he lost the vision in his left eye and optic neuritis was diagnosed. He is a medical doctor, and he consulted because at night he began to see iris halos around lights with the right eye, in which he still had sight.

He showed all the features of pigmentary glaucoma: Krukenberg spindle, typical chamber angle, atrophy of the iris pigment layer, trapezoidal anterior chamber, and slow photomotor reflex.

Gonioscopy showed a wide open angle with very pigmented trabecular meshwork at the height of the Schlemm canal and significant mesodermal remnants reaching the Schwalbe line.

The retina was normal in the left eye, while in the right eye a small bag of detachment was present at 7 o'clock with a tear, as can be seen in Fig. 20.49. I performed photocoagulation at the edge of the detachment, on the undetached retina. Since he was a medical doctor and had nearly lost the left eye, I asked his permission to take out a larger trabeculectomy piece when performing the trabeculectomy in the left eye (Figs. 20.50, 20.51).

	Right eye	Left eye
IOP	27 mmHg	29 mmHg
Visual acuity	20/20 with sph. −4.50	Finger counting
Visual field (Goldmann)	Typical Bjerrum scotoma Rönne step and loss of almost all the inferior nasal quadrant	Temporal remnant 25° in diameter

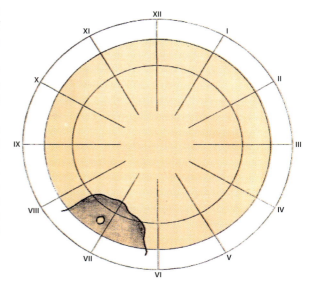

Fig. 20.49 Retinal detachment with small bag

Fig. 20.50 **a** Gonioscopy of the right eye. **b** gonioscopy of the left eye

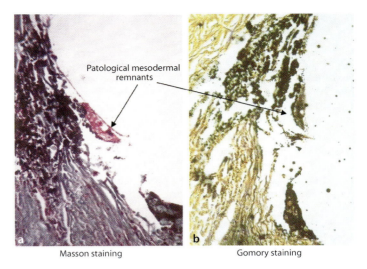

Masson staining   Gomory staining

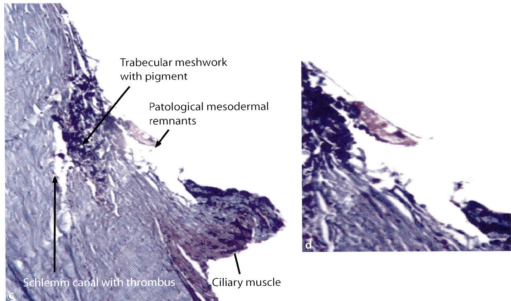

Fig. 20.51a–d Pathological anatomy of the piece of trabeculectomy of the left eye of clinical history no. 14. **c, d** The same piece with a greater enlargement

Clinical History No. 15

This is a 37-year-old man who had suffered from undi-agnosed pigmentary glaucoma for more than 15 years. Despite the open angle, the first clinical manifestation were iris halos around lights, a very marked goniodys-genesis, and the pathological anatomy showed patho-logical mesodermal remnants, such as are found in late pigmentary glaucomas. The patient consulted in 1974. Bilateral glaucoma had been diagnosed in 1967 with ocular pressure at 40 mmHg in the right eye and 30 mmHg in the left eye and no surgery was indicated. At the time of the consultation, with maximum medi-cation, we found the following data:

A trabeculectomy was done in both eyes, which has regulated the ocular pressure to date. The pathological anatomy of the trabeculectomy piece is very interest-ing. We will make a short summary of the following clinical history because we have found the same anato-mopathological sign (Figs. 20.52, 20.53, 20.54).

	Right eye	Left eye
Visual acuity	Light	Finger counting
	<20/100 With sph. −12 cyl −3 to 0°	20/24+++ With sph. −13 cyl. −1 to 0°
Chamber angle	Typical of pigmen-tary glaucoma with goniodysgeneses. Absence of cili-ary body band	Typical of pigmen-tary glaucoma with goniodysgeneses. Absence of cili-ary body band
Optic nerve	Exc. 6/6	Exc. 6/6
Visual field	III	III

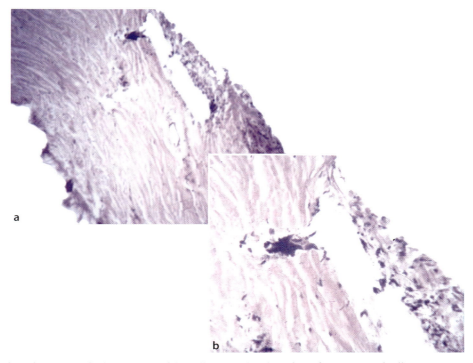

Fig. 20.52a,b Schlemm canal. In the *upper right* the entrance of the collector with a thrombus of pigments and cells

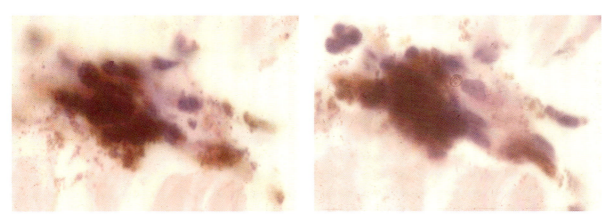

Fig. 20.53 Thrombus formed of cells and pigment focused at pigment level

Fig. 20.54 Thrombus of cells and pigment focused at cell level

Clinical History No. 16

This 46-year-old male presented bilateral pigmentary glaucoma with typical angle. He has two children, a 19-year-old boy and a girl aged 17, both with very pronounced pigmentary glaucoma and goniodysgenesis.

He was operated with bilateral trabeculectomy and his ocular pressure and pressure curve were regulated until 2000. The visual field defects did not progress. We also found a thrombus of pigment within a collector (Figs. 20.55, 20.56).

	Right eye	Left eye
IOP	25 mmHg	25 mmHg
Visual acuity	20/25	20/30
	20/20 with sph. +0.50	20/20 with sph. +1
Visual field	Typical glaucoma defects	Typical glaucoma defects

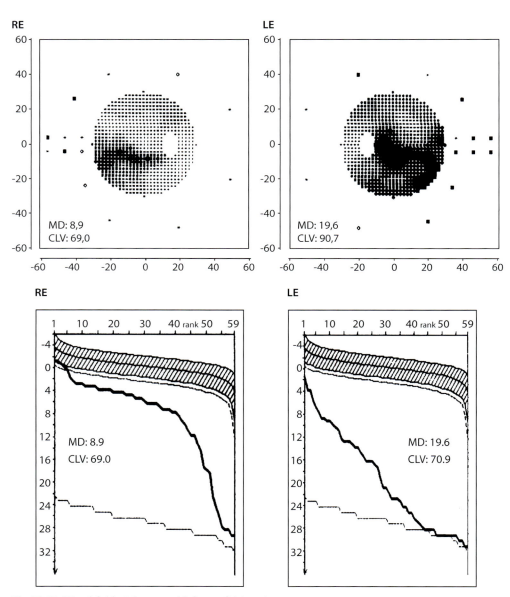

Fig. 20.55 Visual field, right eye and left eye of this patient

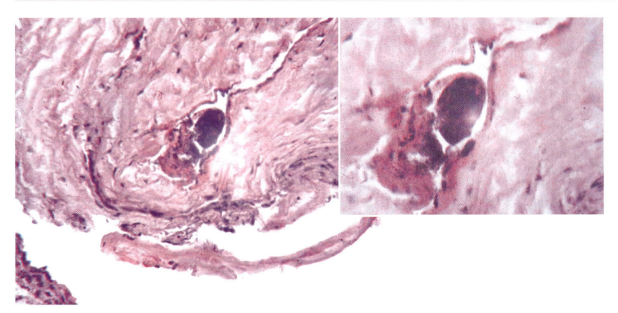

Fig. 20.56 Thrombus in a collector

Clinical History No. 17

This 54-year-old male consulted for the first time in 1974. He was diagnosed in the right eye with retinal detachment operated 15 years earlier, which had not recovered. At the time of the consultation, he had 0 vision and atrophic detached retina. In the left eye, he had pigmentary glaucoma. His mother and brother were myopic, between −3 and −8 D, and his son had bilateral pigmentary glaucoma. He also had esophageal diverticulitis and cervical arthrosis.

As regards his ocular history, he had been operated 16 years before for retinal detachment in the right eye, but he did not recover his sight. Fourteen years before consultation, when he was 40, glaucoma was diagnosed in the left eye and it was treated with pilocarpine 2%, four times daily. Another ophthalmologist changed his treatment to beta-blockers 0.5%, twice daily and pilocarpine 1%, four times a day.

This patient presents pigmentary glaucoma, a disease expressed in a retinal detachment of the right eye. He had lost his sight after surgery. Two years later, glaucoma was discovered and treated erroneously with pilocarpine, which is contraindicated in pigmentary glaucoma for the possibility of provoking retinal detachment. His visual field stopped developing after the surgery, which regulated the daily pressure curve and he now maintains his visual field and his sight.

Left eye	
IOP	23 mmHg, with therapy
Visual acuity	20/80 and 20/25 with sph. −6
Axial length	27.20 mm (Fig. 20.57a)
Lens	Normal, congenital posterior polar cataract and two rings
Zonula	With granules of pigment adhering
Iris	Almost complete peripheral atrophy
Chamber angle	Schlemm canal strongly pigmented 360°, pathological mesodermal remnants cover the ciliary body band and reach up to the Schlemm canal and the pigmented Schwalbe line
Optic nerve	Optic disc with eccentric excavation 5/6
Visual field	Deep scotoma in lower Bjerrum's area and depression of sensitivity in progress (1981) and (1982). (Fig. 20.57b, c)
DPC	With medical treatment: M: 22.1 mmHg and V: 4.4 mmHg pathological A trabeculotomy was made 30/5/83
Funduscopy	Peripheral retina: lesions predisposing to retinal detachment
Postsurgical development	Both eyes the mean defect (MD) and the corrected loss variance (CLV) are completely stabilized
Postsurgery DPC	M: 14 mmHg and V: 2 mmHg

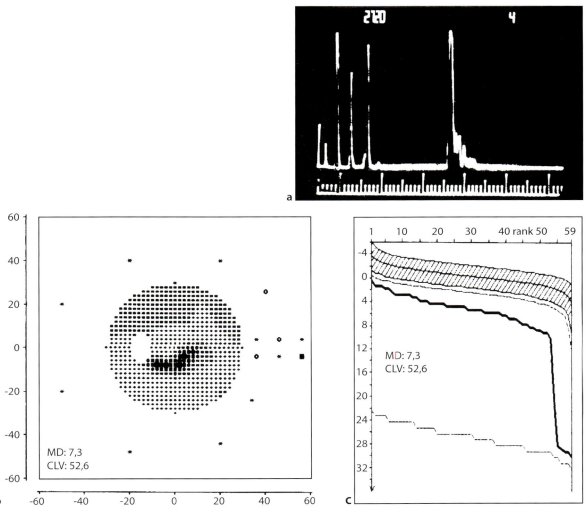

Fig. 20.57 **a** Axial lenght of 27.20 mm. Myopia sph -6. **b** Bjerrum scotom. **c** Bebie curve shows a combined defect, half diffuse and half scotomatous

Clinical History No. 18

This 26-year-old male is the son of the preceding case history.

However, there is a slight diffuse depression, as can be seen in the Bebie cumulative defect curve. With medical therapy, the daily pressure curve was completely regulated and in 7 years of follow-up there has been no visual field defects.

Examining the peripheral retina showed five tears in the right eye, two at 12 o' clock, one at 3 o' clock, one at 4 o' clock, and one at 5 o' clock, and one in the left eye at 12 o' clock, which were photocoagulated.

	Right eye	Left eye
IOP	30 mmHg	30 mmHg
Visual acuity	Finger counting	Finger counting
	With sph. −5.75. cyl. −0.25 to 90° = 20/20	With sph. −6.25 = 20/20
Chamber angle	Open, typical pigmentation. Goniodysgenesis	Goniodysgenesis
Iris	Shows atrophy of the iris pigment layer between 6 and 7 o' clock	Shows atrophy of the iris pigment layer between 6 and 7 o' clock
Optic disc	Exc. 4/6	Exc. 3/6
Visual field	Normal: MD: 1.8	MD: 2.3, Slight defect
	CLV: 1	CLV: 1.6 (Fig. 20.58)

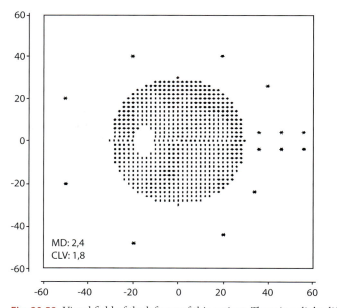
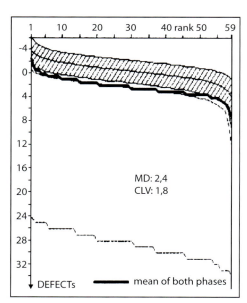

Fig. 20.58 Visual field of the left eye of this patient. There is a slight diffuse defect

Etiopathogeny

Current ideas on the etiopathogeny of this form of glaucoma can be summed up as follows:

- Sugar thinks that the main factor producing the increase in ocular pressure is pigment dispersion. The congenital factor is secondary.
- Nordmann considers that it is above all a congenital anomaly of the iris pigmentary epithelium, which leads to dispersion of the pigment that can obstruct drainage of the aqueous humor. This first anomaly is often associated with a second one, situated in the chamber angle. Briefly, like us, he believes that it is a late congenital glaucoma [66].
- Malbrán describes eight cases in his work. All of these presented an absence of the ciliary body band hidden by the persistence of pathological mesodermal remnants and peripheral atrophy of the iris.
- Based on the cases I have presented in this chapter, I consider that this is late-onset congenital glaucoma (an anomaly in the chamber angle, myopia, dominant heredity). Secondarily, there is a pigment dispersion, which appears late in the progression of the disease.

The cases in which we have shown a great accumulation of pigment in the trabecular meshwork, hiding it completely, as well as the thrombi of pigment in the collectors, suggest that the causes producing the glaucoma are the congenital alteration of the angle and the pigment.

The pigmentary manifestation is a phenomenon that sets in later over the congenital component and, in most cases, demonstrates the disease. Even though this pigmentary manifestation is determined by heredity, it appears later, and its clinical manifestations, such as the pigmented ring of the trabecular meshwork at the Schlemm canal, the Krukenberg spindle, the atrophy of the epithelial layer of the iris, the pigmentation of the zonula, and the pigment rings on the posterior face of the lens are acquired manifestations that occur as the disease develops.

In homage to Jorge Malbrán, who was the first to discover that pigmentary glaucoma was a late congenital glaucoma, we will translate one of the most important parts of his work. Malbrán says:

Pathological mesodermal remnants are seen in nearly all cases of congenital glaucoma. François and Kluyskens take particular note of this and mention other authors observations in agreement. The uveal trabecular meshwork is abnormally developed. The embryonic mesodermal tissue, fibrous or reticular in structure, cottony and silky in appearance, presents variable pigmentation. Galenga and Matteucci's interpretation is little different from that of François, Kluysken and Barkan, recognizing that the peculiarities found at uveal trabecular meshwork level determine a high insertion of the iris with a tissue with the appearance and features of the iris itself, i.e. a completely undifferentiated tissue that, as we said earlier, gives the name of abnormally developed mesodermal tissue. [15]

References

1. Busacca A, Carvalho C (1968) La morphogenèse du sinus camérulaire par la gonioscopie. Ann Ocul 201:400–430
2. Gorin G (1964) Developmental glaucoma. Am J Ophthalmol 58:572–580
3. Kniestedt C, Kammann M, Sturmer J, Gloor B (2000) Dysgenetische Kammerwinkelveränderungen bei Patienten mit Glaukom oder Verdacht auf Glaukom aufgetreten vor dem 40. Lebensjahr Klin Mbl Augenheilkd 216:377–387
4. Jerndal T, Hansson H A, Bill A (1978) Goniodygenesis. A new perspective on glaucoma. Scriptor, Copenhagen
5. Boles Carenini B (1965) Contributo alla conoscenza del cosidetto glaucoma giovanile. Ann Ottal XCI:140–170
6. Kluyskens J (1950) Le glaucome congénital. Rapport présenté à la Société Belge d'Ophtalmologie 94:159–160
7. Sampaolesi R (1962) Nuevo signo gonioscópico en los glaucomas congénitos de aparición tardía. Arch Octal B Aires 37:161–165
8. Sampaolesi R (1968) New gonioscopic signs in congenital glaucoma of late onset. First South American Symposium on Glaucoma, Bariloche 1966. Mod Probl Ophthalmol 6:106–123
9. Rieger H (1934) Verlagerung und Schlitzform der Pupille mit Hipoplasie des Irisvorderblattes. Z Augenheilk 84:98–99
10. Rieger H (1935) Beiträge zur Kenntnis seltener Missbildungen der Iris. II. Über Hypoplasie des Irisvorderblattes mit Verlagerung und Entrundung der Pupille. Albrecht von Graefes Arch Klin Exp Ophthalmol 133:602–635
11. Arnold PH (1911) Veränderungen des Oberflächen-Relief der Iris an der Stelle des Augenblasensplates. Klin Mbl Augenheilk 47:441–560
12. Streiff J (1915) Über eine untere Irismulde und über Iristypen und Übergang zur Anomalie. Klin Mbl Augenheilk 54:33–48
13. Vogt A (1931) Slit lamp microscopy of the living eye, Vol III. Springer, Berlin Heidelberg New York
14. Sugar HS, Barbour FA (1949) Pigmentary glaucoma: a rare clinical entity. Am J Ophthalmol 32:90–92
15. Malbran J (1957) Le glaucome pigmentaire, ses relations avec le glaucome congénital. Probl Act Ophtalmol I, pp 132–146
16. Etienne R (1960) L'atrophie essentielle des couches epithéliales de l'iris et du corps ciliaire. Ses relations avec le glaucome. Ann Oculist 192:224–244
17. Etienne R, Pommie. ML (1957) Contribution à l'étude du glaucome pigmentaire. Ann Oculist 190:491–499
18. Weekers R, Watillon M (1966) Hypertension oculaires attribuables à fraction conjuguée d'une anomalie mésodermique et d'une migration pigmentaire. Bull Soc Ophthalmol France 637–650
19. Di Tizio A, Le Pri L (1963) Contributto clinico allo studio del glaucoma pigmentario. Boll Oculist XLII:435–453
20. Nordmann J, Gerhard JP, Payeur G (1966) A propos du glaucome dit pigmentaire. Bull Soc Ophtal France 651–655
21. Heinzen H, Lueder R (1960) The value of gonioscopy for the diagnosis of pigmental glaucoma demonstrated by 9 personal cases. Ophthalmologica 139:244–2454
22. Shaffer RN, Weiss DI (1970) Congenital and pediatric glaucoma. Mosby, St Louis, pp 107, 117, 119
23. Mauksch H (1925) Über idiopathischen Zerfall des retinalen Pigmentblattes der Iris bei zwei Brüdern. Z Augenheilk 57:262
24. Cavara W (1929) Contributo a la conocenza del fusi di Krukenberg. Boll Ocul 8:1161
25. Koby F (1932) Biomicroscopie du corps vitre. Masson, Paris
26. Focosy M (1933) Su i depositi pigmentati della cristalloide posteriori. Boll Ocul 12:873
27. Bietti G (1934) Weitere Beitrage zur Kenntniss des Retrolentikularen Pigment-Ringes und zu seiner Entstehungsweise. Klin Mbl Augenheilk 93:54
28. Mann I (1937) Developmental abnormalities of the eye. Cambridge: Cambridge University Press
29. Zentmayer W (1938) Association of anular band of pigment on posterior capsule of the lens with a Krukenberg's spindle. Arch Ophthalmol Chicago 20:52
30. Evans WH, Odom RE, Wenaas EJ (1941) Krukenberg's spindles: a study of two hundred and two collected cases. Arch Ophthalmol Chicago 26:1023–1056
31. Cameron W (1941) Krukenberg's spindle associated with megalocornea and posterior pigmentation of the lens. Am J Ophthalmol 24:687–689
32. Bellows JG (1944) Krukenberg's spindle and its relation to anular pigment band on the periphery of the lens. Arch Ophthalmol Chicago 32:480–482
33. Becker B, Shin DH, Cooper DG, Kass M (1977) The pigment dispersion syndrome. Am J Ophthalmol 83:161–166
34. Kaiser-Kupfer MI (1980) Clinical research methodology in ophthalmology. Trans. Am Ophthal Soc LXXCVIII:896–94
35. Farrar SM, Shields MB, Miller KN, Stoup CM (1989) Risk factors for the development and severity of glaucoma in the pigment dispersion syndrome. Am J Ophthalmol 108:223–229
36. Campbelll, DG (1979) Pigmentary dispersion and glaucoma: a new theory. Arch Ophthalmol 97:1667–1672
37. Calixto N (1981) Contribuição para o estudo de alguns aspectos da sindrome de dispersao pigmentaria do segmento interior de olho. PhD thesis. Facultade de Medicina da Universidade Federal de Minas Gerais
38. Calixto N, Cronenberg S (1985) Glaucoma pigmentario sem pigmento. Rev Bras Oftalmol 44:30–40
39. Brachet A, Chermet M (1974) Association glaucome pigmentaire et décollement de rétine. Ann Oculist 207:451–457
40. Sampaolesi (1975) Desprendimiento de retina y glaucoma pigmentario. Arch Oftalmol Buenos Aires 50:370–375

41. Richter CU, Richardson TM, Grane WM (1986) Pigmentary dispersion syndrome and pigmentary glaucoma: a prospective study of the natural history. Arch Ophthalmol 104:211

42. Richardson TM (1989) Pigmentary glaucoma. In: Ritch R., Shields MB, Krupin TS (eds) The glaucomas. Mosby, St. Louis, pp 981–995

43. Rosen E (1962) Microzonuloscopy. In Krukenberg spindles and annular pigment rings of the lens. Am J Ophthalmol 53:845–853

44. Scheie HG, Fleischauer HW (1958) Idiopathic atrophy of the epithelial layers of the iris and ciliary body. Arch Ophthalmol 59:216

45. Mapstone R (1981) Pigment release. Br J Ophthalmol 65:258–263

46. Ritch R, Shields MB, Krupin T (1996) The glaucomas, Clinical Science, 2nd edn. Mosby, St Louis

47. Kaufman PL, Mittag TW (1991) In: Podos SM, Yanoff M (eds) Glaucoma textbook of ophthalmology, Vol. 7. Podos-Yanoff, Mosby, St. Louis

48. Sugar HS (1957) The glaucomas, 2nd edn. Hoeber-Harper, New York

49. Sugar HS (1966) Pigmentary glaucoma: 25 year review. Am J Ophthalmol 62:499–507

50. Bick MW (1957) Pigmentary glaucoma in females. Arch Ophthalmol 58:483–494

51. Krukenberg F (1899) Beiderseitige angeborene Melanose der Hornhaut. Klin Mbl Augenheilk 37:254–258

52. Hansen NR (1923) Über Hornhautverfärbung. Klin Mbl Augenheilk 81:399

53. Francois J (1958) L'hérédité en ophtalmologie. Massos, Paris

54. Shaffer R (1967) Symposium on glaucoma. Transactions of the New Orleans Academy of Ophthalmology. Mosby, St. Louis

55. Anderson JS, Pralea AM, DelBono EA et al (1997) A gene responsible for the pigment dispersion syndrome maps to chromosome 7q35-q36. Arch Ophthalmol 115:384–388

56. Anderson JS, Delbono EA, Haines JL, Wiggs JL (1999) Identification and genetic analysis of pigmentary glaucoma Loci on 7q36 and 18q. Invest Ophthalmol Vis Sci 140:5596

57. Ritch R, Shields MB, Krupin TS (1989) The glaucomas, 1sr edn. Mosby, St Louis, pp. 981–995

58. Sampaolesi R (1995) Amotio retinae und Pigmentdispersionssyndrom. Klim Mbl Augenheilkd 206:29–32

59. Sampaolesi R (1974) Glaucoma, 1st edn. Editorial Médica Panamericana, Buenos Aires pp 735–765

60. Sampaolesi R (1967) El llamado glaucoma pigmentario, su relación con el glaucoma congénito. Arch Oftalmol Argentinos 367–383

61. Sampaolesi R (1968) Le glaucome dit pigmentaire, son rapport avec le glaucome congénitale. Bull Mem Soc Fr Ophtalmol 434–463

62. Brachet A, Chermet M (1974) Association glaucome pigmentaire et décollement de retine. Ann Oculist 207: 451–457

63. Campbelll DG (1994) Pigmentary glaucoma: mechanism and role for laser iridotomy. J Glaucoma 3:173–174

64. Jampel HD (1993) Lack of effect of peripheral laser iridotomy in pigment dispersion syndrome. Arch Ophthalmol 111:1606

65. Lehto I (1997) Läßt sich vom Effekt der Iridotomie beim Pigmentglaukom auf den Pathomechanismus schieben? Universitäts-Augenklinik, Helsinki, Finland

66. Nordmann J (1968) Discusión al trabajo "Le glaucome dit pigmentarie," Sampaolesi. Bull Soc Fr Ophtalmol 434–463

Further Reading

1. Alper JC (1985) Congenital nevi. The controversy rages on. Arch Dermatol 121:734–735

2. Blanco MF; Mazzini MA (1956) Clínica Dermatológica e Sifilográfica.Hachette, Guanabara, RJ, Brazil, pp 104–1075

3. Bourquin J (1917) Angeborene melanose des auges. Zeitschr Augenheilk 37:129

4. Capeans Tomé C (1999) Actualización en tumores intraoculares. Tecnimedia Editorial, pp 127–140

5. Calixto N, Cronemberg S (1989) Glaucoma pigmentário. In: Almeida HG, Almeida GV, Calixto NE, Carvalho CA (eds) Roca, Sao Paulo, pp 277–290.

6. Cu-Unjieng AB, Shields JA, Eagle RC, Shields CL, Marmor M, De Potter P (1995) Iris melanoma in ocular melanocytosis. Córne 14:206–209

7. Elder DE, Murphy GF (1990) Melanocytic tumors of the skin. Atlas of tumor pathology, 3rd Series. Fasc. 2. Armed Forces Institute of Pathology, Washington, DC, p 64

8. Elshaw SR, Sisley K, Cross N, Murray AK, MacNeil SM, Wagner M, Nichols CE, Rennie IG (2001) A comparison of ocular melanocyte and uveal melanoma cell invasion and the implication of alpha 1beta1, alpha4beta1 and alpha-6beta1 integrins. Br J Ophthalmol 85:732–738

9. Friedman SM, Margo CE (1998) Choroidal melanoma and neurofibromatosis type 1. Arch Opthalmol 116:694–695

10. Garrido CM, Arra A (1987) Valve of the S100 protein in the study of nevus and ocular melanomas. Ophthalmologica 194:201–203

11. Gunduz K, Shields J, Shields CL et al (1998) Choroidal melanoma in a 14- year-old patient with ocular melanocytosis. Arch Ophthalmol 116:1112–1114

12. Gunduz K, Shields CL, Shields JA, Eagle RC Jr, Singh AD (2000) Iris mammillations as the only sign of ocular melanocytosis in a chi choroidal melanoma. Arch Ophthalmol 118:716–717

13. Heegaard S, Jensen OA, Prause JU (2000) Immunohistochemical diagnosis of malignant melanoma of the conjunctiva and uvea: comparison of the novel antibody against m with S100 protein and HMB45. Melanoma Res 10:350–354

14. Heegaard S, Jensen OA, Prause JU (2000) Immunohistochemical diagnosis of malignant melanoma in Queensland, Australia. Ophthalmic Epidermiol 7:159–167

15. Hogan MJ, Alvarado JA, Weddell JE (1971) Histology of the human eye. WB Saunders, Philadelphia

16. Honavar SG, Singh AD, Shields CL, Shields JA, Eagle RC Jr (2000) Iris melanoma in a patient with neurofibromatosis. Surv Ophthalmol 45:231–236

17. Honavar SG, Shields CL, Singh AD, Demirci H, Rutledge BK, Shields JA, Eagle RC Jr (2002) Two discrete choroidal melanomas in an eye with ocular melanoma. Surv Ophthalmol 47:36–41

18. Infante de German-Ribon R, Singh AD, Arevalo JF, Driebe W, Eskin T (1999) Choroidal melanoma with oculodermal melanocytosis in Hispanic patients. Am J Ophthalmol 128:251–253

19. Jakobiec FA (1982) Ocular anatomy, embryology and teratology. Harper and Son, Philadelphia, pp 97–119

20. Kadonga JN, Frieden IJ (1991) Neurocutaneus melanosis definition and review of the literature. J Am Acad Dermatol 24:747–755

21. Kaufer G (1969) Nevus melanosis adquiridas y melanomas de conjuntiva. Arch Oftalmol Buenos Aires. TXLIV:177–184

22. Magnin PH (1969) Bases de la melanogénesis humana. Editorial Universitaria de Buenos Aires, Buenos Aires

23. Matthews JL, Martin JH (1971) Atlas of human histology and ultrastructure. Lea and Febiger, Philadelphia

24. McLean W, Burnier MN, Zimerman LE, Jakobiec FA (1994) Tumors of the eye and ocular adnexa. Atlas of tumor pathology, 3rd Series. Fasc. 12. Armed Forces Institute of Pathology, Washington, DC, pp 76–82

25. Meerhoff W, Sanabria D, Bonifaciiino R et al (1995) Melanoma de conjuntiva en melanosis primaria adquirida. Arch Cátedra Oftalmol 2:4–9

26. Nawa Y, Yoshiaki H, Mototuev S (1999) Conjunctival melanoma associated with extensive congenital nevus and split nevus of eyelid. Arch Ophthalmol 117:269–271

27. Neale MH, Myatt NE, Khoury GG, Weaber P, Lamon A, Hungerford JL, Kurbacher CM, Hall P, Corrie PG, Cree IA (2001) Comparison of the ex vivo chosen sensitivity of uveal and cutaneous melanoma. Melanoma Res 11:601–609

28. Offret G, Dhermy P, Brini A, Bec P (1974) Anatomie pathologique de L'oeil et de ses annexes. Masson, Paris, pp 46–54

29. Ota M (1939) Nevus fusco-coeruleus ophthalmo-maxilaris. Tokyo Med. J 63:1243

30. Polak M, Azcoaga JE (1967) Neurohistología. Editorial Universitaría de Buenos Aires, pp 39–40

31. Rehany U, Rumelt S (1999) Iridocorneal melanoma associated with type 1 neurofibromatosis: a clinicopathologic study. Ophthalmology 106:614–618

32. Richardson TM, Hutchinson BT, Grant WM (1977) The outflow tract in pigmentary glaucoma: a light and electron microscopic study. Arch Ophthal 195:1015

33. Streiff J (1926) Pigmentsternchengrupen Auf der hinteren Linsenkapsel als Spur der Membrana Capsularis in einem Fall von einseitiger Aniridie und Retinalpigmentmangel und Vorderblattanomalie der Iris am anderem Auge. Klin Mbl Augenheilk 77:610–617

34. To KW, Rabinowitz SM, Friedman AH et al (1989) Neurofibromatosis and neural crest neoplasms: primary acquired melanosis and malignant melanoma of the conjunctiva. Clin Patholl Re 33:373–3799

35. Vajdic CM, Kricker A, Giblin M, McKenzie J, Aitken J, Giles GG, Armstrong BK (2001) Eye color and cutaneous nevi predict risk of ocular in Australia. Int J Cancer 92:906–912

36. Warmar RE, Bullock JD, Shields JA, Eagle RC (1998) Coexistence of 3 tumors of neural crest origin: neurofibroma meningioma and uveal malignant melanoma. Arch Ophthalmol 116:1241–1243

Contents

Though these glaucomas are usually divided into those having only ocular malformation and those in which ocular malformations are associated with other multiple and extraocular anomalies, the former are typically accompanied with somatic disorders, though of less severity.

Rieger Mesodermal Dysgenesis of the Cornea and Iris

This disease is also known as Hagedoorn mesodermal dysgenesis and Streiff corneal posterior marginal dysplasia. There are different degrees of mesodermal dysgenesis, which we will describe below.

In his *Textbook of Ophthalmology* (1909), Axenfeld used the term "anterior embryotoxon" for an opaque arch located at the periphery of the cornea, thus obscuring the limit between the cornea and the sclera. This anterior embryotoxon, also known as diffuse limbus, is typical of infantile glaucoma. The same author described the posterior embryotoxon later.

The posterior embryotoxon is a whitish ring-shaped line located at the level of the Descemet membrane, fully inside the cornea close to the sclerocorneal limbus and generally at the level of the Schwalbe line. From here to the periphery there is a slight veil-like opacification that hinders visualization of the anterior surface of the iris, unlike the clear view from the latter to the cornea. It is generally identified, as stated by Burian [1], by slit-lamp examination starting from the sclera to the cornea. This white cord is mainly visible at the temporal and nasal part. It is not really white but rather has a yellowish-white or golden color. Sometimes, small filaments emerge from this cord toward the center of the cornea. Other times, the cord detaches from the cornea and attaches to the superficial iris mesenchymal layer and forms a synechia with it. This posterior embryotoxon was masterfully described by Streiff [2]. This disorder, which can be found in healthy patients, may have different degrees of development. It is actually a highly variable malformation, which may in turn have associated malformations depending on whether it involves the sclerocorneal wall, the uveal part of the chamber angle, or both, in addition to the iris superficial mesenchymal layer.

In degree 1 cases, the distal edge in relation to the limbus is marked with a white line, which is a transparent, vitreous cord presenting round concentrations where pigment deposits can be observed with magnification. This cord-like formation creates a protrusion in the anterior chamber, in contrast with what occurs with the Schwalbe line. This first level, which involves only the sclerocorneal wall, is known as Streiff posterior corneal marginal dysplasia (Fig. 21.1).

This transparent, gelatinous cord is sometimes considered to be the Schwalbe line, but in some cases, Busacca [3] found that the Schwalbe line is actually behind it, between this cord and the limbus, like an incomplete circular ring. Sometimes the cord detaches itself from the posterior part of the cornea and hangs like an arch in the anterior chamber. It is rarely associated with glaucoma.

In degree 2 cases, this malformation not only involves the sclerocorneal wall but also the uveal part of the chamber angle, with no iris disorders. In these cases, numerous iris processes begin at the lines of the iris crests, i.e., the apex of the last circular fold of the iris, and end in the shape of a thicker button on this characteristic whitish cord. They sometimes seem to be either triangular or trapezoidal goniosynechiae.

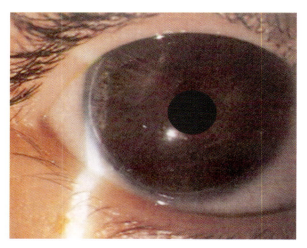

Fig. 21.1 Streiff posterior corneal marginal dysplasia: posterior embryotoxon. Under microscopy, with a 2-mm slit, a whitish, sometimes slightly golden cord forming a protrusion in the anterior chamber, can be observed from the scleral to the corneal part

with the cord, which appears to be the Schwalbe line. This cord may detach from the external wall and descend to the anterior iris surface and remain there supported by the iris, enter, and sink into the superficial mesenchymal iris layer, or else become welded to one edge of the displaced pupil in a slit-shape. Miotic drugs close the pupil, with one of its margins overlapping the other and leaving the patient in total darkness. This set of disorders of the scleral wall, chamber angle, and superficial mesenchymal iris layer, together with the slit-like deformation of the pupil is known as Rieger mesodermal dysgenesis of the cornea and iris [4], which was first described by Rossano [5] (Fig. 21.2a,b). U.S. authors currently call it simply Rieger anomaly.

Ocular hypertension is associated proportionately with these different degrees of the anomaly, but only in 50% of cases according to our own statistics and in 60% as reported by Alkemade [6]. However, it should be stressed that degree 3 malformation is sometimes present in eyes with good visual acuity and no glaucoma (Fig. 21.5). This means that the mechanism responsible for ocular hypertension is unknown and that the morphology of the chamber angle, even if severely anomalous and very different from the normal one, does not correlate well with the rise in IOP. Our experience leads us to think that the etiopathogenesis should be looked for in the fine pretrabecular layer of pathologic mesodermal remnants, which generally covers the trabecular meshwork, rather than considering the rough chamber angle malformation to be responsible for it. This is consistent with Jerndal's reports [7]. However, glaucoma has a high frequency rate and, in this regard, Seefelder stated that this dysplasia may, in some cases, be one of the causes predisposing to

Occasionally, denser remnants of pathological mesodermal tissue can be seen beginning at the root of the iris and continuing up to the external sclerocorneal wall. Some authors call this picture Axenfeld syndrome.

In degree 3 cases, there are additional malformations that involve the superficial iris mesenchymal film. This malformation becomes manifest by iris hypoplasia and by the presence of a series of weldings of the superficial mesenchymal iris layer. Weldings occur particularly

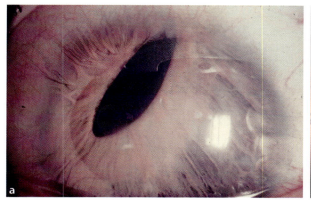
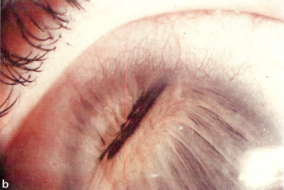

Fig. 21.2a,b Rieger mesodermal dysgenesis of the cornea and iris in a 5-year-old single-eyed boy (the fellow eye was buphthalmic, with absolute glaucoma). The pupil had a slit-like shape (**a**) and the IOP was 38 mmHg. The visual acuity was 0.4. Miotic drugs induced pupil contraction (**b**) and deprived him of vision

glaucoma depending on the severity of degree of the chamber angle disorder. When the degree is highly severe, there may be hydrophthalmos. Seefelder's words reflect our findings from the study of many cases with this malformation (see Clinical history No. 2, of a child with glaucoma whose mother had this malformation with no glaucoma).

In degree 3 disease, corectopia, dyscoria, ectropion of pigment layer, partial colobomas, total coloboma, and partial aniridia are manifestations that may accompany this syndrome. Sometimes, it is associated with the presence of a microcornea, typical when the malformation involves all 360°. We have had cases in which glaucoma had an onset during childhood, adolescence, and sometimes in adulthood, which we were able to follow up.

In Rieger's syndrome, in addition to ocular malformations there are also anodontias, dental anomalies, palate disorders, and other skeletal anomalies. There is almost always a typical facies. There is epicanthus, hypercanthus, hypertelorism, broad nasal bridge, cleft palate, etc. (Fig. 21.6a–c).

The hereditary pattern is autosomal dominant, with strong penetration and broad expression.

The following is a list of highly recommended publications: Seefelder [8], Rieger [4], Axenfeld [9], Streiff [2], Falls [10], Burian [11], Busacca and Pinticart [3], Waardenburg et al. [12], Alkemade [6], Waring et al. [13], and Jerndal [7].

Clinical History No. 1

This 10-year-old male was diagnosed with bilateral Rieger mesodermal dysgenesis. On the first consultation, buphthalmos with absolute glaucoma was found in the right eye. The IOP was 50 mmHg. In the left eye, visual acuity was 20/100 with no spectacle correction and the IOP was 30 mmHg. The cornea showed clearly visible posterior embryotoxon at the temporal and nasal area. In addition to the posterior embryotoxon, there was an anterior embryotoxon or diffuse limbus, which is strongly marked in the left eye. There were six Descemet membrane tears: two originating at the corneal center and heading for 12 o' clock, three horizontal, and one following the limbus in the inferotemporal area. Pronounced hypoplasia of the superficial mesenchymal iris layer, slit-shaped pupil extending from 9:30 to 12 o' clock. There was good contraction and miotics closed it completely (Fig. 21.2).

The chamber angle (Fig. 21.3) showed a cord-shaped Schwalbe line, wide-based goniosynechiae, which are trapezoidal up to the Schwalbe line, a cylindrical piece of the Schwalbe line detaching from its place and coming into the goniosynechiae. At the inferonasal area, the pathologic mesodermal tissue reached the Schwalbe line. At the iris root end and over the corneoscleral wall, where there were no goniosynechiae, there was a pink tissue joining the iris wall with the scleral wall. This is typical of congenital glaucomas and clouds the ciliary body band. A gelatinous whitish cord came out of the lower end of the pupil and ended in the corneal wall. Figure 21.2a is a front view of the eye and Fig. 21.3 illustrates the part of the chamber angle described under the previous figure.

In the evolution the first inferonasal goniotomy was performed in October 1966. The IOP reduced from 30 mmHg to 12 mmHg. However, 1 year later, in December 1967, the IOP rose to 24 mmHg. A second goniotomy was then performed in the inner superior area. The goniotome penetrated exactly up to the level of the pupil insertion and the IOP returned to 12 mmHg. After 4 months, it rose again to 30 mmHg and was regulated between 20 and 22 mmHg with adrenaline 1% and propranolol. The visual field remained unchanged in an examination 4 years later.

Figure 21.4 illustrates another child with Rieger syndrome.

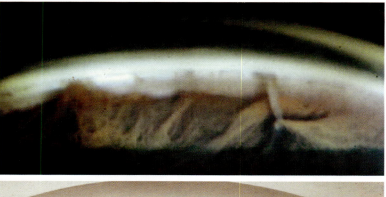

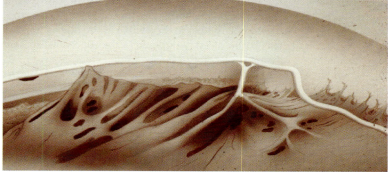

Fig. 21.3 Chamber angle in Rieger mesodermal dysgenesis. This figure corresponds to clinical history No. 1. There is a whitish, round, prominent, transparent cord on the right-hand side of the figure, which detaches from the Schwalbe line and comes down resting on the iris posterior surface. At this part, the iris ends on the posterior corneal surface, in the form of iris processes. In the rest of the chamber angle, there are pathologic mesodermal remnants which, at the *left*, do not reach far enough to cover the full extension of the ciliary body band, but at the center of the figure, cover it completely, as well as the spur. The iris tissue attaches to the whitish cord taking on the shape of a triangular goniosynechia, and, on the right, it is attached to it by means of a less dense whitish cord, which becomes bifurcated in its superior part. A gelatinous cord comes from the edge of the slit-shaped pupil (*bottom left*) and enters the pathologic mesodermal tissue where it can no longer be seen. There are two vertical filaments covered with pigment, which join the whitish cord to the pathologic mesodermal tissue. In brief, the morphology of the chamber angle is severely anomalous

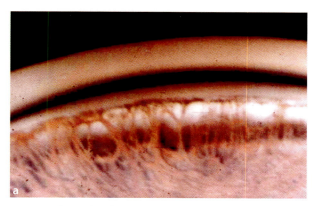

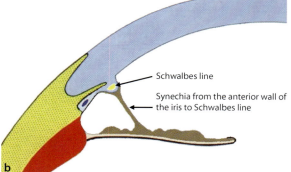

Schwalbes line

Synechia from the anterior wall of the iris to Schwalbes line

Fig. 21.4a,b A chamber angle belonging to another child, 6 years of age. **a** With Rieger syndrome, as in the previous figures. The morphology of is completely different goniosynechiae and anomalies of both chamber angle walls, a large quantity of pathologic mesodermal remnants that stand out in a comb-shape fashion at the anterior iris surface up to the Schwalbe line. The morphologic disorder in Rieger syndrome is severe and has very different gonioscopic pictures. **b** Diagram

Clinical History No. 2

This 3-year-old boy came for his first consultation with the following clinical record: "In 1959 the infant presented with an IOP of 70 mmHg in both eyes, and Rieger's mesodermal dysgenesis of the cornea and iris, associated with partial colobomas. In spite of the coloboma, a bilateral Elliot's procedure was performed successfully, but anterior chamber formation was delayed in both eyes. Postoperative gonioscopy revealed the presence of iris remnants attached to the gap made. Since IOP returned to original values a bilateral cyclodialysis was performed after consultation with other ophthalmologists. The procedure failed and a second bilateral Elliot's operation was performed at 7 o'clock, followed by another bilateral cyclodialysis, because IOP values remained at 45 mmHg."

This means that on the first consultation the child had already undergone four procedures in each eye. Our examination revealed IOP in the right eye, 31 mmHg and in the left eye, 27 mmHg. The corneas were slightly hazy. There were scars from previous surgical procedures at the four iridectomies; one of the eyes appeared to have iridectomy-induced essential atrophy of the iris. He was diagnosed with posterior embryotoxon, Rieger mesodermal dysgenesis of the cornea and iris. Examination of the child's mother revealed Rieger dysgenesis with corneoscleral disorders of the chamber angle and iris with no ocular hypertension. In the mother, the whitish cord, apparently the Schwalbe line, was detached from the corneoscleral wall, falling on the iris (Fig. 21.5).

We performed two goniotomies on the boy's right eye but did not operate the left eye because of the right eye. Six years later the visual field remained unchanged and he was able to start high school. It should be noted that, though both mother and son had pronounced mesodermal dysgenesis, the mother had no glaucoma even though the son did.

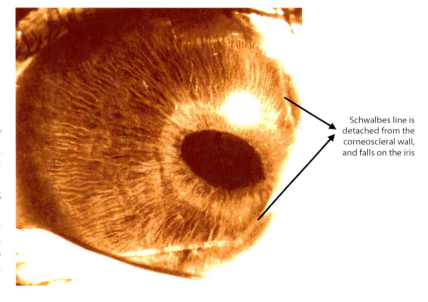

Fig. 21.5 Eye of a normotensive patient with Rieger mesodermal dysgenesis and normal visual field. Image of a slit-shaped pupil displaced toward the temporal side. The hypoplastic iris leaves the constrictor muscle visible. The gelatinous white cord lying on the iris can be seen at the bottom from 7 to 5 o'clock, from 5 to 3 and from 3 to 2. This woman's son had mesodermal dysgenesis of the iris with bilateral glaucoma at birth and 70 mmHg IOP in both eyes

Schwalbes line is detached from the corneoscleral wall, and falls on the iris

Clinical History No. 3

A 3-year-old boy was diagnosed with Rieger mesodermal dysgenesis and bilateral glaucoma. He was referred to us by a colleague.

There was telecanthus (distance between inner canthi: 3.75 cm), a chin recess, dental disorders, etc. (Fig. 21.6). In brief, this is a typical case with all the features described by Rieger.

One month after bilateral trabeculotomy, the IOP was regulated at values of 12–13 mmHg. After 3 months, the right eye remained stable and the IOP of the left eye was regulated with miotic agents.

Postoperative gonioscopy clearly shows the detachment of the whitish cord: it falls toward the anterior chamber in the right eye. The Schlemm canal is open and contains blood. In the left eye, where the anomaly was more pronounced, the trabeculotome was caught in the whitish cord.

	Right eye	Left eye
Corneal diameters	Horizontal: 13 mm	Horizontal: 13 mm
	Both eyes: posterior embryotoxon, clearly visible white cord covering the whole corneal circumference. No iris crypts, the frill of the iris has not developed and the pupils are slightly oval	
Gonioscopy	The superficial mesenchymal layer covers one-fourth of the total iris length. At the periphery, it separates from the deep one and becomes inserted, taking the form of fine spokes in the whitish cord attached to the posterior corneal surface, slightly anteriorly to the usual place at Schwalbe line	Similar picture but the chamber angle anomaly is more marked and the tissue covering its structures, behind the separation of the superficial mesenchymal layer, is much denser
Optic disc	Cup/disc ratio: 5/6, temporal margin: 1/3	Cup/disc ratio: 5/6; temporal margin: <1/3. Optic disc pallor and nasal rejection of the vessels.
IOP	20 mmHg	25 mmHg

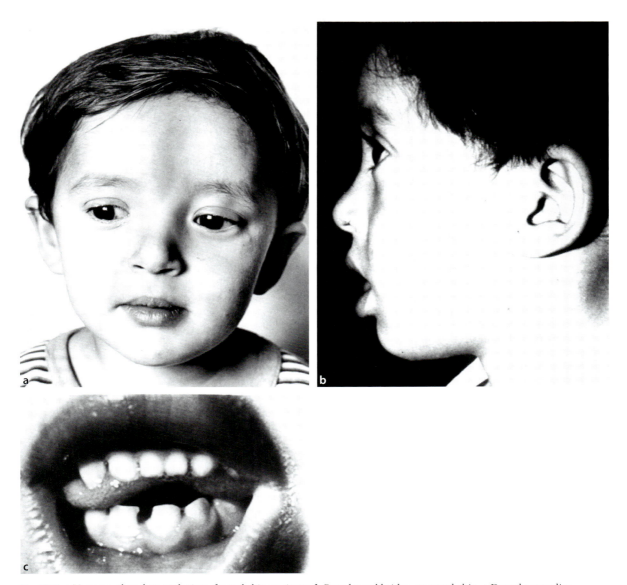

Fig. 21.6 **a** Hypercanthus, hypertelorism, frontal skin angioma. **b** Broad nasal bridge, recessed chin. **c** Dental anomalies

Clinical History No. 4

This is the mother of the 3-year-old child in clinical case no. 2. Given the dominant nature of the hereditary pattern, in these cases we also examined the mother, with the following findings:

	Right eye	Left eye
IOP	30 mmHg	25 mmHg
Visual acuity	20/20	20/20 with no spectacle correction
	Anterior and posterior embryotoxon, the latter more evident	Anterior and posterior embryotoxon
	Oval-shaped pupil with oblique major axis	Oval-shaped pupil with horizontal major axis
Chamber angle	Identical to her child's	
Optic disc	Cup/disc ratio: 2/6; temporal margin: 2/3	Cup/disc ratio: 3/6; temporal margin: 1/3
Visual field	Normal	Normal
DPC with medical therapy	Mean: 18 mmHg Variability: 3.7 mmHg	Mean: 17 mmHg Variability: 5.4 mmHg

As for genetic background, the patient only knows that there is a blind maternal uncle and also a blind maternal grandmother.

The patient's IOP was regulated with medical therapy.

Clinical History No. 5

A 5-year-old male was diagnosed with Rieger mesodermal dysgenesis (degree III) that progressed in a fashion similar to essential atrophy of the iris.

This patient was referred to us by our colleague Rodolfo Laje Weskamp Irigoyen Jr., who has given permission for this case report. Upon routine examination, this ophthalmologist found an IOP of 50 mmHg in both eyes, accommodative esotropia with hyperfunction of the oblique major muscle and facial asymmetry (see Fig. 21.7a, b and compare them with the appearance of the child in Fig. 21.6a, b).

	Right eye	Left eye
Visual acuity	20/30 with sph. +1 × 50°	20/30 +++ with sph. + 1.50
Axial length	23.31 mm	25.22 mm
Normal axial length for age	21 mm	21 mm
Corneal diameter	12 mm	12 mm

Though ocular hypertension typically appears late in Rieger syndrome, in this child it must have appeared early, since, as shown by echometry in Fig. 21.7c, d, the axial length was abnormal.

Gonioscopy shows goniodysgenesis with persistence of mesodermal pathologic tissue up to the Schwalbe line in both eyes. The morphology of this chamber angle evolved to such an extent that synechiae appeared on the posterior corneal surface (Fig. 21.7e) and finally led to polycoria identical to that seen in essential atrophy of the iris (Fig. 21.7f).

There is iris hyperplasia with absence of the frill of the iris in both eyes, thereby leaving the avascular and vascular pillars uncovered.

I have seen this type of progression of a case of Rieger dysgenesis as if it were an essential atrophy only once, and I have found reports by Kwitko [14] and Alkemade [6].

There are no tears either in the Descemet membrane or the endothelium.

This child was started on therapy with beta blockers 0.5% and Pilocarpine 0.5% from May 1982. The IOP went down to 12 mmHg in the right eye and 22 mmHg in the left eye. Since in December 1982 the IOP of the left eye rose to 34 mmHg, he underwent combined surgery (trabeculotomy + trabeculectomy). The IOP was regulated at 12 mmHg in that eye and the visual acuity improved to 20/20. The diurnal pressure curve remained regulated in both eyes.

One year later, in December 1983, the IOP of the left eye remained normal while in the right eye it had risen to 20, 22 and 26 mmHg. This situation continued until September 1984, when the IOP of the right eye rose to 36 mmHg. With combined surgery, the IOP was regulated but only for 1 month. Then, in the left eye, operated on previously and with its IOP regulated, there ap-peared six triangular goniosynechiae, iris resorption, and a new peripheral pupil at 6 o'clock nasally, a picture identical to that of essential atrophy of the iris.

Figure 21.7 g, h, show the visual field examinations of the left eye performed with Program G1 and Bebie curve, which evidence great impairment. The optic nerve had a cup/disc ratio of 4/6 in the right eye and 5/6 in the left eye.

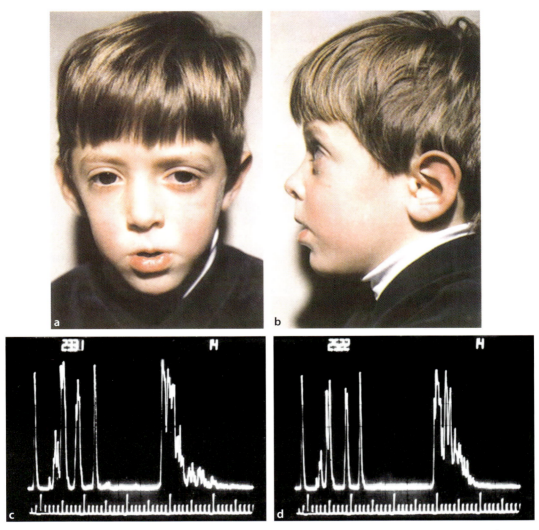

Fig. 21.7a–h Facial asymmetry (**a, b**). This should be compared with the appearance of the child in Fig. 21.6. **c, d** Echograms evidencing pathologic axial length. (*e–h see next page*)

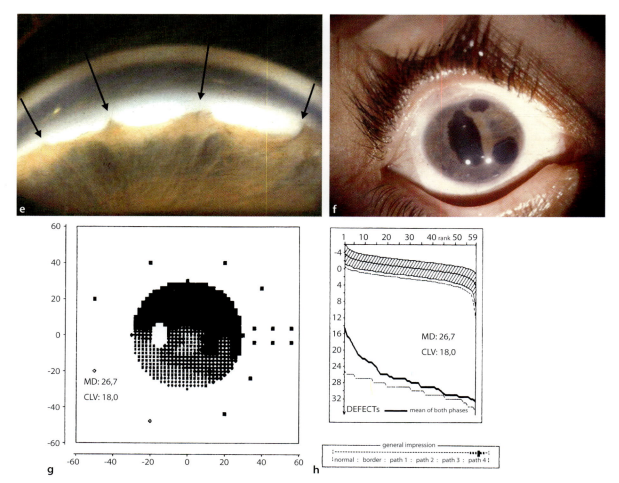

Fig. 21.7a–h (*continued*) **e, f** Gonioscopies showing progression toward the development of goniosynechiae on the posterior corneal surface, which finally led to a polycoria identical to that present in essential atrophy of the iris. **g, h** Gray-scale visual field of the left eye and program G1; the Bebie curve shows a severely impaired retinal sensitivity

Clinical History No. 6

This 18-year-old female consulted for refraction adjustment in December 1980. Her mother had noticed a white thread on the left pupil, and though she had mentioned this to other ophthalmologists consulted previously, they had stated it was not a matter of concern (Fig. 21.8).

	Right eye	Left eye
IOP	60 mmHg	58 mmHg
Visual acuity	20/60 with Sph. +1.25, cyl. +1.25 × 120°	20/200 with sph. +2.75

The visual field examination performed at the time was the Goldman perimetry, which revealed degree 3 damage in both eyes, with a loss in the upper hemifield and concentric isopter narrowing.

The cornea in both eyes had no edema or tears in the endothelium or Descemet membrane.

The patient was started on acetazolamide, four 250-mg pills daily, pilocarpine 1% q.i.d. and levoepinephrine 2% b.i.d. Since the IOP could not be reduced below 40 mmHg in the right eye or below 30 mmHg in the left eye, she underwent bilateral combined surgery, which regulated the IOP as shown by single-spot checks yielding 16 and 18 mmHg, respectively. The diurnal pressure curve was also regulated. The visual acuity remained unchanged and the visual field stopped its progression. There was a follow-up over 8 years starting in 1980.

The diagnosis was Rieger mesodermal dysgenesis (degree 3). This argues in favor of the vital importance of gonioscopic examination of the chamber angle and the interpretation of its results for diagnosis.

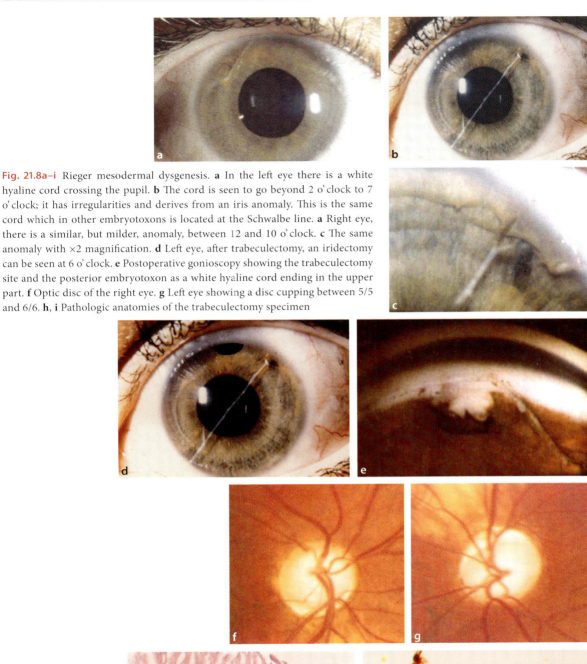

Fig. 21.8a–i Rieger mesodermal dysgenesis. **a** In the left eye there is a white hyaline cord crossing the pupil. **b** The cord is seen to go beyond 2 o'clock to 7 o'clock; it has irregularities and derives from an iris anomaly. This is the same cord which in other embryotoxons is located at the Schwalbe line. **a** Right eye, there is a similar, but milder, anomaly, between 12 and 10 o'clock. **c** The same anomaly with ×2 magnification. **d** Left eye, after trabeculectomy, an iridectomy can be seen at 6 o'clock. **e** Postoperative gonioscopy showing the trabeculectomy site and the posterior embryotoxon as a white hyaline cord ending in the upper part. **f** Optic disc of the right eye. **g** Left eye showing a disc cupping between 5/5 and 6/6. **h**, **i** Pathologic anatomies of the trabeculectomy specimen

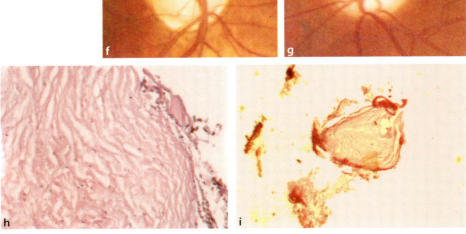

Clinical History No. 7

The 44-year-old female patient came for consultation because she had had far vision difficulties for 3 years. In a previous visit with another ophthalmologist, bilateral ocular hypertension was detected and she was referred to us. She had had hearing problems since she was a child, her nose was normal, the interpupillary distance was 62 mm, and the distance between the inner canthi was 35 mm (Fig. 21.9).

The IOP of the right eye was regulated with miotic agents while in the left eye a trabeculectomy was performed.

Posterior embryotoxon, mesodermal dysgenesis and partial coloboma of the iris were discovered. In some cases of posterior embryotoxon, sometimes associated with mesodermal dysgenesis, in the nasal or temporal area, at the horizontal meridian, there is a small trans-parent crescent-shaped area in the sclera, with its concavity coincident with that of the limbus.

Normally, at the limbus, the sclera comes closer to the cornea at the superficial part than at the deep part and thus covers the structures of the chamber angle. In contrast, in this anomaly, the situation is the opposite. At the crescent, the structures of the chamber angle can be seen through it (Fig. 21.10).

Kraupa [15] was the first to describe this malformation in the nasal and temporal areas. Kayser [16] described the same when he studied a case of posterior embryotoxon with pupillary membrane remnants, and he stated that he could see the chamber angle directly from outside. Ascher [17] coined the name "partial coloboma of the limbus" for this anomaly and said he was able to see the Schlemm canal directly, due to the lack of scleral tissue in that place.

	Right eye	Left eye
Visual acuity	20/30 with Sph +2, cyl −6 × 80°	20/30 with sph −9 × 90°
IOP	21 mmHg	26 mmHg
Visual field	I	II
Chamber angle	Open. At 6 o'clock, the trabecular meshwork over the Schlemm canal was heavily pigmented. Very prominent Schwalbe line with iris synechiae. At 12 o'clock, there is a whitish membrane covering the ciliary area of the iris. Corectopia. The pupil was pulled toward the supertemporal side, tending to adopt a slit-like shape	Gonioscopy revealed the appearance of Rieger mesodermal dysgenesis. At 6 o'clock the whole structure of the chamber angle was abnormal and at the inferonasal area there was a pigment ectropion covering the pupillary area of the iris. All this area, from 11 o'clock to 6, and at 9 o'clock was covered with a transparent nonhyaline membrane, revealing a paler hazel color of the iris. In another area of the chamber angle, there was persistence of pathologic mesodermal tissue up to the Schwalbe line
Cornea	Keratotorus	Keratotorus
Anterior chamber	2.8 mm	2.8 mm
Diagnosis	Rieger mesodermal dysgenesis associated with keratotorus	Rieger mesodermal dysgenesis associated with keratotorus

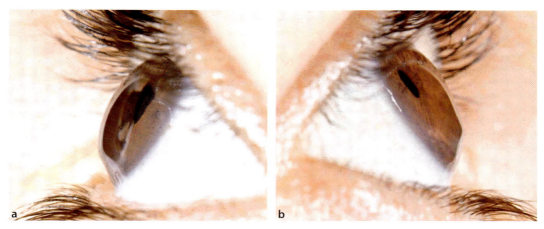

Fig. 21.9 **a** Keratotorus, pupil shifting, chamber angle malformation, pigmentary ectropion and supra-iris membrane. All these elements can be seen in the photograph due to the presence of the keratotorus (clinical history no. 7). **b** Keratotorus and pupil shift in the same patient

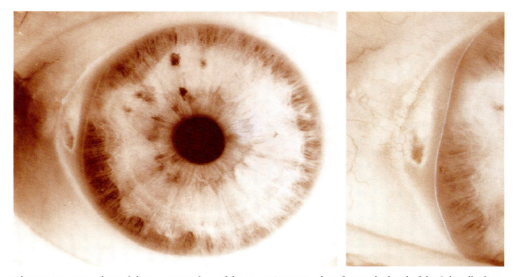

Fig. 21.10 Posterior embryotoxon, mesodermal dysgenesis and partial coloboma of the limbus. In the left nasal area, greater magnification reveals the coloboma and the characteristic cord of the posterior corneal surface at the level of the Schwalbe line. The iris hypoplasia is very marked in the peripheral part, and it uncovers the pupil constrictor muscle at the central part

Clinical History No. 8

This clinical history reports a 49-year-old woman who was referred to me by Dr. Nicoli and Dr. Travi. She was diagnosed with bilateral late congenital glaucoma with retinitis pigmentosa.

	Right eye	Left eye
Refraction	Sph. +3, cyl +1 × 110°	Sph. −2, cyl −2 × 60°
Visual acuity	Finger counting	Finger counting
IOP	24 mmHg	70 mmHg
Anterior chamber depth	2.02 mm	2.12 mm
Optic disc	Cup/disc ratio: 5/6; temporal margin: 1/3	Cup/disc ratio: 0/6; temporal margin: 3/3
Visual field	Typical of pigmentary chorioretinitis	Typical of pigmentary chorioretinitis

As shown by Fig. 21.10, this is a case of posterior embryotoxon with atrophy of the peripheral quarter of the iris, similar to mesodermal dysgenesis but with no pupil deformities. Goniosynechiae up to the Schwalbe line, pronounced iris peripheral atrophy make the pigmentary layer visible and the major arterial circle at some sectors.

Medical therapy regulated IOP in the right eye. In the left eye, filtering iridectomy successfully regulated IOP.

The genealogic tree shows that the patient's parents were first cousins, the maternal grandfather had retinitis pigmentosa and two of the patient's three brothers have retinitis pigmentosa.

Peters Anomaly

This is a congenitally defective formation of the Descemet and endothelium membranes, which, at the center of the cornea, give rise to a ring-shaped iris synechia and consequently to a central leukoma and secondary glaucoma due to athalamia. Diameters of 13–14 mm and corneal central disciform opacity are apparent. The IOP ranges from 25 to 35 mmHg.

This syndrome was described by Peters [18] as a glaucoma secondary to peripheral athalamia caused by an anterior ring-shaped iris synechia at the margins of a congenital formation defect of the Descemet membrane. In his book on glaucoma (1930) [19], in the chapter on hydrophthalmus, Peters quotes his 1906 description as a congenital corneal opacity, the consequence of a formation defect of the Descemet membrane.

In 1899, Von Hippel [20] described it as an internal inflammatory corneal ulcer. These opacities can be very large, as in the case reported by Buck [21], and lead to an enlargement of the eyeball, as observed in a series of cases accompanied by chamber angle and iris disorders.

Meisner [22] found a corneal opacity in a case of hydrophthalmus with defective formation of the Descemet membrane with an absence of crystalline lens. He attributed this to defective closure of the lens vesicle leading to its absence. The absence of normal chamber angle structures has been described by Appelmans et al. [23].

Waring et al. [13] described the different steps that may be involved in this anomaly: posterior keratoconus, corneal tissue defect and leukoma, iris adhesions at the margin of the leukoma, and lens apposition to the leukoma. As regards pathogenesis, the papers by Townsend et al. [24–26] are highly recommended.

Diagnosis

Diagnosis is generally easy, but differential diagnosis with other congenital corneal opacities should be considered, for example:
- Hydrophthalmus with hazy cornea;
- Parenchymatous keratitis;
- Inflammatory leukoma with staphyloma secondary to gonococcal conjunctivitis;
- Epidermoid (corneal mesodermal metaplasia);
- Congenital corneal staphyloma or leukomatous keratectasia.

Demaske and Müller, at the Meeting of the German Society of Ophthalmology, reported the following case [27] (kindly provided by the authors).

Clinical History No. 9

This 18-month-old girl weighed 2.960 kg after a full-term, normal pregnancy and measured 50 cm in length. her mother had a cleft palate. She had a 2.5-year-old healthy brother.

In her right eye, there was spherical congenital corneal staphyloma, with a corneal diameter of 10 mm, absent Descemet membrane (Fig. 21.11a), and anterior iris synechia. In her left eye, there was Peters anomaly, ring-shaped central opacification with an almost circular iris synechia; the iris stroma was visible; corneal diameter was 10 mm.

Ultrasonography in both eyes showed that the vitreous body was free. The left eye had a greater length than normal (5 mm above normal values).

In the right eye, the staphyloma was reduced with cryotherapy and a penetrating keratoplasty 8.5 mm in diameter was performed 15 days later (Fig. 21.11b, c).

At the beginning, the graft was smooth and remained transparent for a few weeks.

Three months later, there were folds on the posterior graft surface and mild parenchymal opacity from the margin.

Four months later, a small staphyloma appeared at the lower part of the graft.

After 9 months, the opacity of the staphyloma was the same size as before surgery.

At month 11 postoperatively, the eye was enucleated due to chronic blepharoconjunctivitis and a very pronounced oculodigital phenomenon. Histology revealed a corneal epithelium of varying thickness with vascular growth in the basal cell layer and Bowman membrane tears. Behind this there was conjunctival tissue that was filled with collagen and vascularized, which included part of the iris and loose pigmentary cells. The Descemet membrane was absent and it was homogeneously PAS-positive.

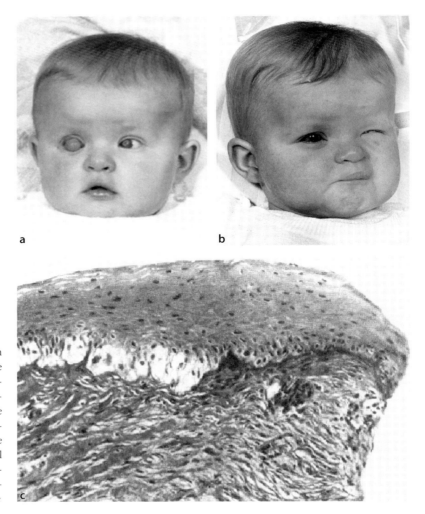

Fig. 21.11 a Congenital staphyloma in the right eye and Peters anomaly in the left eye. From a clinical history reported by Damaske and Müller [27] (reproduced with permission). b Appearance of penetrating keratoplasty after surgery. c Histologic preparation of the corneal staphyloma: edema of the basal epithelial layers. Separation of the layers from their own substance with vascularization; iris with partial synechiae

Clinical History No. 10

This 5-day-old boy was full-term, the child of healthy parents: a 23-year-old father and 22-year-old mother. He had a buphthalmic right eye with a disciform central leukoma.

The corneal diameter of the right eye was 14 mm. There was a white disciform leukoma 9 mm in diameter. At the center of the leukoma, and concentric to it, there was a yellowish 3-mm-diameter disc with a darker center (Fig. 21.12). Slit-lamp examination revealed a bullous keratopathy in its early stages. Outside the leukoma, in the 2.5 mm left on each sides, the cornea was transparent and the peripheral part of the iris with its typical dark triangles can be seen, as well as the area of iris tissue between them and the root insertion, though the latter was larger than usual. The dark triangles form, distally, a festooned line. The whole iris is visible, extending from the periphery of the leukoma to the limbus, and it was attached to the posterior corneal surface. This means that there was peripheral athalamia.

The IOP was 25 mmHg, while in the fellow eye, which was apparently normal, it was 6 mmHg, with a corneal diameter of 10 mm and an incomplete posterior embryotoxon. The chamber angle, with arrested development, showed dark areas continued by a short iris root. There were pathological mesodermal remnants inserted at the Schlemm canal. The iris tissue was not developed, while both the Henle layer and the superficial mesodermal layer were developing. This leaves the whole vascular tree of the iris completely visible: part of the greater arterial circle of the iris, radial vessels and the complete lesser arterial circle of the iris.

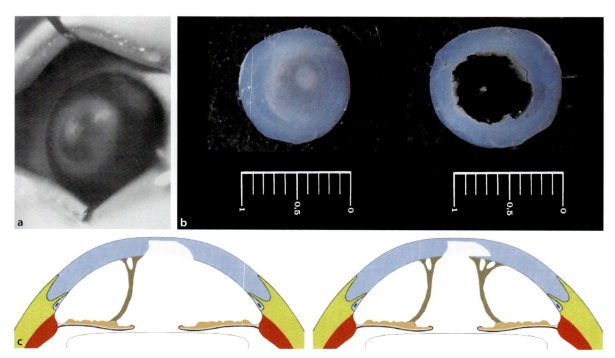

Fig. 21.12 **a** Cornea of a case of Peters anomaly, **b** in a view from its anterior and posterior surfaces. Anatomic piece from the cornea of the patient described in clinical history no. 10. On the anterior surface there is a leukoma. The iris (*dark*) becomes transparent at the pericentral part, and in the central area there is a dehiscent zone. On the posterior surface the iris can be seen, tightly attached to the posterior corneal surface. **c** Diagram of Peters anomaly, posterior corneal ulcer with or without cataract

Therapy

After 2 days, a perforating corneal graft 10 mm in diameter was performed (when the infant was 9 days old). The surgical protocol is the following:

1. A 10-mm trephine is used to cup the superficial corneal layers.
2. The anterior chamber is opened.
3. The section is completed through the full corneal thickness with Troutman scissors.
4. The cornea is attached to the iris around its whole circumference, at the external third, and is verified. A 2-mm surface in the inner corneal wall is left free.
5. A loop is created in the iris with Vannas scissors, close to its insertion in the cornea; a circular section is made by introducing one blade of the scissors through it at this same level.
6. A transparent crystalline lens becomes visible through the wound, with a very small anterior polar cataract. The ocular fundus is illuminated in red. Figure 21.12 shows the piece removed in a view through its anterior and posterior surfaces.
7. The donor cornea is implanted with 4 silk sutures at 3, 6, 9, and 12 o'clock, completed with a nylon continuous suture.
8. Upon completion of surgery, the chamber is fully formed.

Follow-up examinations took place after 5 days.

The graft was transparent, the anterior chamber was formed and the fundus was illuminated in red.

The IOP was 6 mmHg in both eyes. This demonstrates that it was a secondary glaucoma to peripheral athalamia.

Follow-Up Examination After 10 Days

The IOP was 7 mmHg in both eyes. At the inferonasal part of the recipient cornea, there were two small staphylomas. A small incision was placed in them and the margins were attached with virgin silk sutures.

Follow-Up Examination After 20 Days

The graft was transparent, the staphyloma described above was closed. The IOP was 6 mmHg in both eyes.

Follow-Up Examinations After 4 Months

The graft had become hazy and had a tectonic role. The IOP remained at 8 mmHg in both eyes.

Pathologic Anatomy

The cornea shown in Fig. 21.12 was embedded in paraffin and stained with hematoxylin-eosin, PAS, and trichrome stain. The microphotographs were obtained with phase contrast. Later the following findings were made:

Epithelium

The basal layer was edematous (Fig. 21.13). At the central area of the leukoma, there was a yellowish disc with a dark center (Fig. 21.12). Histology revealed that the basal cells and the basement membrane were destroyed, and there was a serious anomaly in the underlying Bowman membrane (Fig. 21.14).

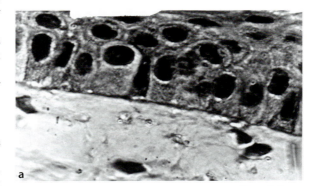

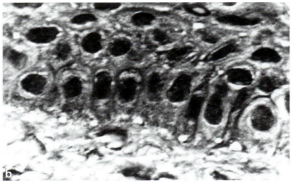

Fig. 21.13a,b Peters anomaly, corneal epithelium (original preparation). **a** Epithelium with preserved basement membrane, absence of Bowman membrane. There is a small aqueous infiltration into basal cells. **b** Another area where the epithelium has lost the basement membrane. The aqueous infiltration (edema) is much more pronounced

In the areas corresponding to the bullous keratitis, a typical histologic image was obtained (Fig. 21.15).

The basement membrane of the epithelium persisted in some areas (Fig. 21.13b). In other areas, the basement membrane was destroyed (Fig. 21.13a).

Bowman Membrane

The Bowman membrane was preserved in the periphery, with a an abnormal area, thinning to fully disappear in the paracentral area (Fig. 21.15). Fig. 21.16, magnified, shows the transition zone to the point where Bowman membrane has fully disappeared.

Stroma

There is an increased number of keratocytes at the central area (Fig. 21.17). Figure 21.18 shows the area where there is an anterior synechia of the iris and where both tissues are difficult to identify.

Descemet Membrane and Endothelium

Figure 21.18 show the persistence of the Descemet membrane and endothelium at the corneal periphery, but then they disappear before the formation of the anterior synechia of the iris.

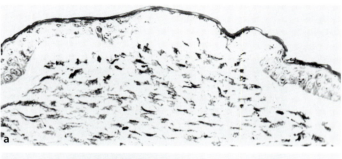
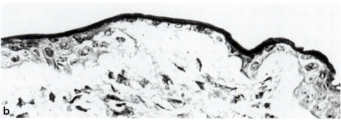

Fig. 21.14a,b Peters anomaly (original preparation). a Central and anterior part of the cornea. b With ×2 magnification. The epithelium is almost completely destroyed in its central part and has become reduced to a cellular layer. Bowman membrane is severely disturbed and the parenchyma shows excessive keratocytes

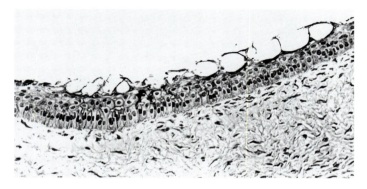

Fig. 21.15 Peters anomaly. Area of the epithelium where there is bullous keratosis. There is no Bowman membrane and an increased number of keratocytes

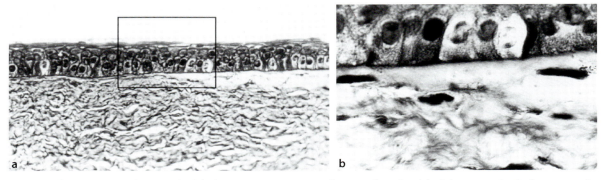

Fig. 21.16a,b Peters anomaly. a On the *left*, there is no Bowman membrane and on the *right*, it is present. In the latter area, the basement membrane of the epithelium persists. b The area enclosed by the rectangle in a, with greater magnification

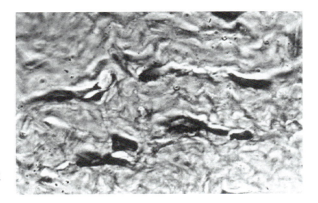

Fig. 21.17 Peters anomaly. Corneal parenchyma, increased number of keratocytes

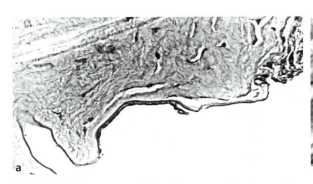

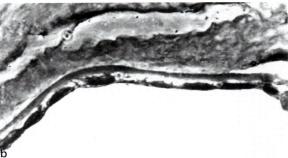

Fig. 21.18a,b Peters anomaly. Posterior corneal surface. a The *left end* corresponds to the area of the incision created with the trephine and at the *right end* there is iris tissue which continues in the corneal stroma. The Descemet membrane is absent. In the *central part of the figure*, the corneal periphery, there are remnants of both Descemet membrane and endothelium, which disappear up to the area of the iris synechia. b With ×4 magnification, disturbances of the Descemet membrane and endothelium. The Descemet membrane is very thin, reduced to one-third of its normal thickness and the endothelial nuclei show pyknosis

Pathogenesis

Von Hippel [20], described the picture as an inner corneal inflammatory ulcer.

Peters [18] believed it was a congenital defect of the Descemet membrane in the center of the cornea, which gave rise to a ring-shaped synechia of the iris at this level, as well as to peripheral athalamia and glaucoma.

Meisner [22], examining a similar case, but associated with congenital aphakia, stated it was a defect in the closure of the crystalline lens vesicle.

Appelmans et al. [23] described the absence of the normal structures of the chamber angle.

Reese and Ellsworth [28] considered it to be a syndrome due to an anterior chamber cleavage disorder.

Alkemade [6] made the distinction between primary and secondary Peters anomaly. The primary form (similar to the case we described above) is quite rare, a developmental defect of the cornea, of recessive heredity; the secondary form is a component that may accompany Rieger mesodermal dysgenesis of the cornea and iris.

Nakanishi et al. [29], with electron microscopy, demonstrated that both Bowman and Descemet membranes, even where they appear as normal at the periphery, are actually not so, and that the Descemet membrane is similar to one formed 3 days after a wound. These authors quoted reports by Hay and Ravel [30], which show that the epithelium is responsible for the embryogenesis of Bowman membrane. Nakanishi et al. [29] state that if this is so, Peters anomaly is an ectodermal disorder, and that the absence of Bowman membrane, as suggested by Alkemade, renders Reese and Ellsworth's description embryologically incorrect, since the part of the cornea involved in Peters anomaly does not develop during anterior chamber formation.

As we can see, each author, on different grounds, supports a pathogenic mechanism. However, since our focus here is on glaucoma, we would like to recommend a paper by Atsushi et al. [31] covering the ultrastructure of sclerocornea.

Figure 21.19, reproduced from this paper, shows a central epithelium in the sclerocornea of eight to ten cell layers with absence of Bowman membrane; there are vessels in the stroma (stained in toluidine blue) and a thinned Descemet membrane (0.8–1.5 µm) one-tenth the thickness of a normal eye. Nath et al. [32] have also researched the same topic. There are similarities in the Bowman and Descemet membrane anomalies revealed by this preparation and Peters syndrome. In addition, in Peters syndrome and sclerocornea, there are general somatic disturbances, cardiac malformations, etc. Bowman membrane is generally absent in leukomas, unlike Descemet membrane, which is always present.

In my opinion, Axenfeld posterior embryotoxon, Rieger mesodermal dysgenesis, sclerocornea, and Peters syndrome are all anterior segment disorders with features in common as well as with distinct characteristics, some which clearly separate them: iris mesodermal dysgenesis, dominant hereditary pattern, Peters anomaly, and recessive heredity. They may be associated with glaucoma, but the case described in clinical history no. 2 should be kept in mind. In this case, mother and son had Rieger dysgenesis with a large malformation of the anterior segment: the child had severe glaucoma, whereas the mother was normal. In contrast, in clinical history no. 4, both mother and child had anterior segment anomalies and they both had glaucoma. Glaucoma in only present when aqueous humor outflow pathways are disturbed. This explains the case described by Appelmans [23], in which he found a fully anomalous chamber angle, or the case we described, where glaucoma was only secondary and with a normal chamber angle.

In my practice, I have seen minor forms of Peters anomalies, a forme fruste of Peters anomaly, with broad-based implantation synechiae corresponding to pericentral leukomas with a flat chamber angle and glaucoma. Leukomas are generally small, and when they are transparent, they reveal the synechiae of the iris with the posterior corneal defect (Fig. 21.20).

Fig. 21.19a,b Sclerocornea (reproduced from [31]). **a** *Ep* epithelium, *St* stroma. Absence of Bowman membrane. *V* small vessels. **b** *DM* Descemet membrane, thinned to one-tenth of its normal size, *En* endothelium, *AC* anterior chamber

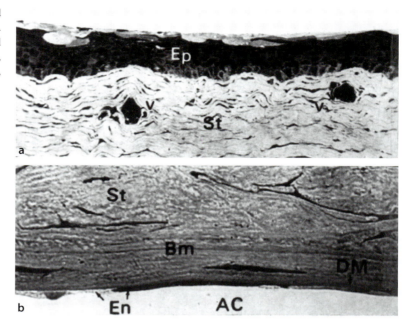

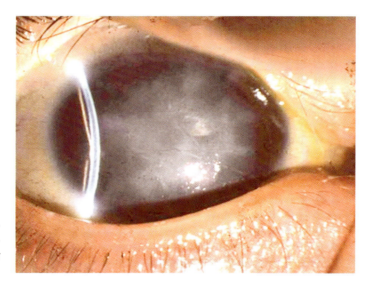

Fig. 21.20 Forme fruste of Peters anomaly. Synechiae which have a broad base where they are implanted with pericentral leukomas. Flat chamber angle and glaucoma

Aniridia

This was described for the first time in 1819 by Barrata [33]. However, the name coined for this entity is only valid in its clinical aspect since in most cases there is a rudimentary iris: irideremia [34]. This rudimentary stump is visible on gonioscopy, since it is behind the corneoscleral limbus, and sometimes is directly visible (Fig. 21.21). It is made up of a fragment of pigmentary epithelium covered by mesodermal tissue (Fig. 21.22).

The features of this malformation have been broadened and improved gradually, and, at present, the condition is much more widely studied. The iris is not the only structure involved. Other ocular and extraocular structures are also anomalous. As a consequence of malformations at the chamber angle, it is associated with glaucoma in two-thirds of cases.

There are no difficulties in clinically diagnosing it and the pediatrician detects it upon the first examination of the newborn. When the eye is illuminated, the whole anterior segment appears in a reddish color.

The presence of aniridia stands out but not the symptoms of glaucoma. We have examined 32 eyes with aniridia.

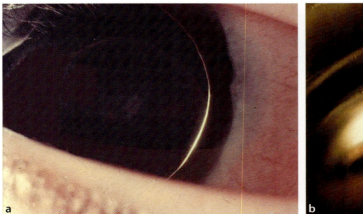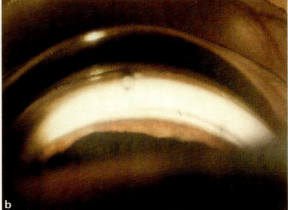

Fig. 21.21 a An eye with bright golden aniridia. The lens equator reflects light and, in front of it, at the left, there is a small iris stump. **b** Gonioscopic image of an aniridia case showing the iris stump in the angle

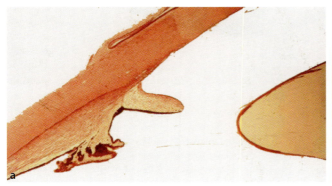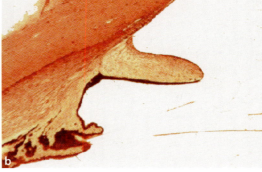

Fig. 21.22a,b Aniridia. **a** Pathologic anatomy (personal observation). **b** The same image as **a** with ×2.5 magnification. The Schlemm canal is seen as a white slit, covered by a thickened trabecular meshwork in some sectors (*left*). Remnants of mesodermal tissue extend from the anterior surface of this stump up to the trabecular meshwork, at the level of the middle of the Schlemm canal. The iris stump at the level of its insertion is dramatically thickened compared to the normal iris root, which is very thin and made up only of a deep mesenchymal layer

Heredity

This is a hereditary disease. The individual suffering from it transmits it in a dominant, regular fashion, even in the absence of a family history [12].

The rate in both genders is the same, so it is present in 50% of the descendants. Sometimes, it may appear in a healthy family by a mutation, when only one individual in the family has the disease, and it is extremely rare in other offspring. This may be useful knowledge for genetic counseling. The genealogic charts of Figs. 21.24 and 21.27 show these two modalities.

There is a genetic relationship between aniridia and iris coloboma. The presence of aniridia is more frequent in children born to parents with iris colobomas [35]. Aniridia, iris colobomas, iris holes, and circumpupillary aplasia are part of a genetic unit. It is the polyphenic effect of the gene. However, it should be remembered that, of this genetic unit, only aniridia is associated with macula aplasia: the other manifestations are not. In our case, the same patient had aniridia and choroidal coloboma (see clinical history No. 16).

Sex

Aniridia has no specific preference for either sex. The sex distribution shows no significance: X2 = 1.0 [36].

Frequency

According to Mollenbach [37], one case occurs per 100,000 births.

Clinical Picture

1. Aniridia is generally bilateral and it is accompanied with other ocular and general manifestations.
2. Usually, there is a marked visual acuity loss. This is due to macular aplasia, when present, to the refractive error (myopia or hyperopia) or to lens anomalies. Macular aplasia is clinically characterized by the absence of the central reflex and of the yellow color upon ophthalmoscopy with green light and causes amblyopia and nystagmus.
3. Glaucoma is present in two-thirds of cases with partially similar characteristics to those of congenital glaucoma. The chamber angle has a similar aspect to that of congenital glaucoma, since there is a good correlation between the filtering scleral trabecular meshwork surface and the intraocular pressure.

The thicker the pathological mesodermal layer covering it, the higher the intraocular pressure. In small children, this tissue is lax and has broad meshes. In adolescents, it is denser, but maintains its characteristic appearance. Sometimes, it extends up to the spur, and in some cases, it reaches the Schlemm canal and even the Schwalbe line.

There are also cases of iris stumps folded against the scleral wall of the chamber angle and attached or forming a synechia with it. In these cases, the intraocular pressure is very high and there is corneal edema. Here we completely agree with the report by Chandler and Grant [38]. There is typical atrophy of the ciliary processes.

In glaucoma with aniridia, the reason for consultation is the aniridia and not the glaucoma. There is generally no corneal edema. There are no tears in the Descemet membrane, the corneal diameters are generally normal, and there is no photophobia. Patients should be examined regularly since, in many cases, ocular hypertension develops later.

Cornea

There is a pannus around the whole corneal circumference, with vessels coming into the center superficially and going deeper in the stroma. Sometimes the cornea is almost completely opacified. This corneal process is part of the same anomaly. Even with very dense opacities, patients maintain some visual acuity allowing them some autonomy.

Crystalline Lens

In three cases, I have found a colobomatous-type lens malformation that may mislead the ophthalmologist into thinking of a lens luxation. Figure 21.23a, b shows this clearly. It should be kept in mind that during adulthood, the lens becomes opacified generally near 40 years of age. Fifty percent of patients develop cataract. In some of them, the lens, whether opacified or not, luxates.

Funduscopy

Peripheral lipidic retinal degeneration appears on funduscopy.

Nystagmus

Nystagmus is almost constant and is a consequence of poor vision or of the myopia due to macular hypoplasia or aplasia. A lack of macular reflex and yellow pigment is common.

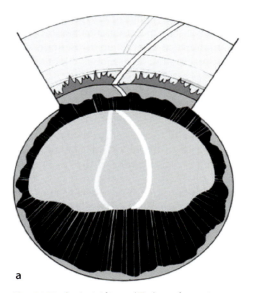
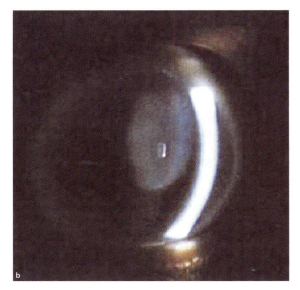

Fig. 21.23a,b Aniridia. **a** (*Top*) a schematic representation of the chamber angle where there is persistence of pathological mesodermal remnants. The crystalline lens is colobomatous. A quick examination of the patient may make the ophthalmologist think of a luxation, which is actually not present. The upper margin is acute and the lower one, blunt, as shown by the optical section (pear-shaped). The lower zonula is less dense and sometimes it is even absent. **a** The lens with a cataract suggests a luxation, but this is not the case. **b** Section with a slit lamp, which shows a lens coloboma and the distended zonula at the bottom (pear-shaped crystalline lens)

Clinical History No. 11

This 18-year-old female was diagnosed with aniridia (Fig. 21.24). She had an alcoholic father.

- Visual acuity. Finger-counting and nystagmus in both eyes.
- IOP. Right eye, 17 mmHg; left eye, 27 mmHg.
- Crystalline lens. As shown by Fig. 21.24, there is a cataract in the lens of the right eye while in the left eye the lens is transparent, though both seem to be luxated towards the top.

However, a thorough examination reveals a small, malformed, and colobomatous lens (Fig. 21.25). This lens has a normal equator and zonule in its upper half. There is a missing and round-shaped lower half. In the inferotemporal area, the zonular fibers are elongated and absent in the nasal sector. The lens of the left eye, even though it is transparent, has no evidence of an intracrystalline structure. There is pigment in its posterior surface and a small opacity in the anterior surface, which protrudes from the capsule like in a pyramidal cataract.

- Right eye. (1) Upper chamber angle: the corneal profile line continues directly into that of the ciliary processes. Between the two, there is an iris stump of apparently 0.5 mm; the pathological mesodermal remnants reach out to the Schwalbe line. (2) Temporal chamber angle: the pathological mesodermal remnants uncover the Schwalbe line. The ciliary processes are atrophic and dark, there is a crest of uveal tissue in front of the ciliary processes and then the iris stump. The pars plana shows a transparent cyst at 11 o'clock and two further cysts at the end of the ciliary processes at 9 o'clock. (3) Inferotemporal chamber angle: at 6 o'clock there is a transparent and oval cyst in the pars plana. The iris is reduced to merely a small elevation. The retinal concretions seem to be calcareous. At the area of the ora serrata, there is a cystic degeneration. The pathological mesodermal remnants reach the Schwalbe line in their fullness. This eye appears to have no pressure because there is atrophy of the ciliary processes. (4) Nasal chamber angle: the scleral trabecular meshwork is free. The pathological mesodermal remnants reach the spur and the heads of the ciliary processes are all inclined in the same direction. In this area, the iris is barely a raised surface. The retinal concretions are on a whiter retina, are smaller, and greater in number. (5) Funduscopy: the optic disc is atrophic, and there is nasal vessel rejection. The macula has no reflexes (aplasia). At the center there is pigment on the pigmentary layer of up to three optic disc diameters. Then at the periphery, the pigment disappears and the choroid becomes visible.

- Left eye. (1) Chamber angle: this is not a lens luxation but an atypical coloboma. The iris is identical to that of the right eye, but there is no anterior formation of ciliary processes. (2) Temporal chamber angle: this is the same as in the right eye; the peripheral retina, at the lower area is full of lipidic concretions, and there is a prominent Schwalbe line; the iris tissue extends up to it. The ciliary processes seem to be less atrophic. (3) Nasal chamber angle: the same as in the right eye. There are no cysts in the ciliary body. (4) Funduscopy: the retina is in the same condition as in the right eye.

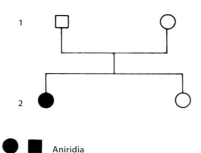

Fig. 21.24 Genealogical tree of case no. 11

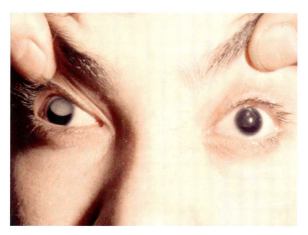

Fig. 21.25 Aniridia with a lens cataract malformation: coloboma as described in clinical history no. 11. The right eye has a cataract, but not the left. There appears to be a lens luxation, but it is actually a coloboma

Clinical History No. 12

This 17-year-old female was the only family member of five siblings with the disease (Fig. 21.26).

	Right eye	Left eye
Best spectacle visual acuity	20/200 with sph −2.50 cyl, −1.50 × 35°	20/200 with sph −2.75, cyl −1.75 × 150°
IOP	6 mmHg	18 mmHg
Anterior segment	Anterior and posterior embryotoxon and aniridia	Posterior embryotoxon and aniridia
Crystalline lens	Star-shaped posterior cortical cataract	Hypoplastic ciliary processes
Chamber angle	Aniridia associated with a posterior embryotoxon; the pathologic mesodermal remnants cover only the ciliary body band	
Funduscopy	Peripheral lipidic degeneration	

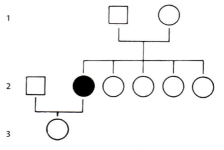

Fig. 21.26 Genealogic tree of clinical history no. 12

Clinical History No. 13

This 36-year-old male was the only family member with aniridia in a family of five normal siblings and normal parents. He has one boy and one girl born to a normal wife. His daughter has aniridia. A daughter born from his wife's previous marriage is normal (Fig. 21.27).
- Visual acuity: finger-counting in both eyes.
- IOP: 27 mmHg in both eyes.
- Crystalline lens: both eyes show an iris stump with a pigment ectropion. The pathological mesodermal remnants are very aplastic and reach up to the spur. In some parts, the Schwalbe line is protruded.
- Funduscopy: both eyes show peripheral lipidic retinal degeneration and disc cupping of 5/6. Temporal margin less than 1/3.

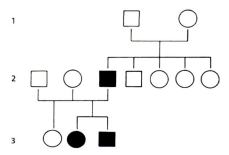

Fig. 21.27 Genealogic tree of clinical history no. 13

Clinical History No. 14

This is a 3-month-old female (daughter of case history no. 13) (see Fig. 21.27).

	Right eye	Left eye
IOP	36 mmHg	30 mmHg
Corneal diameter	13 mm	14 mm
Anterior segment	Bilateral corneal edema	Bilateral papillary membrane remnants
Crystalline lens	Pyramidal cataract	Pyramidal cataract
Chamber angle	The iris stump is attached to the external scleral wall of the chamber angle and forms a synechia with it, up to the cornea; Schwalbe line is not visible	
Funduscopy	There is no peripheral retinal disturbance and there is marked optic disc pallor	

Clinical History No. 15

This 18-month-old male is the son of case history no. 13 (Fig. 21.27).

	Right eye	Left eye
IOP	17 mmHg	17 mmHg
Corneal diameter	11 mm	11 mm
Anterior segment	Papillary membrane remnants	
Chamber angle	Iris stump. The pigmentary epithelial layer does not correspond with this stump and extends above it as in the previous cases. Small amount of pathological mesodermal remnants which leave the filtering trabecular meshwork free	
Funduscopy	No retinal disorders	

Clinical History No. 16

This child is a 3-month-year-old male whose genealogic tree is shown in Fig. 21.28.

This is a mutation in a healthy family. The couple is concerned about the likelihood of the presence of the disease in future children. Our genetic advice was that they could have more children, and indeed three healthy boys were born. The mother has a brother with Down syndrome and her father is an alcoholic.

	Right eye	Left eye
IOP (1962)	16 mmHg	16 mmHg
IOP (1967)	19 mmHg	24 mmHg
Crystalline lens	Anterior polar cataract, hypoplastic ciliary processes	
Chamber angle	Iris stump is visible, not only by gonioscopy but also directly if seen frontally. The pathological mesodermal remnants reach the posterior part of the scleral trabecular meshwork. In some sectors, the iris stump has the morphology of the atrophic iris of congenital glaucoma, with vascular handles that end in the anterior greater circle of the iris	
Vitreous body	Persistence of the hyaloid artery	
Funduscopy	Partial bilateral choroidal coloboma and pale optic discs; there is no macular reflex. There is atrophy of the pigmentary epithelium that uncovers the image of the choroidal vessels	

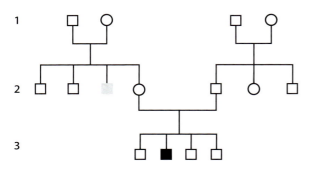

Down syndrome

Aniridia

Fig. 21.28 Genealogic tree of clinical history no. 16

Therapy

Preoperative pharmacotherapy generally fails and surgery is required. Surgical therapy is successful in 30% of cases, but the addition of pharmacotherapy is required in two-thirds of them. The procedure used is combined surgery: trabeculectomy and trabeculotomy, with, in most cases, added pharmacotherapy; Ocusert is found to be very effective.

In aniridia, the use of contact lenses preventing the passage of light, with the iris drawn inside them, improves photophobia and nystagmus [39].

Pathologic Anatomy

In cases associated with glaucoma, the gonioscopic findings are confirmed by the presence of pathologic mesodermal tissue obstructing the trabecular meshwork, which is positive for Gomori's stain. Figure 21.29 evidences this.

These specimens are from a child who was operated, before he turned 1 year of age, by myself and Dr. Alezzandrini. When glaucoma appears so early in aniridia cases, which is rare, we believe it to be a different clinical form.

Etiopathogenesis

The first descriptions of the area of the chamber angle in aniridia cases can be traced back to Pagenstecher [40], De Benedetti [41], and Lembeck [42]. These authors describe eyes with congenital aniridia and glaucoma in which the chamber angle is occluded by the iris stump (Fig. 21.23). They describe this formation and also affirm that the Descemet membrane unfolds into two layers at the periphery, one going to the trabecular meshwork and the other to the iris. In 1962, Hogan and Zimmerman [43] confirmed these findings.

Rindgleisch [44] and Collins [45] describe eyes with aniridia not associated with glaucoma, in which this anomaly is not confirmed by histology.

Barkan [46] and Higgitt [47] described a displacement of these pathological mesodermal remnants that occurs with time and that cover the trabecular meshwork, thus giving rise to late glaucoma.

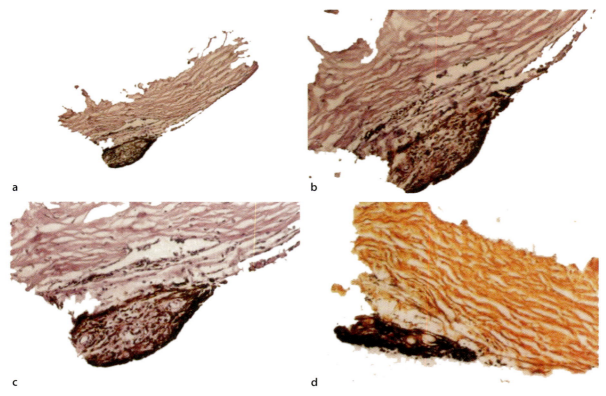

Fig. 21.29 a Trabeculectomy specimen of an aniridia case with glaucoma. H-E (×40). There is a corneoscleral flap, the Descemet membrane is visible, as well as the iris stump, which is attached to the trabecular region. **b** The same case as above (H-E, ×200). Iris stump attached to the trabecular meshwork. Between both structures there are pathologic mesodermal remnants. **c** Posterior part of the trabeculectomy specimen (H-E, ×100). The structures visible are the Schlemm canal, trabecular meshwork, which is compressed, close to the mesodermal remnants and the iris stump. **d** Semiserial section of the same case as above (Gomori's stain, ×100). The iris stump stroma and mesodermal remnants are dyed *black*

Comments and Conclusions

Of the 14 eyes with aniridia we have just described, glaucoma was present in 50%. The chamber angle anomalies were visible. Figure 21.30 is a summary of this sample, with the inclusion of IOP values and schematic chamber angle representations: the part in black represents the topography of the pathological mesodermal tissue. There is a good correlation between IOP values and the filtering surface occluding the pathological mesodermal remnants.

In their book on glaucoma, Chandler and Grant [38] were the first to correlate gonioscopic findings with rises in IOP. Grant [48] quotes Sampaolesi and Reca's paper [49] as the first to verify this finding.

When the pathological mesodermal remnants occlude more than half the circumference, thus passing the spur line, ocular hypertension develops. If the scleral trabecular meshwork remains free, this condition does not occur. There are cases in which ocular hypertension cannot be accounted for by the presence of pathologic mesodermal remnants, as in the case of the patient described in clinical history no. 13 (Fig. 21.30).

The appearance of the chamber angle changes over the years, and hypertension typically develops late.

The pathogenesis may be due to arrested development of the optical vesicle in embryos measuring 65–85 mm, between weeks 11 and 12 of gestation. The neural ectoderm has, by this time, differentiated the retina but not the fovea. There is only a primitive iris. The eye, then, stops its retinal and iris development [8].

Ocular complications are listed in Table 21.1. The complications without a number are those described by us, and on which we have not found any related literature.

As regards the crystalline lens, it has colobomatous lesions, not luxations.

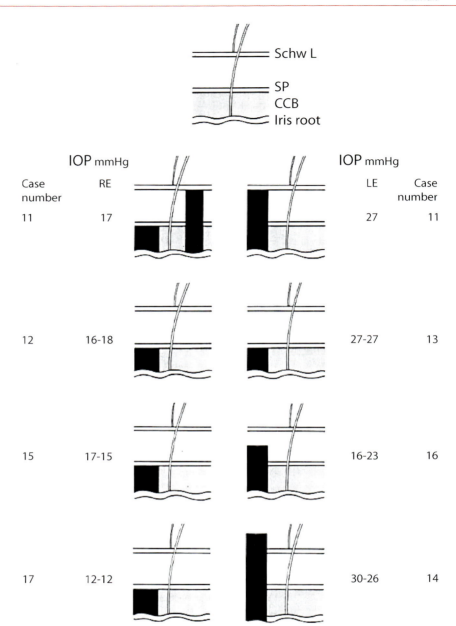

Fig. 21.30 The chamber angle in aniridia. *Schw L* Schwalbe line, *SP* spur, *CCB* ciliary body band, the part in *black* represents the topography of the pathological mesodermal tissue. There is a good correlation between IOP values and the filtering surface occluding the pathological mesodermal remnants. *IOP mmHg* IOP in mm of mercury, *RE* right eye, *LE* left eye

Table 21.1 Ocular manifestations of patients studied in Fig. 21.30

Case number	Age	Chamber angle	IOP		Crystalline lens	Pupillary membrane	Macular aplasia and nystagmus	Retina, choroid and vitreous body
			RE	LE				
11	18 Years	In half the circumference, the pathological mesodermal remnants reach Schwalbe line; in the other half, the spur	17	27	Pyramidal catara ct	Yes	Yes	Lipidic peripheral degeneration and ciliary body cysts
12	17 Years	Pathological mesodermal remnants cover the ciliary body band and the anterior and posterior embryotoxon	16	18	Stele cataract	–	–	Lipidic peripheral degeneration
13	36 Years	Aplastic pathological mesodermal remnants reach the spur. Prominent Schwalbe line	27	27	Anterior and posterior pyramidal cataract	–	Yes	Lipidic peripheral degeneration
14	3 Months	Blocked chamber angle due to attachment of the iris stump to posterior corneal surface	30	26	Pyramidal cataract	Yes	Yes	–
15	18 Months	The pathological mesodermal remnants reach the spur	17	17	–	Yes	Yes	–
16	3 Months	The pathological mesodermal remnants cover the upper half of the scleral trabecular meshwork	16	16	Anterior polar cataract	Yes	Yes	Incomplete choroidal coloboma and persistence of the hyaloid artery
17	4 Months	Normal chamber angle	12	12	–	–	–	–

Aniridia and Wilms Tumor

Miller et al. [50] evaluated 440 children with nephroblastoma (Wilms tumor), six of whom had aniridia. Children with aniridia may have Wilms tumor. None of the children included in this sample with Wilms tumor and aniridia had a family history of aniridia. The syndrome is associated with mental retardation as well as with other anomalies.

One in every five sporadic cases develops Wilms tumor [51].

The descriptions above are the classical knowledge of the disease and our clinical experience. Present research into aniridia will provide further elucidations of the disease. The paper by Hitner [52], where he divides aniridia into three genetic types according to their genetic prevalence, is highly recommended (Table 21.2).

Aniridia comes in three types: aniridia type I (85%), aniridia type II (13%), and aniridia type III (2%). Type I is an isolated form of aniridia, of dominant autosomal heredity with complete penetration and variable expressiveness. Aniridia type II has a dominant hereditary pattern, and is accompanied by Wilms tumor, genitourinary anomalies, and mental retardation. In type III, there is recessive autosomal heredity with cerebellar ataxia and mental retardation.

The author also relates, though more distantly, this syndrome with Rieger and Peters syndromes.

Sclerocornea and Flat Cornea

This occurs when the cornea becomes hazy and has the appearance of the sclera. This haziness starts at the periphery, which may become involved fully or in a sector. In the former, the corneoscleral limbus can no longer be identified. Sometimes this haziness covers the whole cornea. When this happens, its curvature is usually altered, since it mimics the shape of the sclera. This is known as flat cornea [75]. The anterior chamber also flattens.

Adrogue and Wolff [55] described a case associated with aniridia. François and Neetens [54] thought that it might be associated with aniridia, lens ectopia, or iris, lens, choroidal, and retinal coloboma, and optic nerve and retinal aplasia.

Manzitti [74] described a flat cornea associated with a choroidal and retinal coloboma and ectopic lens.

Bloch [75] studied 42 cases and found 21 with iris hypoplasia and anterior synechiae.

Table 21.2 Ocular and general complications of aniridia

Hydrophthalmus [53]

Cornea	Microcornea [54], Sclerocornea [55], Keratoconus, megalocornea, embryotoxon [52], flat cornea [54]
Sclera	Blue sclerotics [51, 52]
Chamber angle	Open [34], closed with persistence of pathological mesodermal remnants up to the spur or not, posterior and anterior embryotoxon [2, 57]
Pupil	Papillary membrane [58]
Crystalline lens	Anterior polar cataract [59], posterior polar cataract, luxation [60–62]
Choroid	Coloboma
Vitreous	Persistence of hyaloid artery [58]
Retina	Lipidic peripheral degeneration [63], ciliary body cysts, atrophic pigmentary layer, aplastic ciliary body [64]
Macula	Aplasia [65, 66]
General complications	Craniofacial dysostosis [67], polydactyly [68], atrial malformations [69]

This picture occurs sometimes in association with ocular hypertension. In these cases, the hypertension should be regulated with trabeculectomy. Visual acuity can be enhanced subsequently with keratoplasty. It has a recessive dominant hereditary pattern.

We have had two cases. One of them was a boy with no light perception and the other one was an adult. In the latter, the sclerocornea was partial. We performed a filtering iridectomy, which successfully regulated the IOP.

Differential diagnosis should also be made with congenital endothelial dystrophies.

Clinical History No. 17

This was a 70-year-old female diagnosed with partial sclerocornea with late congenital glaucoma, corticonuclear cataract, and posterior embryotoxon.

	Right eye	Left eye
Visual acuity	Sph. –5.50; cyl. 0.75 × 120° = 20/200	Sph. –5; cyl. –0.75 × 60° = 20/200
IOP	29 mmHg	29 mmHg
Tonographic test: CL3-7	0.07	0.07
Anterior chamber depth	3.59 mm	3.59 mm
Cataract	Yes	Yes
Chamber angle	Posterior embryotoxon with goniosynechiae reaching up to a thickened Schwalbe line	

Therapy was a filtering iridectomy on the left eye. When the conjunctiva was selected, a subconjunctival lipoma was found in the temporal area. It was removed and sent for analysis. The surgical limbus was not located at the usual level because of the shifting of the sclera over the cornea at 12 o'clock (anterior embryotoxon). The Minsky maneuver enabled the incision to be located properly, 4 mm behind the apparent limbus. The iris cleaved spontaneously. The follow-up examination revealed that the IOP was regulated.

Summary

Corneal and iris mesodermal dysgeneses are typically associated with anomalies in the external, inner, and intermediate chamber angle wall. Most often, late congenital glaucoma is also present, but this does not enlarge the anteroposterior axis of the eye substantially since, being late glaucoma, when it appears, the sclera is no longer distensible. However, it should be kept in mind that sometimes there may be no glaucoma, even in the presence of marked chamber angle lesions. However, the mere presence of a posterior embryotoxon warrants consideration of glaucoma.

Goniotomy or trabeculotomy are barely effective, and trabeculectomy or combined surgery should be performed instead. These are included in the current classification of goniodysgeneses.

Peters anomaly becomes manifest with a central leukoma limited by an anterior ring-shaped synechia of the iris, associated with glaucoma and, sometimes, with megalocornea. Glaucoma is present from birth and requires filtering procedures and corneal grafting.

Aniridia is actually apparent, since there is always an iris stump present. Glaucoma appears late and its presence is related to the degree of obstruction of the filtering trabecular area caused by pathological mesodermal remnants. Surgery is not very effective and supplementation with pharmacotherapy is often required.

Sclerocorneas and flat corneas may be associated with glaucoma.

Of all the ocular anomalies described above, the most benign one is Rieger dysgenesis. In Peters anomaly associated with glaucoma, the eye is generally lost, and in aniridia, eye fundus anomalies lead to severe visual loss.

Goniodysgeneses may appear in generalized malformations such as Ehler Danlos syndrome, homocystinuria, Marfan syndrome, neurofibromatosis, Pierre Robin syndrome, Turner syndrome, etc.

References

1. Burian HM, Rice MH, Allen L (1957) External visibility of the region of Schlemm's canal. Report on a family with developmental anomalies of the cornea, iris and chamber angle. Arch Ophthalmol 57:651–658

2. Streiff EB (1949) Dysplasie marginale postérieure de la cornée (Embriotoxon postérieure Axenfeld) dans le cadre de malformations irido-cornéennes. Ophthalmologica 118:815–822

3. Busacca A, Pinticart WE (1948) Étude gonioscopique d'un cas de embriotoxon corneae posterius. Ophthalmologica 115:283

4. Rieger H (1891) Über Hypoplasie des Irisvorderblattes mit Verlaegerung und Entrundung. Graefes Arch Ophthalmol 37:192

5. Rossano R (1934) Absence presque complète du feuillet mésodermique de l'iris dans deux générations. Hypertensión oculaire et polycorie dans un cas. Bull Soc Ophtalmol Paris 3–12

6. Alkemade PH (1969) Dysgenesis mesodermalis of the iris and the cornea. A study of Rieger's syndrome and Peter's anomaly. Van Goreum, Assen

7. Jerndal T, Hansson HA, Bill A (1978) Goniodysgenesis. A new perspective on glaucoma. Scriptor Bogtrykkriet Forum, Copenhagen

8. Seefelder R (1906) Klinische und anatomische Untersuchungen zur Pathologie und Therapie des Hydrophthalmus congenitus. Graefes Arch Ophthalmol 63:204–280; 481–556

9. Axenfeld TH (1920) Embriotoxon corneae posterious. Ber Dtsch Ophthalmol Ges 42:301

10. Falls HF (1949) Agents producing various effects on the anterior segment of the eye. Am J Ophthalmol 32:4152

11. Burian HM, Braley AE, Allen L (1955) External and gonioscopic visibility of the ring of Schwalbe and the trabecular zone: an interpretation of the posterior corneal embryotoxon and the so-called congenital hyaline membranes on the posterior corneal surface. Trans Am Ophthalmol Soc 51:398–428

12. Waardenburg PJ, Francheschetti A, Klein D (1961) Genetics and ophthalmology, Vol. 1. Blackwell, Oxford

13. Waring G, Rodriguez MM, Laibson PR (1975) Anterior chamber cleavage syndrome. A Stepladder classification. Surv Ophthalmol 20:3–27

14. Kwitko ML (1999) Surgery of the internal eye. Appleton Century Crofts, New York

15. Kraupa E (1920) Fehlen des Lederhautbandes in Sichelform als Abweichung vom gewöhnlichen Verhalten der Hornhaut-Lederhautgrenze. Klin Mbl Augenheilkd 64:698–700

16. Kayser B (1922) Über Embryotoxon corneae posterious nebs einem Befund von persistierenden Resten der Membrana capsula-pupillaris lentis. Klin Mbl Augenheilkd 68:82–88

17. Ascher KW (1941) Partial coloboma of the scleral limbus zone with visible Schlemm´s canal. Am J Ophthalmol 24:615–619

18. Peters A (1906) Über angeborene Defektbildung der Descemetschen Membran. Klin Mbl Augenheilkd 24:27–40, 105–119

19. Peters A (1930) Das Glaukom Handbuch der Augenheilkunde Dritte Auflage. Springer, Berlin Heidelberg New York

20. Von Hippel V (1899) Geschwür der Hornhauthinterfläche. Festschrif f A V Graefe

21. Buck (1918) Hydrophthalmus. Am J Ophthalmol 11:683

22. Meisner (1923) Hydrophthalmus und angeborene Hornhauttrübungen. Ebenda 112:433

23. Appelmans M, Michels J, Forez J (1950) Malformations symétriques du segment antérieur de l'œil (syndrome de Peter). Bull Soc Belge Ophtalmol 94:283–289

24. Townsend WM (1974) Congenital corneal leukomas. I. Central defect in Descemet's membrane. Am J Ophthalmol 77:80–86

25. Townsend WM, Font RL, Zimmerman LE (1974) Congenital corneal leukomas. II. Histopathologic findings in 19 eyes with central defect in Descemet's membrane. Am J Ophthalmol 77:192–206

26. Townsend WM, Font RL, Zimmerman LE (1974) Congenital corneal leukomas. III. Histopathologic findings in 13 eyes with paracentral defect in Descemet's membrane. Am J Ophthalmol 77:400–412

27. Damaske E, Müller KM (1972) Angeborones Hornhautepitheliom und Peter's Anomaly. Ber Dtsch Ophthalmol Ges 71:601–609

28. Reese AB, Ellsworth RM (1966) The anterior chamber cleavage syndrome. Arch Ophthalmol Chicago 75:307–318

29. Nakanishi I, Brown SI (1971) The histopathology and ultrastructure of congenital central opacity (Peter's anomaly). Am J Ophthalmol 72:801–812

30. Hay ED, Ravel JP (1969) Fine structure of the developmental biology. Karger, Basel

31. Atsuchi K, Wood TC, Polack FM, Kaufman HE (1971) The fine structure of sclerocornea. Invest Ophthalmol Vis Sci 10:687–694

32. Nath K, Nema HV, Shukla BR (1964) Histopathology in a case of unilateral microcornea plana. Acta Ophthalmol Kbh 42:609–615

33. Barrata (1961) Cited in Waardenburg PJ, Franceschetti A, Klein D (eds) Genetics and ophthalmology, Vol. I. Blackwell, Oxford, p 741

34. Sampaolesi R, Reca R (1968) El glaucoma en la aniridia (aparente) o irideremia, Arch Oftalmol B Aires 43 31–38

35. Theobald S (1988) A case a double congenital iridemia in a child whose mother exhibited a congenital coloboma of each iris. Trans Am Ophthalmol Soc 5:99–100

36. Paganelli VX (1951) L'antiride bilatérale associée a la forme frustre de la maladie de Crouzon (dysostose cranio-faciale). PhD disseration, Unviersity of Geneva

37. Mollenbach GJ (1947) Congenital defects in the internal membrane of the eye. Opera Ex Domo Biologier Hereditariane Humane Universitatis Harfniesis, Vol. 15. Einer Munksgaard, Copenhagen

38. Chandler PA, Grant WM (1965) Lectures on glaucoma. 1965. Lea and Febiger, Philadelphia

39. de Freitas H (1984)

40. Pagenstecher H (1871) Pathologisch-anatomische. Mitteilung Sitzungsberichtes Ophthal Gest Klin Mbl Augenheilkd 9:427

41. De Benedetti A (1886) Irideremia totale congénita. Ectopía lentis congénita con lusazione spontanea del cristalino e glaucoma consecutivo. Ann Ottalmol 15:184–399

42. Lembeck H (1890) Über die pathologische Anatomie der irideremia totalis congenita. PhD disseration. Openning presentation, Halle

43. Hogan MJ, Zimmerman LE (1962) Ophthalmic pathology, 2nd edn. Saunders, Philadelphia

44. Rindfleisch G (1891) Beitragung und Entstehungsgeschite der angeborenen Missbildungen des Auges. Graefes Arch Ophthalmol 37:192

45. Collins ET (1983) Congenital defects of the iris and glaucoma. Trans Am Ophthalmol Soc UK 13:128

46. Barkan O (1953) Goniotomy for glaucoma associated with aniridia. Arch Ophthalmol 49:1

47. Higgitt AC (1976) Secondary glaucoma. Trans Ophthalmol Soc UK 76:73

48. Grant M, Walton DS (1974) Progressive changes in congenital aniridia with development glaucoma. Am J Ophthalmol 78:842–847

49. Sampaolesi R, Reca R (1968) El glaucoma en la aniridia (aparente) o irideremia. Arch Oftalmol B Aires 43:31–38

50. Miller RM, Fraumeni JF, Manning MD (1964) Association of Wilms tumor with aniridia, hemihypertrophy and other congenital malformations. New Engl J Med 270:922–927

51. Fraumeni JF (1969) The aniris. Wilms' tumor syndrome. Birth defects. 5:198

52. Hitner HM (1989) Aniridia. In: Ritch R, Shields MB, Kruppin T (eds) The glaucomas, vol. 2 Mosby, St. Louis, pp 869–884

53. Marchesini E (1933) Sopra un caso di anoftalmo e microftalmo con coloboma irideo. Contributo alla conoscenza delle malformación congenita oculari. Boll Ocul 12:226–244

54. Felser (1888/1964) Aniridia utriusque oculi completa congenita. Klin Mbl Augenheilkd 26:296. Cited in Duke Elder S (ed) System of ophthalmology, Vol. 3. Henry Kimpton, London, pp 565–573

55. Adrogue E, Wolf JA (1948) Aniridia bilateral con ptosis y embriotoxon. Arch Oftal B Aires 23:141–148

56. François J, Neetins A (1955) Microcornée associée a une hydrophtalmie et a d'autres anomalies héréditaires. Acta Genet Med Rome 4:217–229

57. Beattie PH (1947) A consideration of aniridia, with a pedigree. Br J Ophthalmol 31:649–676

58. Mohr W (1895) Über hereditere Irideremie. Inaug Diss Jena (Wagenmann)

59. Chandler PA, Grant WM (1965) Lectures on glaucoma. Lea and Febiger, Philadelphia

60. Streiff EB (1949) Dysplasie Marginale postérieure de la cornée (Embriotoxon postérieure Axenfeld) dans le cadre de malformations irido-cornéennes. Ophthalmologica 118:815–822

61. Brailey WA (1890) Double microphthalmos with defective development of the iris, teeth and anus. Glaucoma at an early age. Trans Ophthalmol Soc UK 10:139–140

62. Siliato F (1954) La gonioscopia in alcune alterazioni congenite del globo oculare (critica alla teoria della filtrazione nell'idroftalmo). Ann Ottal 80:349–356

63. Marin Amat M (1925) Aniridie, nystagmus, hypermetropischer Astigmatismus, und vordere Polarkatarakt beider Augen. Arch Oftal Hisp Am 24:140

64. Samelson (1873) Traumatic aniridia and aphakia. In: International Ophthalmological Congress 4: 1872. Savill Edwards, London, p 131

65 Goldzieher (1897/1964) Zbl prakt Augenheilk 21:114. Cited in Duke Elder S (ed) System of ophthalmology, vol. 3. Henry Kimpton, London, pp 565–573

66. Grove JH, Shaw MW, Bourque G (1961) Arch Ophthalmol 65:81–84

67. Siliato F (1954) La gonioscopia in alcune alterazioni congenite del globo oculare (critica alla teoria della filtrazione nell'idroftalmo). Ann Ottal 80:349–356

68. Orsetti (1960) Ann Ottal 86:136

69. Jesberg DO (1962) Aniridia with retinal lipid deposits. Arch Ophthalmol 68:331–336

70. Vogt A (1925) Die Ophthalmoskopie im rotfreien Licht. In: Graefe A, Saemisch T (eds) Handbuch der gesammten Augenheilkunde. Untersuchungsmethoden, 3rd edn. Verlag von Wilhelm Engelman, Berlin, pp 1–118

71. Vogt A (1941/1958) Scheweiz Med Wschr 71:432. Quoted by François J (1958) In: Hérédité en ophtalmologie. Masson, Paris, pp 170–175

72. Bornstein MB (1952) Aniridie bilateralé avec polydactylie. J Genet Hum 1:211–266

73. Pfändler UJ (1954/1958) Génét Hum 3:149. Quoted by François J (1958) In Hérédité en ophtalmologie Masson, Paris, pp 170–175

74. Rubel E (1912) Kongenitale familiäre Flachheit der Kornea (cornea plana). Klin Mbl Augenheilkd 50:427–438

75. Manzitti E (1951) Córnea plana congénita. Arch Oftalm B Aires 26:222–225

76. Bloch N (1961) Les différents types de sclerocornée. Leurs modes d´hérédité et les malformations congénitales concomitants. J Gen Hum IV:133–172

Contents

Phakomatosis

The phakomatoses are a clinical entity within genetic disorders. The term was coined because Van der Hoeve in 1933 [1] classified them into four diseases characterized by the presence of phakomas (spots), which are tumors (hamartomas, tumor-like malformations caused by congenital and developmental tissue anomalies, with an excess of one or more of these tissues [2]) located in the skin, nervous tissue, and eyes. These spots can be café-au-lait-type, pigmentary nevi, facial angiomas, etc. These diseases are transmitted by a dominant hereditary pattern. They are known as von Recklinghausen neurofibromatosis, encephalotrigeminal angiomatosis, Sturge-Weber-Krabbe syndrome, Lagleyze-Von Hippel-Lindau cerebroretinal angiomatosis, and Bourneville tuberous sclerosis. The first three may be associated with glaucoma.

Von Recklinghausen Neurofibromatosis

Von Recklinghausen neurofibromatosis [3] is characterized by the presence of neurofibromas in the central nervous system, cranial nerves, peripheral nerves, and sympathetic nervous system. The lesion has a diffuse proliferation of Schwann cells in the peripheral nervous fibers, as shown by Fig. 22.3. In addition, these tumors are located in the skin and mucosa. In the skin, they form vermiform nodules, hard to the touch skin neuromas. These neuromas sometimes take on a plexiform appearance, thickening the skin. When these lesions are close to bony parts, they produce dystrophies or hypertrophies. In other cases, the lesion is a neurofi-

bromatous disorder located in the bone. In the skin of the neck and trunk, there may be café-au-lait-colored spots (phakomas) that are oval-shaped and have neat margins.

The cranial nerves, typically the acoustic and optic nerves, may be involved.

Its hereditary pattern is dominant.

The ocular manifestations are upper lid neurofibroma leading to palpebral ptosis (Figs. 22.1, 22.2), in which the free margin adopts the shape of an italic "S". If the upper eyelid is held between the fingers, its vermiform nature can be felt. Figure 22.3 shows its biopsy sample.

Sometimes the eye may be enophthalmic or exophthalmic. When there is exophthalmos, it is generally unilateral, pulsatile, with no murmur and may be caused by a glioma of the optic nerve which, though it has no Schwann cells, is actually an oligodendrocytoma. According to del Rio Ortega [4], oligodendroglia corresponds to Schwann cells of the peripheral nerves. Meningiomas of the optic nerve sheaths and any other orbital neurofibroma may also be present. These are the causes of exophthalmos. The orbital x-ray in Fig. 22.4 shows a completely enlarged orbit. Sometimes, the disease may progress to orbital erosion and brain herniation (pulsating exophthalmos). The eyeball may have neurofibromas of the ciliary nerves, as well as uveal thickening, micronodules of the iris that may also be present in the chamber angle, and iris heterochromia. Retinal phakomas are seen only rarely.

Two years after the description of the syndrome by von Recklinghausen, Schiess-Gemuseus [5], described glaucoma as a complication of the disease for the first time. There is abundant literature on glaucoma in von Recklinghausen disease: Lieb et al. [6], François and Katz [7], Maggi [8], Toselli and Volpi [9], Wolter and Butler [10], Chandler and Grant [11] and Grant and Walton [12]. The last paper dealt particularly with the chamber angle in glaucomatous eyes.

Glaucoma occurs unilaterally and it is due to obstruction of the outflow pathways by neurofibromatous tissue. It occurs on the same side where the upper eyelid neurofibromatosis is located. It should be kept in mind that all glaucomatous cases described in the literature had upper eyelid neurofibromatosis, though glaucoma is present in only 50% of upper eyelid neurofibromatoses.

In 1968, Grant and Walton [12] summarized the three possible causes of glaucoma:

1. Chamber angle obstruction due to the presence of neurofibromatous tissue;
2. Angle closure due to the presence of the neurofibroma, which increases the volume of the ciliary body and choroids (diffuse uveal neurofibromatosis);
3. Secondary vascularization associated with a gelatinous membrane, finally leading to chamber angle

blockage, similar to diabetes-induced chamber angle rubeosis, etc.

An example of the first mechanism is described in the cases histologically analyzed by François [7]. The disease may also be identical to congenital glaucoma with persistence of pathologic mesodermal remnants, as evidenced by Lieb and Worth's histological preparations [6]. In these cases, glaucoma appeared within the first two years of life. The second type may develop later. The third mechanism generally occurs during adulthood [10]. Our two cases had no glaucoma, the same as the two cases reported by Calixto and Carvalho [13].

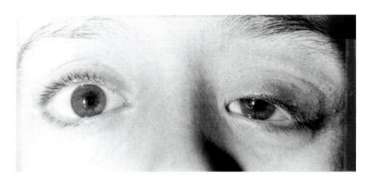

Fig. 22.1 Von Recklinghausen neurofibromatosis. Left eyelid with increased volume and lower border shaped like an italic "S"

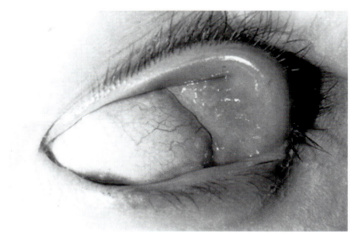

Fig. 22.2 Everted eyelid of the same patient as in Fig. 22.1

Fig. 22.3 Biopsy of the same eyelid (original preparation)

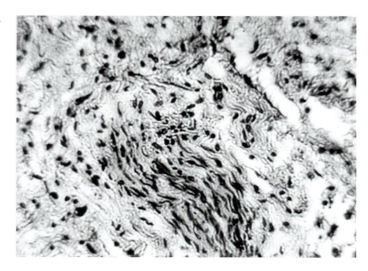

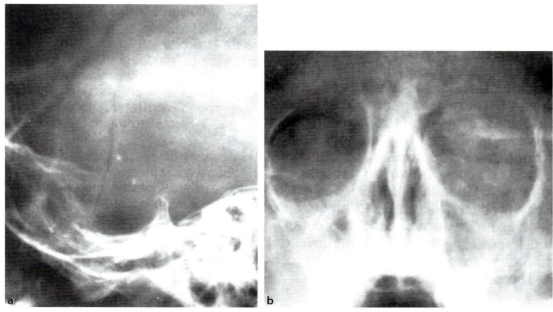

Fig. 22.4a,b X-ray of the patient depicted in Fig. 22.1. **a** Very enlarged sella turcica; **b** larger left eye orbit

Encephalotrigeminal Neuroangiomatosis or Sturge-Weber-Krabbe Syndrome

This disease is also included in the angiomatoses (retinocerebellar hemangioblastomatosis or Von Hippel-Lindau syndrome, retino-optical-mesencephalic aneurysmatic syndrome or cirsoid aneurysm, Coats retinosis).

Schirmer [14] was the first to report the association of a facial skin angioma with congenital glaucoma.

Sturge [15] associated the signs derived from a nervous system lesion (meningeal angioma), such as convulsions, paresis, etc., with the picture described above.

Weber [16] and Krabbe [17] described the typical x-ray anomalies: parallel lines calcified by brain lesions.

Bergstrand et al. [18] coined the name Sturge-Weber disease for this condition.

Van der Hoeve [19] included it in the group of phakomatoses. In most cases, the disease is unilateral.

The manifestations are facial angioma, choroidal angioma, meningeal angioma, intracranial calcifications, and glaucoma. The lesion is identical in the skin, meninges, and uvea.

Facial Angioma

Facial angioma is a nevus flammeus, which may be unilateral or bilateral and may be accompanied by facial hypertrophy. It is a flat angioma that may present in different degrees; sometimes it is manifested by small telangiectasias, while in other cases, it may have massive involvement and it has the appearance of a wine-color spot. When it is unilateral, it does not pass the middle line and the area involved is generally the first two trigeminal branches (Fig. 22.5).

Palpebral Angioma

Palpebral angioma is limited to the eyelid skin, but it also involves vascular anomalies in the conjunctiva and episclera.

Choroidal Angioma

Choroidal angioma is typically too deep to be identified during funduscopy. In most cases, the lesion is located between the optic disc and the macula, generally juxtapapillary. It has the appearance of a grayish-white spot, generally long or circular, with quite neat edges. It is never pigmented, but sometimes has shining spot-like deposits on its surface. It coexists with facial angioma and conjunctival telangiectasias. In this regard, it should be stressed that its differential diagnosis with melanomas may not be easy and many eyes have been enucleated for melanomas that turned out to have choroidal angiomas. The same occurs with retinoblastomas [19].

Stokes [20] reported that the neck compression test can be of help for differential diagnosis with malignant melanoma. Upon compression of the neck veins, in hemangioma cases, IOP will rise markedly, whereas this does not occur with melanomas.

Intrascleral and Episcleral Angioma

When cases of Sturge-Weber are operated on, after dissecting the conjunctiva, in almost all cases the surgeon finds an episcleral angioma that has been described very well by Phelps as not limited only to the episclera but extending over the sclera up to more than half its thickness (Fig. 22.6).

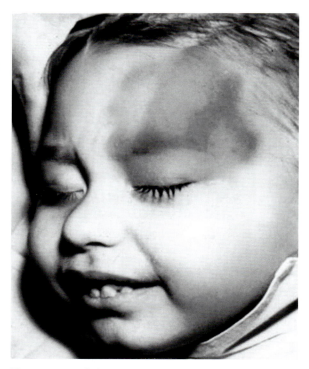

Fig. 22.5 Encephalotrigeminal neuroangiomatosis. Facial angioma on the left eye involving the upper eyelid, eyebrow, and forehead, with the lower eyelid free of the disease. Crying produces great congestion

Meningeal Angioma

This is capillary angioma on the encephalic surface, involving the dura mater but extending deep inside in the shape of a wedge. It generally develops on the same side as the skin angioma and it preferentially locates on the occipital area, always involving brain substance.

Intracranial Calcifications

These calcifications are usually found in children. In general, they increase with age and manifest mainly in the occipital area. In adults, they are present in 80% of cases.

To these central disorders are attributed the psychological manifestations of the disease, which may even lead to dementia and epileptic-like seizures, as well at to neurological disorders such as homonymous hemianopsia, hemiplegia, etc. In these cases, carotid artery angiography, electroencephalography, and cisternography are very useful.

Glaucoma

In nearly 70% of cases, glaucoma is seen in a similar form to that of congenital glaucoma, and in the remaining 30%, it appears as primary open-angle glaucoma, even in the presence of vascular disorders, sometimes in the iris and at others in the chamber angle. Therefore, knowledge of the chamber angle is vital for the indication of surgical therapy when necessary, since, if its morphology is that of congenital glaucoma, goniotomy or trabeculotomy will be mandatory, and if not, any type of procedure can be performed.

The pathogenesis of this type of glaucoma is controversial, since if the chamber angle has the characteristics of congenital glaucoma, the cause lies with the tissues at the level of the trabecular meshwork. Otherwise, episcleral vascular disorders would mean including this glaucoma among those with extraocular causes. Its mechanism needs further elucidation. Chandler and Grant [11] reported that when blood reflows in the Schlemm canal upon neck compression, this is seen usually bifurcated or displaced from its usual position.

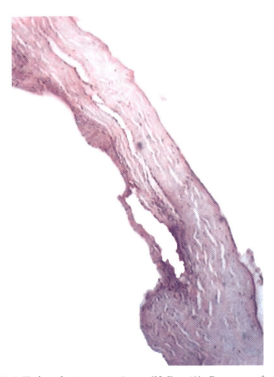

Fig. 22.6 Trabeculectomy specimen (H-E, ×40). Presence of intrascleral vascular ectasias up to the external part of the scleral flap of the specimen. This is remarkable since, in this case, there were not only episcleral ectasias showing on the scleral cover, but also, as can be seen in the figure, on the inner half. These morphological changes are determinants of hypertension

General Lesions

Angiomas can also be present on the neck, trunk, limbs, and digestive mucosa. Sometimes, the facial hypertrophy described above is also associated with body hemihypertrophy. From the point of view of pathological anatomy, it is a capillary hemangioma or a hemangioblastoma, which is a true vascular neoplasm with proliferation of endothelial cells.

Clinical Forms

Different clinical forms have been described, which can be divided according to symptoms: trisymptomatic, bisymptomatic, and monosymptomatic.

There are two trisymptomatic clinical forms: Sturge-Weber-Krabbe syndrome, which presents with facial angioma, nervous disorders, and glaucoma, and Janken syndrome, which is characterized by the presence of facial angioma, nervous disorders, and choroidal angioma with no glaucoma.

The bisymptomatic forms include Schirmer syndrome, which is a facial angioma with congenital glaucoma, and Lawford syndrome, a facial angioma with late congenital glaucoma.

Monosymptomatic forms may present either with isolated congenital glaucoma or with isolated choroidal angioma, with no glaucoma.

Prognosis of the disease may be serious due to the nervous lesions, which may lead to death or to the visual damage produced by glaucoma.

It has a dominant hereditary pattern.

We will now describe a clinical history which will be useful.

Clinical History No. 1

This 22-month-old male weighed 4.6 kg at birth. He had a facial angioma involving the left side of the face, particularly the upper eyelid, eyebrow, and forehead, and all the skin surrounding the inner and outer angles of the eye, but not the lower eyelid (Fig. 22.5). This angiomatous lesion swelled significantly when crying. The left eye had exotropia and the IOP was 20 mmHg in the right eye and 35 mmHg in the left eye.

He had seizures as early as his 2nd day of life, which were of clonic-tonic type on the right side in the arm and leg, three to four times a day, though he had some seizure-free days. They disappeared at 4 months of age.

Funduscopy of the left eye revealed a tortuous superior temporal vein, which failed to end at any vascular formation. The optic disc of the left eye was whitish-gray. This eye was exotropic 12°. The IOP of the left eye decreased to 20 mmHg with the use of miotic agents. The chamber angle was normal in the right eye and it had pathological mesodermal remnants in the left eye, which covered the ciliary body band up to where the Schlemm canal was located; there were small vessels at 10 o' clock. The parents refused to have the child operated on.

In other children, it is not unusual to find the angioma on one side while the glaucoma is bilateral.

The papers authored by Tosti [21] and Manzitti [22] are highly recommended for this entity.

Clinical History No. 2

This 29-year-old woman had unilateral Sturge-Weber-Krabbe syndrome in the right eye (Figs. 22.7, 22.8, 22.9). At the age of 23, she was found to have IOP at 36 mmHg. Laser trabeculoplasty was performed and then she was treated with prostaglandins. She arrived for the appointment with hypertension in the right eye.

This case shows a poor result in terms of regulating pressure. Nonpenetrating deep sclerectomy (NPDS) is not a good indication for Sturge-Weber syndrome.

	Right eye	Left eye
IOP	27 mmHg, with prostaglandins ×1, Cosopt ×3	13 mmHg
Visual acuity	20/100, sph. +3, cyl. +0.75 105° V20/80	20/25, sph. +1.25, cyl. −2.5 160°
Biomicroscopy anterior segment	Angiomatosis of episcleral vessels, subconjunctival 360°	Normal
Gonioscopy	Goniodysgenesis pathological, mesodermal remnants that pass the scleral spur and cover 360° of the ciliary body band; goniosynechiae possibly secondary to trabeculoplasty	Slight goniodysgenesis
Optic nerve	HRT phase IV (Fig. 22.8a)	HRT normal
Visual field		
Conventional perimetry	Stage V	Normal
Nonconventional perimetry	Stage V	Normal
Surgery	1. Non penetrating deep sclerectomy (10/2005)	
	2. Laser goniopuncture (10/2005)	
	3. Trabeculotomy, choroidal detachment (3 bags) reabsorbed in 3 days	
IOP	22 mmHg	14 mmHg

Fig. 22.7a,b Unilateral facial angiomas and conjunctival angiomas

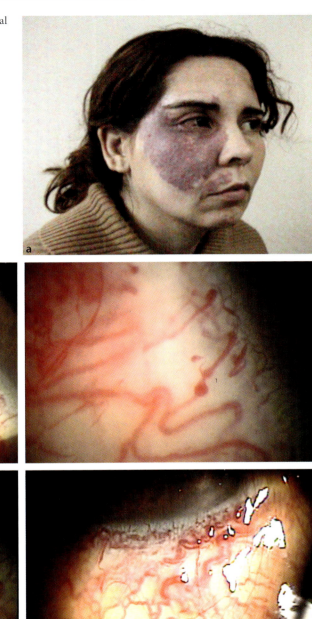

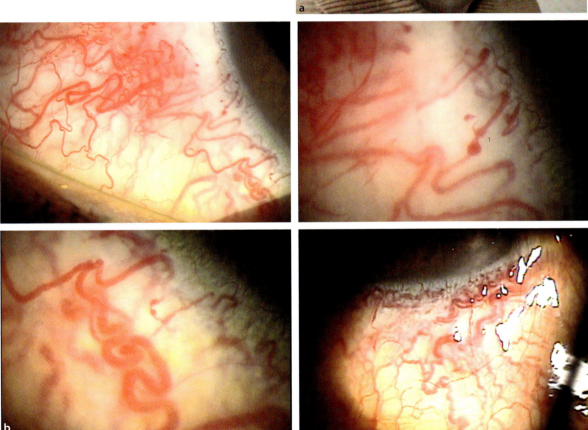

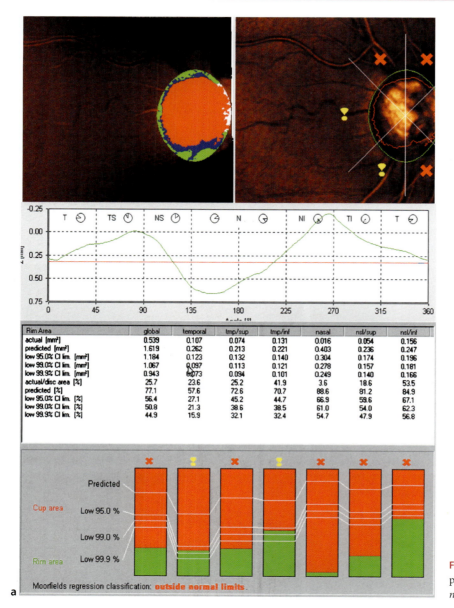

Rim Area	global	temporal	tmp/sup	tmp/inf	nasal	nsl/sup	nsl/inf
actual [mm²]	0.539	0.107	0.074	0.131	0.016	0.054	0.156
predicted [mm²]	1.619	0.262	0.213	0.221	0.403	0.236	0.247
low 95.0% CI lim. [mm²]	1.184	0.123	0.132	0.140	0.304	0.174	0.196
low 99.0% CI lim. [mm²]	1.067	0.097	0.113	0.121	0.278	0.157	0.181
low 99.9% CI lim. [mm²]	0.943	0.073	0.094	0.101	0.249	0.140	0.166
actual/disc area [%]	25.7	23.6	25.2	41.9	3.6	18.6	53.5
predicted [%]	77.1	57.6	72.6	70.7	88.6	81.2	84.9
low 95.0% CI lim. [%]	56.4	27.1	45.2	44.7	66.9	59.6	67.1
low 99.0% CI lim. [%]	50.8	21.3	38.6	38.5	61.0	54.0	62.3
low 99.9% CI lim. [%]	44.9	15.9	32.1	32.4	54.7	47.9	56.8

Fig. 22.8 a Confocal tomography, right eye. Stage IV (*b see next page*)

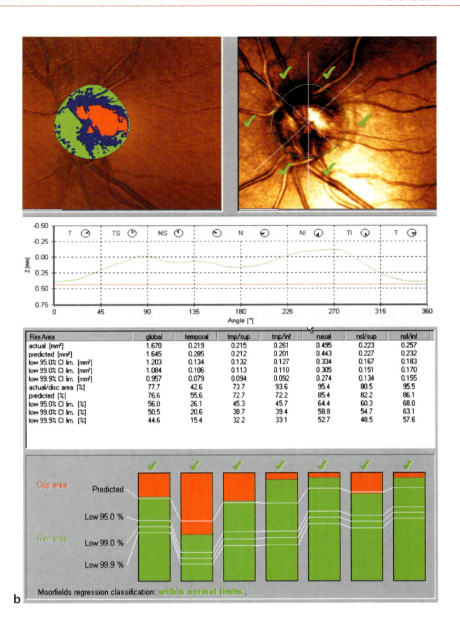

Rim Area	global	temporal	tmp/sup	tmp/inf	nasal	nsl/sup	nsl/inf
actual [mm²]	1.670	0.219	0.215	0.261	0.495	0.223	0.257
predicted [mm²]	1.645	0.285	0.212	0.201	0.443	0.227	0.232
low 95.0% CI lim. [mm²]	1.203	0.134	0.132	0.127	0.334	0.167	0.183
low 99.0% CI lim. [mm²]	1.084	0.106	0.113	0.110	0.305	0.151	0.170
low 99.9% CI lim. [mm²]	0.957	0.079	0.094	0.092	0.274	0.134	0.155
actual/disc area [%]	77.7	42.6	73.7	93.6	95.4	80.5	95.5
predicted [%]	76.6	55.6	72.7	72.2	85.4	82.2	86.1
low 95.0% CI lim. [%]	56.0	26.1	45.3	45.7	64.4	60.3	68.0
low 99.0% CI lim. [%]	50.5	20.6	38.7	39.4	58.8	54.7	63.1
low 99.9% CI lim. [%]	44.6	15.4	32.2	33.1	52.7	48.5	57.6

Fig. 22.8 (*continued*) **b** left eye. Stage normal

b

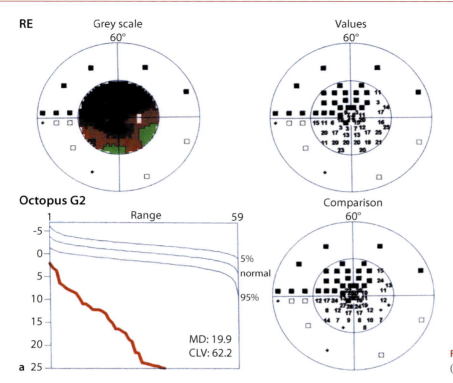

Fig. 22.9 a Visual field, right eye (*b see next page*)

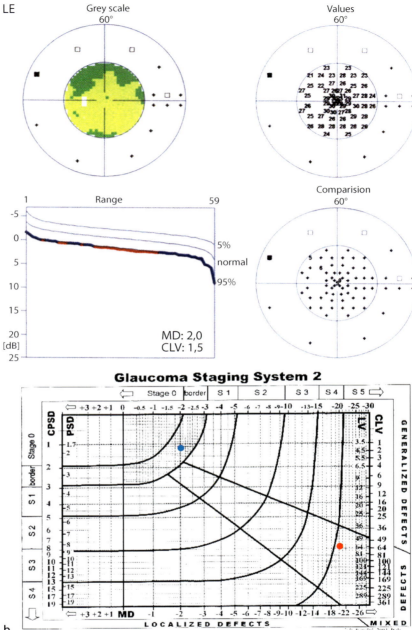

Fig. 22.9 (*continued*) **b** left eye   **b**

Klippel-Trenaunay Syndrome

Clinical History No. 3

This patient, a 12-year-old girl who was followed up from 1993 to 1998, had been operated twice in each eye (trabeculectomies) by other colleagues when she was small. Pressure was regulated perfectly in the left eye, but not in the right eye. The diagnosis was Klippel-Trenaunay syndrome. The patient presented with a bilateral facial angioma, which, as can be seen in Fig. 22.10, affects the right side of the face, but passed the mid-line of the nose and affected the chin and the lower part of the left cheek. A hemangiomatosis in the leg on the same side accompanied this lesion with a hypertrophy and edema that can affect the genitals. In this case, the hypertrophy and edema were reduced in size and the patient, 16 years old, presented 35-mmHg glaucoma (Fig. 22.10a–c) 360°. There was angiomatosis of episcleral and subconjunctival vessels (Fig. 22.10d).

	Right eye	Left eye
IOP	26 mmHg (with medication)	10 mmHg
Chamber angle	Type I	Type I
Visual acuity	Sph. –1.5, cyl. –0.50, 80° 20/40	Cyl. –0.50, 120°, 20/25
Surgery	Trabeculectomy (with mitomycin)	
1994	Panophthalmitis	
IOP (1996)	12 mmHg	
Visual acuity (1998)	Sph. –1, cyl. –2, 20°, 20/200	Cyl. –0.50, 120°, 20/25
Optic nerve	Megalodisc (D. area: 3.160 mm²)	Megalodisc (D. area: 3.32mm²)
Visual field (Fig. 22.11)	MD: 2.9 CLV: 2.4 (Figs. 22.12, 22.13)	MD: 0.3 CLV: 3.2
	Normal	Normal

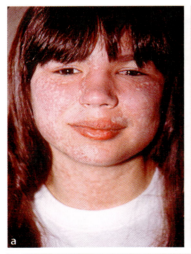
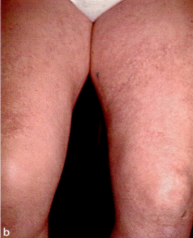
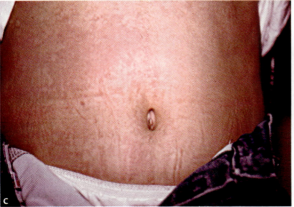
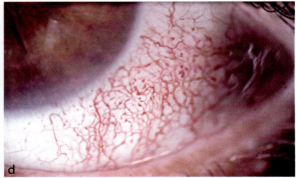

Fig. 22.10 a Bilateral angioma of the face, b bilateral angioma of the legs, c bilateral angioma of the abdomen. d Angiomatosis of episcleral and subconjunctival vessels

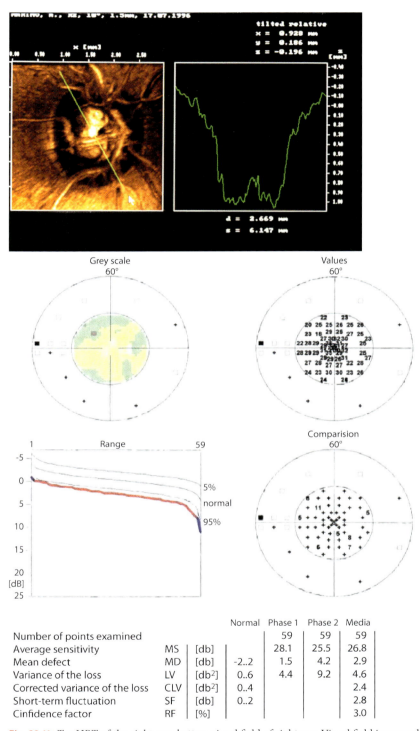

			Normal	Phase 1	Phase 2	Media
Number of points examined				59	59	59
Average sensitivity	MS	[db]		28.1	25.5	26.8
Mean defect	MD	[db]	-2..2	1.5	4.2	2.9
Variance of the loss	LV	[db²]	0..6	4.4	9.2	4.6
Corrected variance of the loss	CLV	[db²]	0..4			2.4
Short-term fluctuation	SF	[db]	0..2			2.8
Cinfidence factor	RF	[%]				3.0

Fig. 22.11 *Top* HRT of the right eye; *bottom* visual field of right eye. Visual field is normal

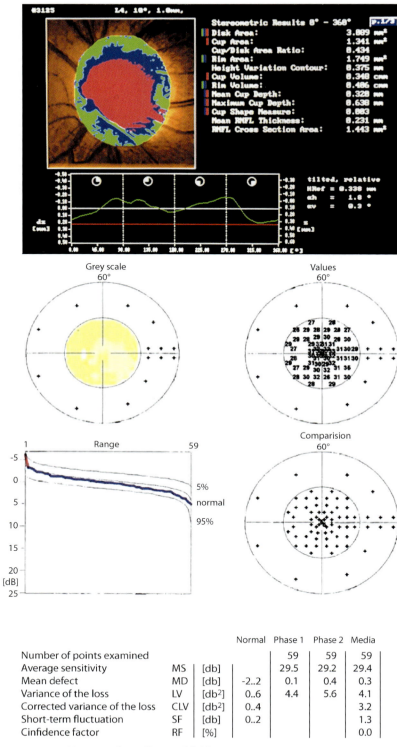

			Normal	Phase 1	Phase 2	Media
Number of points examined				59	59	59
Average sensitivity	MS	[db]		29.5	29.2	29.4
Mean defect	MD	[db]	-2..2	0.1	0.4	0.3
Variance of the loss	LV	[db²]	0..6	4.4	5.6	4.1
Corrected variance of the loss	CLV	[db²]	0..4			3.2
Short-term fluctuation	SF	[db]	0..2			1.3
Cinfidence factor	RF	[%]				0.0

Fig. 22.12 HRT LE megalopapilla visual field octopus normal

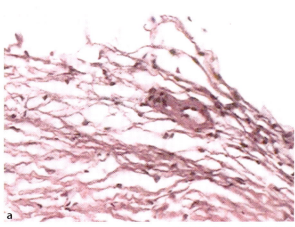

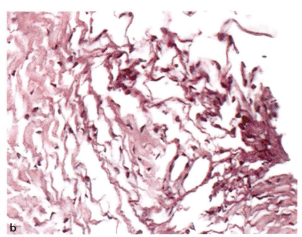

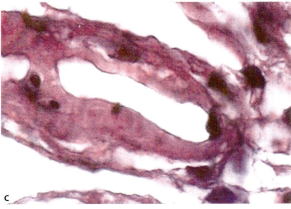

Fig. 22.13 a Trabeculectomy piece (H-E, ×100). The trabecular meshwork can be seen, modified by the presence of pseudo-diverticular structures that merge and distort the trabeculae. **b** Trabeculectomy piece (H-E, × 100). In another histological section, the diverticular formations looking like cirsoid vascular structures. **c** Trabeculectomy piece (H-E, ×1000). One of the pseudodiverticula, coated with an endothelium in its space and with a collagen-type wall

- Macroscopy:
  – Whitish fragment, 3×2×1 mm.
- Histopathological diagnosis;
  – Trabeculectomy, biopsy;
  – Ideal surgical limits;
  – Mesodermal remnants (diffuse and ligamentous);
  – Embryotoxon;
  – Vascular anomaly;
- Technique: material included in paraffin prior to MOS observation. Semiserial sections. Stain with H-E, Masson's trichrome, PAS, reticule, and PAP.

- Microscopy: partial sinusectomy piece of ideal surgical limits including corneoscleral flap, Descemet membrane, Schwalbe line, trabecular meshwork, and Schlemm canal. Abundant (uveal) trabecular meshwork, with presence of melanic pigment in relation to ligamentous structures, where hyaline thickening can be seen in leaves (embryotoxon). Segmented Schlemm canal and numerous vascular-type structures in juxtacanalicular meshwork and scleral furrow. Actually, is a vascular goniodisgenesis.

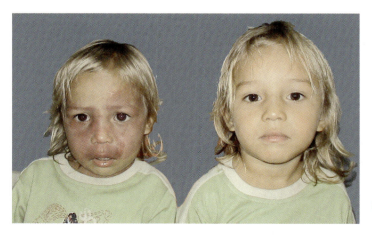

Fig. 22.14 Klippel-Trenaunay syndrome in one of the twins

Von Hippel-Lindau's Retinocerebellar Hemangioblastomatosis

Glaucoma has been described in some cases of this disease, but as a glaucoma secondary to severe hemorrhagic or exudative-type retinal lesions together with uveitis and cataract.

Summary

Glaucoma may present in the neurofibromatoses when the chamber angle is blocked by the neurofibromatous tissue that may also be found in the ciliary body or when a secondary rubeosis in the chamber angle blocks the outlet pathways.

In Sturge-Weber-Krabbe syndrome, glaucoma may be due to alterations in the chamber angle, just as in congenital glaucoma. At other times, the chamber angle is seen without alterations or with vascular alterations. In the latter case, it is suspected that the interscleral outlet pathways are affected.

Nevus of Ota

Oculodermal melanocytosis was described by Ota in 1939 [23] as an ocular melanocytosis associated with increased pigmentation of the skin in the distribution of the ophthalmic, maxillary, and the mandibular divisions of the fifth cranial nerve. Histologically, the ocular component (melanosis oculi) is increased pigmentation of the uveal tract, sclera, and episclera. The skin component does not consist of true nevus cells; it is composed of dendritic or fusiform cells containing granules of melanin found deep in the dermis. Its incidence is 0.1%–0.5% (Fig. 22.15, Fig. 22.16).

It is generally accepted that ocular melanocytosis is associated with increased uveal melanoma. This asso-

ciation has also been reported with oculodermal melanocytosis and melanomas of the skin, nervous system, and orbit.

Nevus of Ito is histologically similar to nevus of Ota, but involves the area of innervation of the lateral supraclavicular and lateral brachial nerves in the shoulder.

Nevi of Ota may be classified into various types based on extent, ranging from mild ocular involvement only to ocular, periocular, zygomatic, cheek and temple involvement, which can be unilateral or bilateral.

The lesions present as nonpalpable cutaneous pigmentations (black, purple, blue, and brown). The intensity of the pigmentation may appear to vary from day to day.

The first reported case of nevus of Ota associated with choroid melanoma was in 1981 by Hulke [24]. The incidence of nevus of Ota in the white population in general is 0.04% and uveal melanoma has been detected in 1.4% of patients with nevus of Ota in the same population [25, 26]. Using Bayes' theorem, Singh et al. [27] estimated the risk of developing a melanoma among the white population with ocular and/or oculodermal melanosis as 1 in 400 vs 1 in 13,000 in the general population, and in 90% of cases the uveal melanoma is diagnosed between 31 and 80 years of age.

The glaucoma present in nevus of Ota may be related to the hyperpigmentation of the whole anterior segment, including the trabecular meshwork and the outflow of aqueous humor, including the ciliary pathway. The constant movement of melanic pigment here is also interesting, since this could determine the blockage of the endothelial cells of the trabecular meshwork, following the idea we described about its belonging to Aschoff and Kiyono's reticuloendothelial system or the Davenport mononuclear phagocytic system. It could thus be recognized as similar to pigmentary glaucomas, from functional saturation of the cells responsible for filtering the aqueous humor.

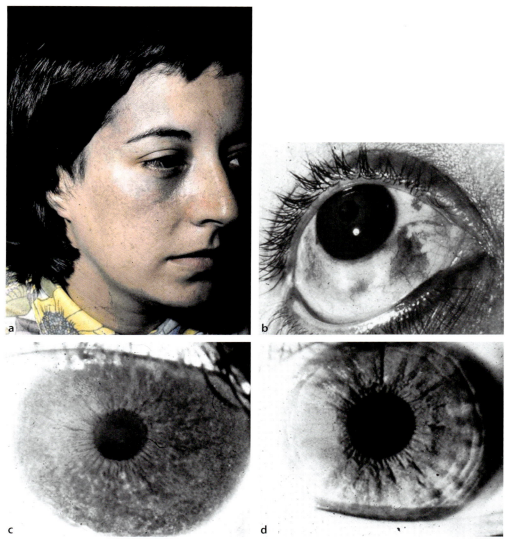

Fig. 22.15a–d Right periorbital pigmentation of the skin (**a**). On the lower eyelid, it reaches the rim. **b** Right eye: pigmentation in ocular globe. This is seen at scleral, episcleral, and conjunctival level **c** Iris of the right eye. The morphology of the iris of the right eye has a similar appearance to that of congenital glaucomas, as there are few crypts and those that exist are full of pigment. No circular contraction folds are seen. **d** Iris of the left eye. The left eye is completely normal in appearance and the circular contraction folds can be seen clearly

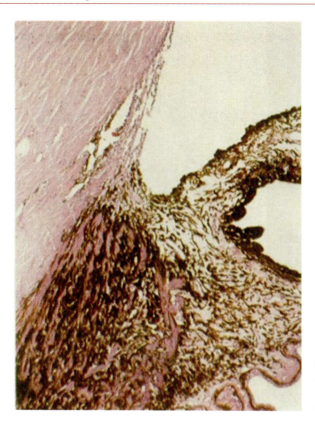

Fig. 22.16 Enucleation piece (H-E, ×40). Chamber angle, part of sclera, iris and ciliary body. The marked melanocytosis of the ciliary body and iris can be recognized. The trabecular meshwork and the Schlemm canal show melanic pigment overload

References

1. Van der Hoeve J (1933) Le phakomatoses de Bourneville, de Recklinghausen et de von Hippel Lindau. J Belge Neurol Psychiat 33:752–762
2. Willis RA (1958) The borderline of embryology and pathology. Butterworth, London
3. Recklinghausen FD (1882) Über die multiplen Fibrome der Haut und ihre Beziehungen zu den Neuromen. Festschrift f. R. Virchour. Hirschwald, Berlin
4. Del Rio Ortega P (1928) del: Tercera participacion al conocimiento morfologico y su interpretación funcional de la oligodengroglia. Mem Soc Españ Hist Anat 14:5–121
5. Schiess-Gemuseus H (1884) Vier Fälle angeborener Anomalie des Auges. Grafes Arch Ophthalmol 30:191
6. Lieb WA, Wirth WA (1959) Geeraets. Hydrophtalmus and neurofibromas. Confin Neurol 3:230–247
7. Francois J, Katz C (1961) Association homolatérale d'hydroptalmie, de la névrome plexiforme de la paupière supérieure et d'hémihypertrophie faciale dans la maladie de Recklinghausen. Ophthalmologia 142:549–571
8. Maggi C (1962) Neurinoma palpebrale plessiforme e buftalmo. Boll Ocul 41:398–414
9. Toselli CE, Volpi D (1963) Gigantismi parziali e facomatosi; l'ipertrofia emifacciale neurofibromatosa con buftalmo omolaterale. Ann Oual 89:791–799
10. Waiter JR, Butler RG (1963) Pigment spots of the iris and ectropion uveae with glaucoma. In: Neurofribromatosis. Am J Ophthalmol 56:964–973
11. Chandler PA, Grant WN (1965) Lectures on glaucoma. Lea and Febiger, Philadelphia, pp 354–356
12. Grant WN, Walton ES (1968) Distinctive gonioscopic findings in glaucoma due to neurofibromatosis. Arch Ophthalmol Chicago 79:127–134.
13. Calixto NE, Carvalho CA (1969) Semiologia do glaucoma congenito. XV Congr Brasil Tal Porto Alegre, pp 105–174
14. Schirmer R (1860) Ein Fall von Te1eangiektasie. Arch Ophthalmol 7:119
15. Sturge WA (1879) A case of partial epilepsy apparently due to a lesion of one of the vasomotor centres of the brain. Clin Soc Transoct 12:162
16. Weber PP (1922) Right sided hemi-hypotrophy resulting from right-sided congenital spastichemiplegia with a morbid condition of the left side brain, revealed by radiograms. J Neurol 3:134–139
17. Krabbe KH (1934) Facial and meningeal angiomatosis associated with calcifications of the brain cortex, a clinical and an anatomopathologic contribution. Arch Neurol Psychiat Chicago 32:737–755
18. Bergstrand H, Olivechona H, Tonnis H (1936) Gefäßmissbildungen und Gefäßgeschwülste des Gehirns. Thieme, Leipzig
19. van der Hoeve J (1937) Phakomatoses. Ned T Geneesk 82: 4418–4425
20. Stokes JJ (1957) The ocular manifestations of the Sturge-Weber Syndrome. South Med J 40:82–80
21. Tosti E (1959) Considerazioni su 4 casi da angiomatosi neuro oculo cutanea. Soc Mal Logic A Tauana 17:
22. Manzitti E, Cocucci D, Mayorga EC, Carrion R (1972) El síndrome de Klipper-Tranaunay y su vinculación con la angiomatosis encefalo-trigeminada de Sturge-Weber. Pren Med Arg 59:340
23. Ota M (1939) Nevus fusco-coeruleus ophthalmo-maxilaris. Tokyo Med J 63:1243
24. Hulke JW (1861) A series of cases of carcinoma of the eyeball. R Lond Ophthal Hosp Rep 3:279–286
25. Gonder JR, Ezell PC, Shields JA, Augsburger JJ (1982) Ocular melanocytosis. A study to determine the prevalence rate of ocular melanocytosis. Ophthalmology 89:950–952
26. Gonder JR, Shields JA, Albert DM et al (1982) Uveal malignant melanoma associated with ocular and oculodermal melanocytosis. Ophthalmology 89:953–969
27. Singh AD, De Potter P, Bonnie AF et al (1998) Lifetime prevalence of uveal melanoma in white patients with oculo (dermal) melanocytosis. Ophthalmology 105:195–198

Contents

Hyperaminoaciduria: Löwe's Oculocerebrorenal Syndrome

This is a syndrome which in 50% of cases is accompanied by glaucoma. It was described for the first time in 1952 by Löwe et al. [1]. It is defined as congenital insufficiency of the renal tubules, with mental retardation, nanism, congenital cataract, and glaucoma.

- Pathological anatomy. Primary congenital nephropathy with secondary rachitism.
- General manifestations. This disease manifests from birth through digestive symptoms: anorexia, vomiting, constipation, and repeated intestinal infections. The children are pale, blond, hypotrophic, and hypotonic. As well as rachitism, the ocular signs are very noticeable: the eyes are sunk in the orbits, bilateral cataract is nearly always present, and it is accompanied by glaucoma in 55% of cases. The rachitism is resistant to the administration of vitamin D and there is renal nanism with osteomalacia.
- Renal manifestations. Renal anomalies are characterized by deficient ammonia production and hyperaminoaciduria, as a consequence of a reduction in absorption at the renal tubules. There is also a drop in the reabsorption of phosphorus and a loss of calcium by urine that gives rise to secondary hyperparathyroidism, osteomalacia, etc. This loss of organic acids opens the way to a reduction of the alkaline reserve.
- Laboratory tests. There is hyperaminoaciduria with normal amino acid values in the plasma. Sometimes there is also glycosuria. These signs appear after 3 or 4 months of age.
- Ocular manifestations. These basically consist of a congenital cataract accompanied by congenital glaucoma in 55% of cases. The cataract is generally bilateral. The pupil dilates badly from hypertrophy of the iris, the response to mydriatics is poor, and at times there is nystagmus. The lens may be small (microphakia). Glaucoma generally accompanies the cataract and needs treatment. The chamber angle may appear in the various forms in which it is seen in congenital glaucoma.
- Heredity. This is recessive and sex-linked [2, 3], making it an exclusively male disease. The mothers, who are the carriers, sometimes present a punctate cataract. The disease gives the impression that the gene causing the metabolism error has a polyphenic effect that opens the way to the malformation of the chamber angle and of the crystalline lens.

Clinical Case No. 1

A 10-month-old male was brought to the hospital with gastroenteritis. As well as all the general symptoms and the positive laboratory results, he was found to have bilateral cataract and glaucoma. The cataract was extracted in both eyes and the IOP regulated itself spontaneously, remaining the same for 4 years after the operation, when the last check-up was done. A complete description of the clinical picture can be consulted in Elizalde et al. [4]. Figures 23.1, 23.2, and 23.3 illustrate this case.

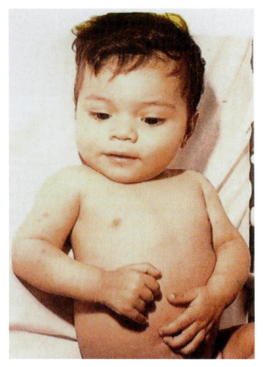

Fig. 23.1 Hyperaminoaciduria, Löwe's oculocerebro-renal syndrome

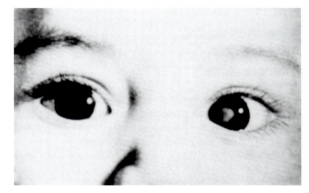

Fig. 23.2 A 10-month-old child with cataract and glaucoma

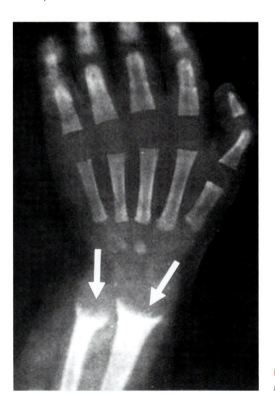

Fig. 23.3 X-ray of the bones of the wrist joint. The epiphysis of the radius and the cubit look like a champagne glass, characteristic of rachitism

Differential Diagnosis

Differential diagnosis should be made especially first with Abderhalden-Fanconi syndrome (cystinosis) [5]. This is an error in amino acid metabolism, which may or may not be accompanied by cystine deposits, aminoaciduria, rachitism resistant to vitamin D administration, and generalized and ocular cystinosis.

Ocular cystinosis can be seen by the deposit of birefringent crystals in the cornea, conjunctiva, uvea, sclera, and episclera. Generally, the cornea is cloudy because of the presence of cystine crystals. In one case that was kindly passed to us by Dr. Manzitti for chamber angle puncture, I was able to show the presence of cystine crystals in the aqueous humor. The aqueous humor showed the pentagonal crystals typical of cystine (Fig. 23.4). We made a solution of cystine in alcohol to test their identity, as well as a chromatography.

This is a primary enzyme defect that is inherited recessively. Differential diagnosis should then be made with De Toni syndrome [6]. This is an idiopathic renal acidosis with nephrocalcinosis, late rachitism, and adiposogenital dystrophy. It manifests in aminoaciduria, glycosuria and albuminuria, nephritis, and renal nanism.

The fact that the first of these syndromes contains cystine in the aqueous humor and that in Löwe's syndrome the aqueous is normal is an additional factor to think about in the polyphenic action of the gene that produces the error in the metabolism in Löwe's syndrome.

Therapy

If the cataract is bilateral it should be operated. The glaucoma will always be treated surgically if the ocular pressure values are high. In this case, the glaucoma will be operated first. Otherwise the cataract will be operated first.

If glaucoma surgery has to be performed, goniotomy or trabeculotomy will be chosen. Whenever a very young child is found with glaucoma and cataract, the ophthalmologist should think first about Löwe's syndrome, secondly about an embryopathy (generally rubeola-related), and thirdly glaucoma secondary to an operated congenital cataract. In the first situation, it is hereditary congenital glaucoma, in the second nonhereditary congenital glaucoma, and in the third secondary infantile glaucoma.

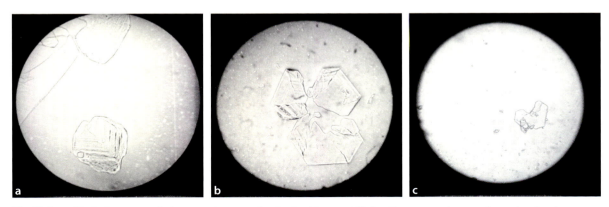

Fig. 23.4a–c Typical pentagonal-shape cystine crystals, obtained by crystallizing the aqueous humor, drawn by chamber puncture of a patient with cystinosis. **c** Cystine crystal obtained from the crystallization of a cystine solution in alcohol

Homocystinuria

Homocystinuria is a congenital error of the metabolism for a defect of the cystathionine-synthetase, transmitted by recessive autosomic heredity and shown from infancy fundamentally by luxation of the crystalline lens, reddening of the cheeks, and alterations in the hair and long limbs. A rather deeper analysis enables the manifestations of this disease to be divided as follows:

- General manifestations. These include neurological disorders such as mental retardation; skeletal alterations such as long limbs (dolichostenomelia) and arachnodactyly; cardiovascular alterations such as dilatation of the arteries and medium-caliber veins; potentially lethal thromboembolisms, which can also occur in small blood vessels from trauma; increased homocystine in urine and blood and reduced cystathionine-synthetase in the liver (puncture biopsy); fine, pale, dry, very altered hair; and reddening of the cheeks.
- Ocular manifestations. Luxation of the lens, in general, spherophakic and microphakic, that enables secondary glaucoma, atrophic, fine and translucent iris, colobomas, cystoid degeneration of the retina, retinal detachment, optic atrophy, and strabismus.

After studying this clinical picture, it is clear that it is important to make a differential diagnosis with Marfan's syndrome. This requires remembering that in homocystinuria heredity is autosomic and recessive and there are mental disorders. In the discussion on alcaptonuria, we presented a picture of differential diagnosis that also contains Marfan's syndrome and homocystinuria. For this reason, laboratory diagnosis is also important. Bickel and Cleve's [7] troprussiate test is used. Since homocystine is found only in small quantities in urine, it is detected by placing 3–5 ml of the patient's urine at room temperature with three to four drops of a fresh solution of 5% sodium nitroprussiate; 2 ml of sodium or potassium cyanide are added at 10%. A positive reaction gives a dark red color. Electrophoresis is also used for the diagnosis.

Medical treatment is currently made with pyridoxine. All the manifestations of the disease improve. When this treatment is used, there is a remarkable difference in the hair before and after, a clear dividing line.

Hurler Syndrome

Hurler syndrome is also known as Pfaundler–Hurler disease, dating from 1920 [8]. This is a metabolism disorder of the mucopolysaccharides, transmitted by recessive inheritance. It is a hyaluronidase deficiency

set off by the accumulation of dermatan sulphate and heparan sulphate, which, as Spellacy et al. [9] show, are deposited in the trabecular meshwork. Its pathogenesis is through deposits of dermatan and heparan sulphate on the trabecular meshwork. The disease manifests itself in the 2nd year of life with lumbar kyphosis and by the grotesque appearance of the face and extremities.

- General manifestations. The clinical signs are disproportionate nanism, alterations in bones and joints, and short stature with a large head. The face has thick lips, a flat nose, broad nostrils, a large tongue, and small teeth. This gives a grotesque appearance, known as gargoylism, from the gargoyles of Gothic cathedrals. There is also hepatosplenomegaly, with voluminous abdomen and inguinal or umbilical hernia.
- Ocular manifestations. These are mainly at the level of the cornea where superficial and deep whitish-gray cloudiness appear. The epithelium and endothelium remain intact. Ellis et al. [10] also describe chorioretinal degeneration, similar to the pigmentary degenerations, atrophy of the optic nerve, and megalocornea. The gargoylism is at times accompanied by moderate glaucoma and at others by buphthalmos. They generally do not survive beyond puberty.

Summary

Löwe's oculocerebrorenal syndrome, homocystinuria, and Hurler syndrome may be accompanied by glaucoma. In the first case, this is congenital glaucoma, in the second secondary glaucoma, and in the third the cause is unknown.

Endogenous Ochronosis (Alkaptonuria). Glaucoma Secondary to Luxation of the Lens

Among the metabolic diseases affecting the ocular system is alkaptonuria, or ochronosis. The first person to call it ochronosis and to study its pathological anatomy was Virchow, in 1866, and then, in 1904, Osler completed the study and description of the clinical picture.

It is thought that this disease occurs because there is a congenital incapacity to metabolize phenylalanine and tyrosine beyond the homogentisic acid state. This oxidizes, probably from tyrosinase, and becomes melanin or a similar substance that is partly eliminated in urine, with the rest deposited in various tissues, mainly in cartilages, and then in ligaments, tendons, conjunctiva, and sclera.

One of the characteristics of this disorder is that alkapton or homogentisic acid (2-5 dihydrophenylacetic) is found in the urine, which has given rise to various tests to detect this substance, the most common of which are:

- The ferric chloride test, which gives a bluish green color.
- The Fishberg test: a drop of urine on a developed photographic plate, dark brown in color.
- The Momers and Katsch test: the urine alkalinized with ammonia takes on a red color when drops of hydrogen peroxide are added; it later turns brown.

For more details on the varieties of the clinical picture, consult the complete work of Dr. R.H. Cambiaso [11].

The following clinical history is particularly interesting because it shows the possible consequences of the infiltration of homogentisic acid on the tissues: spontaneous lens luxation and secondarily ocular hypertension [12].

Clinical Case No. 2
Endogenous Ochronosis (Alkaptonuria)

Clinical case no. 2, aged 63, was a male who consulted for pain and reduced sight in the right eye in February 1966. Ocular hypertension was found and it was treated with miotics. In April he returned with the same problem and the examination gave this result:

	Right eye	Left eye
IOP	76 mmHg	16 mmHg
Visual acuity	20/200; Does not improve with correction	20/20 Without correction

Biomicroscopy showed small brown or ochre-colored deposits in the deep planes of the conjunctiva of both eyes, in the form of commas and rings that move when the conjunctiva is moved at the insertion of the internal and external rectus muscles. There are also deposits below in the sclera, in the tendon insertion region of the internal and external recti, but these are bluish-black in color, as well as in the limbus at 3 and 9 o'clock, in the form of small yellowish-brown drops. These accumulations are subepithelial. Greater magnification shows that beside each drop there are smaller drops that look like oil (Fig. 23.5).

The chamber angle is open but narrow.

The right eye showed edematous cornea. The anterior chamber was irregular in depth, flatter in the lower part. Dilating the pupil of the right eye showed the luxation of the lens upward and forward, letting a tongue of vitreous penetrate through the lower part of the pupil. The Berger space was also positive, as was the Wieger capsulohyaloid ligament.

At the height of the insertion of the external rectus, the dark color of the deposits of ochronotic pigment can be seen. Immediately after this region, toward the cornea, the deposits typical in conjunctiva can be seen, some of them in the form of complete rings and others in half-rings. In the cornea, next to the limbus, deposits of the same substance can be clearly seen as yellow-brown drops.

	Right eye	Left eye
Funduscopy:	Normal	Normal
Tonography: CL3-7	0.04	0.15
Visual field	Normal	Normal

X-rays of the dorsolumbar spine showed generalized osteoporosis with calcification of the intervertebral ligaments. There were multiple discopathies with ossification. Rhizomelic spondylitis (Betcherev disease) was diagnosed. The hips showed slight signs of bilateral arthrosis and ossification of the muscle tendon insertions in the iliacs.

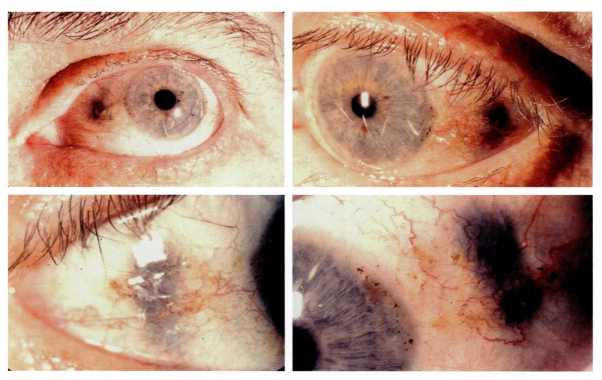

Fig. 23.5 Cornea and conjunctiva at the height of the external rectus, in the horizontal meridian in a glaucoma secondary to luxation of the lens from alkaptonuria and endogenous ochronosis

Progression and Treatment

The progressive results (Fig. 23.6) show the first IOP measurement at 75 mmHg for the right eye and 16 mmHg for the left eye, with visual acuity 20/200 for the right eye and 20/20 for the left eye. The patient returned 1 month later, on May 10, 1966, and the IOP was still high: 62 mmHg. With miotics and Diamox treatment, it only decreased to 55 mmHg, so glycerol was tried orally, and on May 12 the IOP was checked three times at 5:30, 7:30, and 10:30 to find the best time for performing surgery. On May 13, the lens was extracted, after administering glycerol, using cryoextractor. During surgery, a piece of conjunctiva was removed for a biopsy. The postoperative period was normal and, 1 year later, on June 12, 1967, the IOP was normal in both eyes – 16 mmHg in the right eye and 18 mmHg in the left eye – and visual acuity has increased in the right eye from 20/200 to 20/40 using a contact lens.

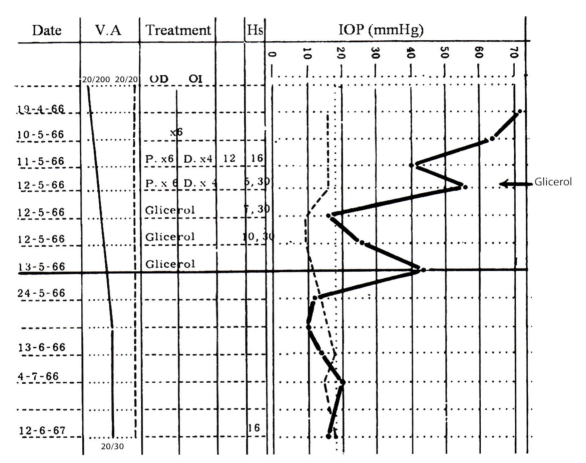

Fig. 23.6 Chart of the progression of ocular pressure of the patient with endogenous ochronosis before and after lens extraction. After lens extraction, the intraocular pressure drops to normal values. Actually it is a secondary glaucoma to luxation of the lens provocated by the deterioration of the sonula caused by alkaptonuria

Anatomopathological Examination of the Biopsy

- Macroscopy. The material sent was a grey-colored piece measuring 4×3×1 mm and was fixed in formol.
- Microscopy (after paraffin embedding and staining with hematoxylin-eosin). The conjunctival stroma contained accumulations of homogeneous yellowish-brown material, varied in shape, some shaped like commas. There was extensive degeneration of the collagen fibers of the stroma, with abundant formation of hyaline-looking material. The epithelium of the conjunctiva was absent in some areas of the section, but the rest was normal (Fig. 23.7).

Seitz [13], made the first histopathological description of a biopsy of conjunctiva obtained from a patient with ochronosis. Since then, the work of Rodenhäuser [14], Rones [15], Allen et al. [16], and Ashton et al. [17] have confirmed and broadened Seitz's observations. The conjunctival biopsies described by Seitz and Rodenhäuser are practically identical to ours: degeneration, homogenization and fragmentation of the elastic and collagen fibers, with deposit of hyaline material similar to that seen in pingueculae, as well as the presence of yellowish-brown ochronotic pigment, without definite structure or form (comma, ring, etc.).

The nature of ochronotic pigment, although it is not finally clarified, is probably the same as melanin. This is confirmed by studies made with the electron microscope by Cooper and Moran [18], as well as the special stains used by Rones (depigmentation, stains for melanin, iron, and fats) and Allen (Fontana, Nile blue sulphate, Variant 1, Variant 2, Masson's trichromic, periodic acid-Schiff, cresyl violet, Mallory's aniline blue).

According to Allen, the ochronotic pigment should be thought of as unleashing a process of destruction, either by altering the physical properties of the tissues with the consequent reduction of their resistance, or by directly producing their necrosis. In the sclera, Ashton has described degeneration of the elastic fibers, elastic degeneration of the collagen fibers, and disappearance of the tissue cells. Duke Elder's [19] opinion on this is similar to that of Allen and Ashton.

As yet there is no satisfactory explanation to justify the preference of the ochronotic pigment for the region of the interpalpebral opening. Anderson considers it may stem from the influence of the light easing the enzymatic activity of the tyrosinase.

Analyzing the ocular manifestations of the case we have just presented, this spontaneous lens luxation in a disease stemming from a metabolism error, similar to other clinical pictures or syndromes that also have lens luxation and metabolism error.

In conclusion, it is remarkable that:

1. In homocystinuria there is an error in the metabolism of methionine, as the cystathionine-synthetase does not act to change it into cysteine with the appearance of homocysteine in urine. In the first and the second of the histological preparations of Henkind and Ashton, a thickened basal membrane of the ciliary epithelium with marked atrophy of the unpigmented epithelium can be seen, which leads to a degeneration of the zonula with lens luxation and iridodonesis. The hyaline layer covering the atrophic epithelium is typical of this disorder. The electron microscope shows atrophy of the unpigmented epithelial layer, thickening of the basal membrane, the zonula with its granular appearance, and the normal pigment layer. The deficiency of the zonula stems from the alterations in the development of the ciliary epithelial cells that contain cysteine and are responsible for the formation of these fibers (Table 23.1).

2. In Marfan disease, hydroxyproline appears in the urine [20], and there are modifications in the mucoproteins and in the electrophoretic picture of the proteins, and lens luxation. In Marchesani disease, it is still not known whether there is a metabolism error.

3. In alkaptonuria, there are alterations in the uvea and in the ciliary body. Allen et al. described deposits of alkapton (Fig. 23.8).

For these reasons, we believe that the degeneration of the fibers of the zonula is possible in endogenous ochronosis and that this opens the way to the spontaneous luxation of the lens and secondarily to ocular hypertension.

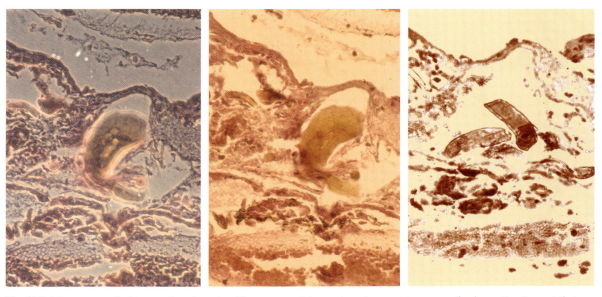

Fig. 23.7 Microscopy of a biopsy of conjunctiva. The stroma of the conjunctiva contains areas of ochronotic pigment that are seen as crystal-like comma shapes. There is degeneration of the collagen fibers of the stroma. Original preparation made by G. Kaufer

Table 23.1 Diseases stemming from metabolism error with lens luxation

	Carson–Neill homocystinuria	Marfan	Marchesani	Endogenous ochronosis
Metabolism error	Methionine	Collagen proteins	?	Phenylalanine and tyrosine
Heredity	R	D	DR	R
Urine	Hemocysteine	Hydroxyproline	?	Alkapton (homogentisic acid)
General manifestations	Mental retardation, pale face and hair, muscular weakness	Iris hypoplasia, (glaucoma)	Spherophakia, microphakia (glaucoma)	Dark deposits, in conjunctiva, sclera and corneal limbus
Ocular pathology	Atrophy of unpigmented ciliary epithelium with degeneration of the zonula			Deposits in ciliary body, conjunctiva, and sclera

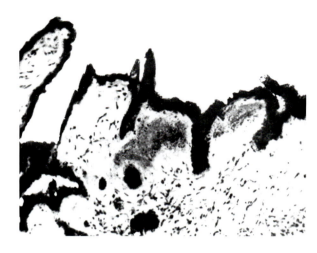

Fig. 23.8 Deposits of alkapton at the level of the ciliary body at the height of the source of the zonular fibers. This may explain the reason for the lens luxation. Courtesy of Allen O' Malley and Straatsma

Summary

In alkaptonuria and endogenous ochronosis, glaucoma is caused by a luxation of the lens from alterations in zonula at its insertion in the ciliary body where cysteine accumulates. It is actually secondary glaucoma, and its treatment consists in extracting the luxated lens, thus curing the glaucoma.

References

1. Lowe CH, Terrey M, MacLachlan EA (1952) Organic aciduria, decreased renal ammoniac, production, hydrophthalmos and mental retardations. Am J Dis Child 83:164–184

2. Streiff EB, Straube G (1958) Les manifestations du syndrome de Lowe. Ophthalmologica 135:632–639

3. Lowe CH (1960) Oculo-cerebral renal syndrome. Maandschr Kindergeneesk 28:77–80

4. Elizalde E, Cambiano C, Gravano JC, Musso M, Beraldi MV, Y Reca R (1970) El Sindrome De Lowe. Arch Argent. Pediat LXVIII:6–19

5. Abderhalden E (1903) Familiäre cystindiathese. Z Phys Chern 38:557–561

6. Toni G de (1954) Un nouveau syndrome dysmetabolique et dysendocrine: acidose rénale idiopathique avec néphrocalcinose et pseudo-paralysie hypopotassemique, nanisme, rachitisme tardif, dystrophie adiposogenitale. Ann Paediat Basel 182:63–76

7. Bickel H, Cleve H (1967) Ein kurzes Hanbuch der Humangenetik V:243

8. Hurler G (1920) Über einem Tip multipler Abartung, vorwiegend am Skelettsystem. Z Kinderheik 24:220–234

9. Spellacy R, Bankes JLK, Crow J, Dourmashkin R, Shah D, Waits RWE (1980) Glaucoma. A Case Of Hurler Disease. Br J Ophthalmol 64:773–778

10. Ellis RW, Sheldon W, Capon NB (1936) Gargoylism (chondro-osteodystrophy) corneal opacities, hepato-splenomegaly, and mental deficiency. Q L Med 29:119–139

11. Cambiaso RH (1953) Ocronosis ocular con alcaptonuria y osteoartritis (Observación personal). Arch Oftal B Aires 38:456–474

12. Sampaolesi R; Reca R, Kaufer G (1967) Alcaptonuria y ocronosis endógena con luxación de cristalino y glaucoma secundario. Arch Oftalmol B Aires 42:165–169

13. Seitz R (1954) Über Die ochronosischen Pigmentierungen am Auge. Klin Mbl Augenheilk 125:432–440

14. Rodenháuser JH (1957) Über Die Augenpigmentierungen bei Alkaptonurie (Ochronosis Oculi). Klin Mbl Augenheilk 131:202–215

15. Rones B (1960) Ochronosis oculi in alkaptonuria. Am J Ophthalmol 49:440–446

16. Allen RA, O'Malley C, Straatsma BR (1961) Ocular findings in hereditary ochronosis. Arch Ophtha Chicago 65:657–668

17. Ashton N, Kirker JG, Lavery FS (1964) Ocular findings in a case of hereditary ochronosis. Br J Ophthalmol 48:405–415

18. Cooper JA, Moran TJ (1957) Studies on ochronosis. I. Report of case with death from ochronotic nephrosis. Arch Path Chicago 64:46–53

19. Duke-Elder S (1965) System of ophthalmology, Vol. VIII, Part 2. Henry Kimpton, London, pp 1064–1068

20. Sjoerdsma A, Davidson JD, Udenfriend S, Mitoma C (1958) Increased excretion of hydroxyproline in Marfan's syndrome. Lancet 2:994

Contents

The congenital mesodermal dystrophies are systemic diseases and essentially consist of Marfan syndrome (arachnodactyly and dolichostenomelia) and Marchesani syndrome (spherophakia and brachymorphia). Both diseases, as well as their somatic manifestations, affect the eyeball. The basic manifestation is seen in alterations in the position and shape of the lens which, added to other ocular malformations can, secondarily, produce glaucomas. It is transmitted by autosomal dominant inheritance. There are great differences in gene penetrance and expressivity [1].

Marfan Syndrome

General Manifestations

Marfan syndrome [2] is characterized by a lanky appearance (dolichomorphism) and long limbs (dolichostenomelia), particularly long-boned hands and feet. The third phalanx and the metacarpals in the hands are overlong. This, added to the retraction of the flexor tendons, creates a spider-like aspect, which is why it has been called arachnodactyly, or spider fingers. The thorax is pigeon-shaped, and there is kyphoscoliosis and dolichocephaly. These patients also present muscular hypotonia resulting from wastage of the muscles. The tendons are hyperextensible. This looseness of the ligaments favors luxations (congenital hip luxation). These are accompanied by heart and large blood vessel problems: interauricular and interventricular communication and dissecting aortic aneurysm. Marfan syndrome, then, is a malformation deriving from problems in embryo development of the mesoderm with localized manifestations in the bone and muscle system and in the elastic conjunctive tissues.

Ocular Manifestations

The main symptom of Marfan syndrome is ectopia of the lens: 78% of the syndromes show this luxation or subluxation of the lens [3]. This problem was first described by Borger [4]. In most cases, the lens luxates upward and outward, but it can also do so toward the interior of the eye, and in these cases is accompanied by retinal detachment, or toward the anterior segment, accompanied by acute glaucoma. The eye may also present axial myopia. At other times, the myopia is caused by anterior luxation of the lens or by spherophakia.

At times there is spherophakia and microphakia [5–7]. These basic ocular manifestations may occur with coloboma of the lens [5]; coloboma of the iris [8, 9]; miosis, poor reaction to atropine, and aplasia of the pupil dilator [10–12]; aniridia [13]; pupillary membrane [14–16]; megalocornea [17]; buphthalmia [18]; coloboma of the optic nerve [19]; heterochromia iridis; and sometimes tapetoretinal degeneration [20, 21]. Marfan syndrome may also be found with Lobstein–van der Hoeve syndrome [22], blue sclerotics, bone fragility, and lung alterations.

Glaucoma

In some cases, glaucoma may be caused by the luxation of the lens to the anterior chamber, i.e., phacogenic glaucoma that is cured by extracting the lens, and in others by the presence of alterations to the chamber angle, with marked persistence of congenital mesodermal remains. The chamber angle in Marfan syndrome is very similar to that of congenital glaucoma, with very thick pathological mesodermal remnants. Reeh and Lehman [23] present the pathological anatomy of the chamber angle. They show how the superficial mesodermal layer of the iris continues at the angle with the outer wall, an iris lacking crypts, without collarette, and an endothelial membrane that covers the anterior surface of the iris. Other authors such as Burian and Allen [24] and Wachtel [25] describe alterations in the shape and size of the Schlemm canal.

A Case of Marfan Syndrome

Clinical history No. 1 refers to a 35-year-old female.
After extracting the lens, the glaucoma continued (Fig. 24.1).

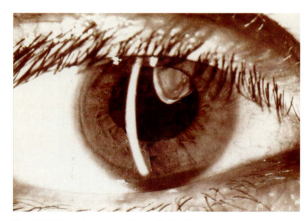

Fig. 24.1 Luxation of the lens, clinical history no. 1

	Right eye	Left eye
	Amaurosis from perforating wound	Superoexternal lens luxation
IOP	29 mmHg	–
Tonography $C_{1.7-3}$	0.03, luxation of the lens	–
Chamber angle	Gonioscopic absence of the band of the ciliary body from persistence of pathological mesodermal tissue that reaches the spur	

Marchesani Syndrome

- General manifestations. Marchesani syndrome [26] is marked by brachymorphia. As opposed to Marfan syndrome, here the patient has a short stature, with a well-developed muscular system, good adipose panicle, and a pyknic constitution. Brachymorphia can be seen, as in Marfan syndrome, in the hands and feet, which are brachycephalous. Weill [8] was the first to describe ectopia of the lens in a 42-year-old patient who presented these clinical features (small hands and fat fingers). Heredity may be dominant or recessive, depending on the case.
- Ocular Manifestations. The basic manifestation is seen in the alteration of the shape of the lens: spherophakia, spherical lens, sometimes accompanied by microphakia. There may be luxation of the lens. There are some alterations of the chamber angle seen in the persistence of pathological mesodermal remnants with similar features to those of congenital glaucoma or late congenital glaucoma. The shape of the lens predisposes to high myopia, its luxation to phacogenic glaucoma, and the alteration of the angle to a late congenital type glaucoma.

Duke Estrada [27] presented a patient with glaucoma: in one eye the ocular hypertonia was secondary to an anterior luxation of the lens with pupillary blockage, while in the other eye, without lens luxation, there was marked ocular hypertension. The therapy in the first eye was extraction of the lens and in the second eye was goniotomy. The author describes the persistence of pathological mesodermal remnants in the chamber angle, extending beyond Schwalbe's line.

N. Calixto (personal communication) has kindly provided Fig. 24.4, where a microphakic and spherophakic lens can be seen.

The glaucoma may occur through two mechanisms, either from pupillary block, by spherophakic lens (in-verse glaucoma because the ocular pressure diminishes with mydriatics), or through lens luxation. However, Calixto has shown that despite extracting the lens, ocular hypertension persists.

Even though the lens has an ectodermic origin, the alterations it undergoes in these two syndromes stem from alterations of the ciliary muscle, which is generally very hypotrophic.

The clinical histories above on Marfan syndrome and the following two on Marchesani syndrome show how difficult it is to attribute glaucoma to the deep alterations of the anterior segment and the existence of lens luxation.

A Case of Marchesani Syndrome Without Glaucoma

Clinical history No. 2 involves a 42-year-old male with a very deep anterior chamber in both eyes.

	Right eye	Left eye
Visual acuity	20/25	20/25
IOP	13 mmHg	15 mmHg
Tonography: C_{L3-7}	0.19	0.15

In the iris, atrophy of the peripupillary pigmentary layer can be seen, and in its ciliary zone there is peripheral iridodonesis, seen with transillumination. Both eyes have microphakic and spherophakic lenses. Varying the size of the pupil with eyedrops does not alter the IOP. The daily pressure curve is normal in both eyes. The chamber angle on both the right and left sides shows persistence of pathological mesodermal tissue with a picture similar to that of congenital glaucoma in children. The shape of the anterior chamber is trapezoidal.

A Case of Marchesani Syndrome with Glaucoma

Clinical history No. 3 involves a 35-year-old male. In 1956, he was seen for glaucoma in the left eye, with pain and colored halos. In 1962, he experienced temporary hemiplegia because of congenital arterial problems (thrombosis of the right brachiocephalic trunk, with no radial and carotid pulse and basilar trunk aneurysm). In 1966, a colleague operated the left eye for glaucoma. Today he shows the following features.

	Right eye	Left eye
Visual acuity	Sph. −3, Cyl. −3 to 10°= 20/200	Hand movements, lens completely luxated at 6 o'clock, detachment of retina, the tear cannot be found
IOP	30 mmHg	7 mmHg

In the right eye, gonioscopy shows wide open angle, pigmented Schlemm canal. There is atrophy of the superficial and deep mesenchymal layer that reveals the epithelial pigmentary layer in triangular zones with an appearance identical to that of the chamber angle of the newborn child. The pathological mesodermal remnants are dysplastic and reveal the upper half of the ciliary body band, whitish in color, where the greater arterial circle of the iris runs and is visible at times. There is peripheral iridodonesis and deep atrophy of the iris pigmentary layer that enables the equatorial edge of the lens to be seen by transillumination. The diagnosis of microspherophakia can therefore be made. The atrophy of the pigmentary layer shows in two zones, one peripheral and one central next to the frill of the iris. The iris parenchyma is atrophic from the frill of the iris to the periphery. The left eye shows a similar picture in the anterior segment, plus a total iridodonesis from the complete luxation of the lens (Fig. 24.2).

	Right eye	Left eye
Funduscopy	Excavation of optic disk 3/6, Medication with pilocarpine, every 4 h and adrenaline 2% once a day regulates the IOP	Retinal detachment
IOP	14 mmHg	
Visual field	Stage I (Fig. 24.3)	

A year and a half later, the patient returned because the lens in this eye had luxated. The extraction was made with cryo with no complications.

	Right eye	Left eye
Visual acuity	20/30++ with correction, Sph. + 10, Cyl. + l.50 to 95° = 20/25	Light vision, detached retina, no tear found
IOP		28 mmHg
Visual field	Same condition; 1 year later the patient returned with the same visual acuity in the right eye and his IOP regulated	

One year later, the patient returned with ocular hypertension of 28 mmHg in the right eye and surprisingly with the retina attached, with no surgery and a visual acuity of 20/30. The visual field can be seen in Fig. 24.3. The pressure was regulated with medication.

N. Calixto (personal communication) has kindly provided Fig. 24.4, where a microphakic and spherophakic lens can be seen.

Fig. 24.2 Chamber angle of the right eye

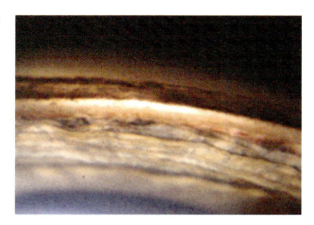

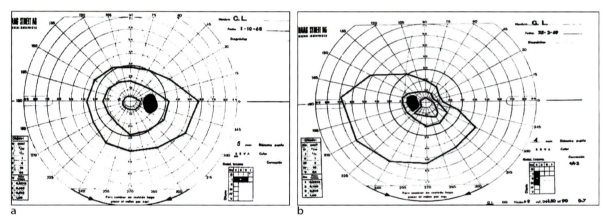

a   b

Fig. 24.3 **a** Right eye; **b** left eye

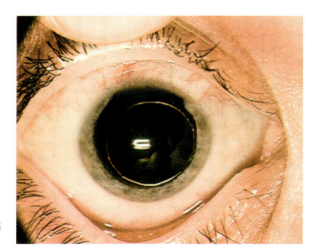

Fig. 24.4 Microphakic and spherophakic in Marchesani syndrome (courtesy of N. Calixto)

Summary

In Marfan and Marchesani syndromes, the cause of glaucoma is generally an alteration in the chamber angle similar to that in congenital glaucoma. However, when the alterations of the position or shape of the lens give way to hypertension, this is secondary.

References

1. Waardenburg PJ, Franceschetti A, Klein N (1961) Genetics and ophthalmology. Blackwell, Oxford

2. Marfan AB (1896) Un cas de déformation congénitale de quatre membres plus prononcée aux extremités characterisée para l'allongement des as. Bull Soc Mm Paris 13:220–226

3. Last U, Vogel F (1957) Bemerkungen zum Marfan-Syndrom. Dtsch Med Wschr 82:746–747

4. Börger F (1914) Demonstration eines 9 jährigen Knaben mit Arachnodaktylie. Mschr Kinderheilk 13:355–356

5. Weve H (1931) Uber Arachnodaktylie (Dystrophia Mesodermalis Congenita-Typus Marfan). Arch Augenkeilk 104:1–46

6. Franceschetti A (1932) Marfanscher Syndromenkomplex und Coloboma Lentis. Klin Mhl Augenheilk 88:686–687

7. Waardenburg PJ (1932) Das menschliche Auge und seine Erbanlagen. Nighoff, The Hague

8. Weill G (1932) Ectopie du cristallin et malformations générales. Ann Oculist 169:21–44

9. Godl H (1937) Arachnodaktylie mit Kongenitalem Uvea-Linsenkolobom. Klin Mhl Augenheilk 98:396

10. Theobald DG (1940) Histologic study of an eye from a child with arachnodactyly. Arch Ophthalmol Chicago 24:1046

11. Theobald DG (1941) Histologic eye functions in arachnodactyly. Am J Ophthalmol 24:1132–1137

12. Rambar AC, Denenholz EJ (1939) Arachnodactylia. Report of a case with autopsy including histologic examination of the eye. J Pediatr 15:844–852

13. Nobecourt P, Cathala J, Temerson (1938) Subluxation congénitale bilatérale du cristallin chez un prématuré. Dolichostenomelie. Bull Soc Pediatr Paris, 36:21–24

14. Neresheimer R (1916) Über Arachnodaktylie. Arch Kinderheilk 65:391–408

15. François J (1935) De la pathogénie et de l'origine hypophysaire du syndrome de Marfan. Bull Soc Fr Ophthalmol 48:157–197

16. Grosser, Igersheimer (1927) Über Arachnodaktylie mit typischem Augenbefund. Klin Wschr 5:1116

17. Franco R, Marin EM, Salvador A (1948) Un Syndrome de Marfan. Rev Din Esp 29:357–364

18. Weve H (1931) Über Arachnodaktylie (Dystrophia Mesodermalis Congenita-Typus Marfan). Arch Augenkeilk 104:1–46

19. Malbran J, Picoli HR (1937) Arachnodactilia (Syndrome De Marfan). Arch Oftalmol B Aires 12:3–17

20. Ellis RWB (1931) Blue sclerotics apparently inherited by the mother arachnodactyly by the father. Proc R Soc Med 24:1054–1057

21. Reeh MJ, Lehman W (1954) Marfan's Syndrome arachnodactylia ectopia lentis. Trans Am Acad Ophthalmol Otolaryng 58:212–216

22. Burian HM, Allen L (1961) Histological study of the chamber angle of patients with Marfan's syndrome. Arch Ophthalmol Chicago 65:323–333

23. Wachtel JG (1966) Ocular pathology of Marfan's syndrome. Arch Ophthalmol Chicago 76:512–522

24. Marchesani O (1939) Brachydaktylie und Angeborene Kugellinse Als Systemerkrankung. Klin. Mhl Augenheilk 103:392–406

25. Duke Estrada W (1961) L'hypertension oculaire dans les syndrome de Weill-Marchesani. Bull Soc Fr Ophthalmol 74:729–733

Nonhereditary Congenital Glaucomas

Contents

Embryopathies: Rubella

This embryopathy is a phenocopy, i.e., a nonhereditary congenital glaucoma that phenotypically copies hereditary congenital glaucoma. This is why differential diagnosis between the two is very difficult. It should be borne in mind that when the mother has rubella in the first 3 months of pregnancy, either openly or sometimes in a subclinical form, this can open the way to an embryopathy. We should remember that this syndrome has cardiac, auditory, and ocular manifestations. The latter occur in the retina, leading to rubella retinitis pigmentosa, or in the anterior segment, causing cataract or glaucoma.

The child is born small. The glaucoma appears in the first 6 months and its production mechanism may be related to an inflammatory infiltration affecting the chamber angle, which shows pigment deposits in small but scattered accumulations.

In general, either cataract or glaucoma are present, but they are rarely present together. Nowadays, to make a confirmed diagnosis, it is necessary to isolate the virus of the organism.

In this embryopathy, glaucoma is less common than cataract. The ophthalmologist should always remember that in rubella embryopathy a diffuse corneal edema usually appears in the early days, and disappears within 1 week, so it should not be confused with glaucoma. The basic elements of the diagnosis will always be ocular pressure and echometry. In addition, in these cases, the pigment accumulations seen in the angle are caused by the depigmentation of the iris, which is easier to see by transillumination.

Leukocoria

Before discussing the topic, it is worth reviewing the concept of leukocoria.

In 1817, Beer [1] gave the name amaurotic cat's eye to an ocular condition seen in newborns and children, characterized by a white or yellowish-white pupil reflection, caused by alterations behind the lens similar to a tumor, which were seen in the examination with oblique lateral illumination.

In 1955, Reese [2] suggested the name leukocoria, including among these the retinoblastomas, the pseudogliomas, and all the other cases, even those which, for lack of a better name, had previously been catalogued as pseudogliomas, even when no tumor was suspected. The best studies on this subject are those of Dolfus and Auvert [3], Badtke [4], Hamburg [5], and Babel [6].

There are three well-known types of leukocoria that may present glaucoma secondary to the process originating them. Knowledge of these and of their differential diagnosis is very important for the practicing oculist.

1. Persistent hyperplastic primary vitreous;
2. Retrolental fibroplasia;
3. Coats disease.

Fetopathies: Persistent Hyperplastic Primary (Hyaloid) Vitreous

The hyaloid circulatory system disappears progressively at the 4th month, as retina vascularization begins, as is described in the Sect. 2.6 and in Chap. 8.

The vitreous has three periods. In the primary vitreous, the hyaloid vascularization fills the fetal vitreous until it approaches and makes contact with the lens, forming the tunica vasculosa lentis and the fetal pupillary membrane. It then gives way to the appearance of a secondary vitreous, which is intimately related to the internal limiting membrane of the retina. Finally, at the zonula, the tertiary vitreous is formed (see Chap. 8). The complete or incomplete persistence of this hyaloid vascular system may be present in postnatal life.

One characteristic of this disease is persistent hyperplastic primary vitreous, present in full-term babies, mostly in an eye that is microphthalmic. Clinically it manifests itself as leukocoria. It may present:

1. In an isolated form;
2. In Patau–Bartholin syndrome (trisomy 13);
3. In Reese dysplasia;
4. In Norrie disease.

Isolated

This is the most common ocular malformation. The transparent secondary vitreous does not develop. The primary vitreous persists as well as remains of the posterior tunica vasculosa of the lens.

The tunica vasculosa lentis is a layer of vessels surrounding the crystalline lens. These blood vessels come from two sources: from in front – the major arterial circle of the iris coming from the anterior ciliary arteries – and from behind – the hyaloid artery. These two systems are reabsorbed before birth: the posterior in the 7th month and the anterior in the 8th month.

Howard [7] cites Heidenreich, who was the first to describe this entity. Reese [2] made the first systematic description of it and gave it its name. Manschot [8] recognized the correctness of this designation.

It is seen in healthy, full-term children. The pupil seems white in color. Careful examination shows the following elements: the ciliary processes are elongated by a mass that, as it retreats, draws them to the center of the posterior face of the crystalline lens. This mass is pinkish-white because of the presence of blood vessels. At this point, the lens is transparent. The anterior chamber is generally flat because the retrolental mass pushes the lens and the iris forward. Close observation shows that there is discrete microphthalmia. There were only two cases out of 59 where Reese did not find this. Small dilated blood vessels can sometimes be seen in the iris, passing the pupil and ending in the anterior face of the lens. The lens may be smaller than normal. At the start, as we said, it is transparent but quickly becomes opaque. This haziness always starts from the posterior pole as a posterior polar cataract. Sometimes the imbibition of the lens is violent and provokes acute glaucoma. The retraction of the retrolental fibrous tissue causes stretching of the ciliary processes. The retraction is more pronounced than that occurring from retrolental fibroplasia (Fig. 25.1).

The edge in the upper arch corresponds to the edge of the dilated pupil. The dark, opaque zone in the lower right corresponds to the haziness of the lens that started as an aqueous imbibition through its posterior face. Between two dark zones, the negative image of the very stretched ciliary processes can be seen, converging toward the center of the posterior face of the crystalline lens. Between them, the white zones correspond to the light coming from the greyish-white mass occupying the background.

It is usually accompanied by secondary glaucoma similar to the congenital glaucoma, but resulting from a very flat anterior chamber or a retrolental vitreous hemorrhage. Sometimes, depending on the child's age, it leads to a buphthalmia with or without corneal hazing. There are three phases to its development: active, regressive, and cicatricial. It may be complicated by a hemorrhage in the vitreous body and it sometimes ends in phthisis bulbi. Its histology has been well described by Friedenwald [9] and Reese [2]. It shows remnants of the hyaloid artery and of the tunica vasculosa lentis.

It should be remembered that it is a monocular disease (90% unilateral).

When the persistence of the primary vitreous does not present in an isolated form, the possibility should be considered that it is accompanying trisomy 13, Reese dysplasia, or Norrie disease.

Figure 25.2 shows the histological image of one of our cases. This microphotograph clearly shows that this is a case of secondary glaucoma, since the morphology of the ciliary body and especially of the ciliary muscle do not correspond to the morphology of congenital glaucoma.

Pathological Anatomy

The characteristic is retrolental fibrovascular membrane. It sometimes covers only the posterior pole of the lens and at others it extends as a discoid membrane covering the posterior chamber backward as from the ciliary processes. If it is partial, it tends to be located toward the nasal side. The tissue making up this membrane is quite heterogeneous: it may be cartilage, glia, fat, smooth muscle, calcium, neuroepithelium, or undifferentiated.

In addition, the ciliary processes seem to be dragged by this membrane toward the posterior face of the lens (Fig. 25.1). This appearance seems to be caused by greater growth of the eye than of the retrolental membrane. The ora serrata is also displaced forward and there are filaments extending from the retrolental mass toward the retina. There are occasionally retinal folds. The crystalline lens generally has alterations. It may show posterior capsule rupture and a continuation of the epithelium behind the equator.

The retrolental membrane may invade the lens and

this may become edematous and cause glaucoma from the flattening of the anterior chamber. The hyaloid artery is frequently seen penetrating the retrolental mass.

We recommend consulting the studies reported by Wátzhold [10], von Hippel [11], Sanders [12], Reese [2], Manschot [8], and Jensen [13].

The ideal treatment is an aspiration of the lens and an extraction or a discission of the fibrillar membrane. This treatment should be carried out before the imbibition of the crystalline lens provokes secondary glaucoma. One very common complication is hemorrhage.

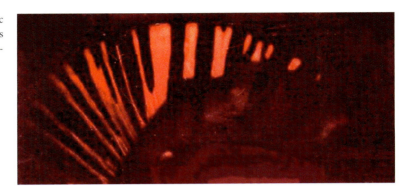

Fig. 25.1 Persistent isolated hyperplastic primary vitreous. The ciliary processes seem to be dragged by the membrane toward the posterior face of the lens

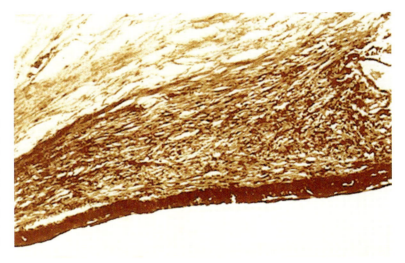

Fig. 25.2 Histological preparation in a case of persistent isolated primary vitreous. This shows that the glaucoma is secondary, as the morphology of the ciliary body, and especially of the ciliary muscle, do not correspond to that of congenital glaucoma. The inner face of the ciliary muscle forms a right angle with the anterior face; in congenital glaucoma, however, this angle is clearly acute

Clinical History No. 1
Leukocorias (Fetopathies: Persistent Hyperplastic Primary Vitreous)

This 10-month-old female was born full-term with normal weight.

	Right eye	Left eye
Corneal diameter	9 mm (Microcornea)	11 mm
IOP	25 mmHg	20 mmHg
	The leukocoria started from a greyish-white mass coming from the optic disc and also surrounding the temporal and inferior blood vessels, pulling on them. There are neoformed vessels. The start of aqueous imbibition of the lens can be seen in its posterior part	Similar picture but much less so. Remains of the tunica vasculosa lentis can be seen in the inferior temporal part. It is X-shaped. The ciliary processes are under traction. Diagnosis: persistent primary vitreous

Clinical History No. 2
Leukocorias (Fetopathies: Persistent Hyperplastic Primary Vitreous)

This is the case of a 1-year-old girl.

	Right eye	Left eye
Corneal diameter	11 mm	10 mm
IOP	18 mmHg	10 mmHg
	A whitish mass was found behind the crystalline lens with haze of the capsule at the same place and the beginnings of cataract. The ciliary processes are being pulled completely toward the center of the posterior face of the lens. Diagnosis: persistent hyperplastic primary vitreous and glaucoma	

Trisomy 13 or Patau–Bartholin Syndrome

This is one of the more common trisomies after trisomy 18 and 21. These are children who have an extra chromosome in the 13-15 pair. These eyes are found fundamentally with Reese dysplasia together with persistent primary vitreous. It was described as dyscrania-dysphalangia by Ullrich [14] and Meyer-Schwickerath et al. [15]. It can sometimes be accompanied by cryptophthalmia and anophthalmia. It occurs in males and females. The children die very soon.

Reese Dysplasia

This was first described by Krause [16] with the name of encephalophthalmic dysplasia.

Reese studied this topic between 1950 and 1958 [17, 18]. He believed it to be a binocular congenital malformation that occurs in newborns. It is characterized by microphthalmic or sometimes normal-sized eyes with a flat anterior chamber with posterior synechiae and persistent pupillary membrane.

There is a white retrolental membrane here, sometimes vascularized, elongated ciliary processes and sometimes with hemorrhages between them. The cornea as well as the crystalline lens may become hazy. There may also be glaucoma.

From the histopathological point of view, persistent hyperplastic primary vitreous and severe retinal malformations may be seen in these cases. The retina shows folds and is formed of primitive, disorganized cells, sometimes ordered in rosettes with several retinal layers in them. The folds are sometimes falciform and there may be a larger one extending from the optic disc to the lens.

This type of Reese dysplasia malformations are found in eyes with coloboma, microphthalmia, or in children who have received x-ray radiation. They are often associated with other malformations such as harelip, ogival palate, encephalocele, meningocele; lung, cardiac, urogenital, or skeletal malformations; and the presence of supernumerary digits. These children die within the first year of life.

Zimmerman [19] and Hunter and Zimmerman [20] consider that the name Reese dysplasia is not really correct, because a number of retinal dysplasias from different diseases are included under it.

Norrie Disease, or Progressive Oculoacoustic Cerebral Degeneration

Historical Background

Gordon Norrie [21] described a congenital disease with blindness that he named congenital ocular atrophy. In 1971, Fradkin [22] reported Norrie disease, or congenital progressive oculoacoustic cerebral degeneration. He defined it as a rare type of progressive, degenerative congenital disease of the eyes, ears, and brain.

Warburg [23, 24] published the first Danish pedigree and suggested the name of Norrie for this syndrome. Her paper presents the case of a white child. In the commentary, she mentions X-chromosome-linked syndromes with retinal malformations, deafness, and mental retardation. Among the components she cites are opaque cornea, obliterated angle, atrophic iris, uveal ectropion, and anterior and posterior synechiae. The disease also presents vitreous vascularization. Mental retardation is present in half the patients, and deafness in one-third, with some ending in the existing phthisis bulbi.

In 1973, Townes and Roca reported on an American family [24]. The authors stress that, as Norrie described, only males are affected (sex-linked). They describe a retrolental membrane, cataract, and glaucoma.

The pathogenesis of glaucoma in this syndrome may be directly related to the presence of the Barkan membrane. In 1998, Richter et al. [26] published an interesting paper describing an experimental model in which they point out the vascular alterations in this syndrome.

This is a form of blindness seen shortly after birth. Behind the transparent crystalline lens, a yellowish-white vascularized mass can be seen. The lens becomes hazy (cataract) after a few months and the cornea progressively loses its transparency. The eyes, which were normal in size, begin to shrink. This condition is reached before school age. Posterior synechiae and atrophies of the iris are also seen. The picture becomes stable at 10 years of age. The anterior chamber may be normal, disappear, or be very deep. In adulthood, the eyes are sunken, atrophic, and small, with band keratitis.

The extraocular symptoms are mental deficiency in one-third of cases (35%), another third have moderate mental retardation, and the rest are normal. Hearing problems of varying degree may arise in one-third of cases, appearing later, between 9 and 45 years of age.

Histology

Almost complete aplasia of the myelin sheaths and axons in the optic nerve are found. Briefly, the histology shows that the vision loss is attributable to a malformation of the retinal layers, the sensory cells, the optic nerves, and the tract to the geniculate body. In the eye itself, the alterations are seen in persistent primary vitreous; there are also intraocular hemorrhages and synechiae. The mental deficiencies can be attributed to malformations of the cerebral cortex.

Heredity

This is a sex-linked recessive inheritance with complete penetration.

Pathogenesis

The pathogenesis of Norrie disease is unknown. Eventually a common biochemical aberration may be demonstrated that provokes a malformation of the 21 and 31 neurons of the optic pathway, the sensory cells, the cerebral cortex, and the mesencephalus. There are also lesions of the VIII (auditory) pair.

Differential Diagnosis

Differential diagnosis depends on the time the patient is examined and the following diagnosis is made based on whether the lens is transparent, when there is cataract, when there is phthisis bulbi, retinoblastoma and pseudoglioma, hereditary congenital cataract, malformative cataract, secondary cataract, microphthalmia, old iridocyclitis, xerophthalmia, or keratomalacia.

We now describe the complete pathological anatomy of a case studied by Zárate et al. [27], which was the first publication to present a complete autopsy. The case presented is that of a male newborn with facial dysmorphias, general dysmorphias in the limbs, macrocephaly, primitive neuroectoderma tumor, pachymicrogyria and polymicrogyria (thickening and increase of the cerebral convolutions) with foci of cerebral calcification.

In the ocular globes, all the characteristics of this disease described in the various publications were seen: Barkan membrane, posterior embryotoxon, hyperplasia of the constrictor muscle of the iris, absence or hypoplasia of the iris dilator muscle, edema and corneal vascularization, cataract with tunica vasculosa lentis, retinal dysplasia with rosettes, displacement of retinal layers, reduction of the outer segments of rods and cones, and abnormal vascularization of the developing retina.

In summary, Norrie disease is a recessive disorder, linked to the X chromosome, characterized by congenital blindness, and associated with a loss of hearing and central nervous system alterations. One of the genes related with Norrie disease is Xp11.4 (Figs. 25.3, 25.4, 25.5, 25.6, 25.7, 25.8, 25.9).

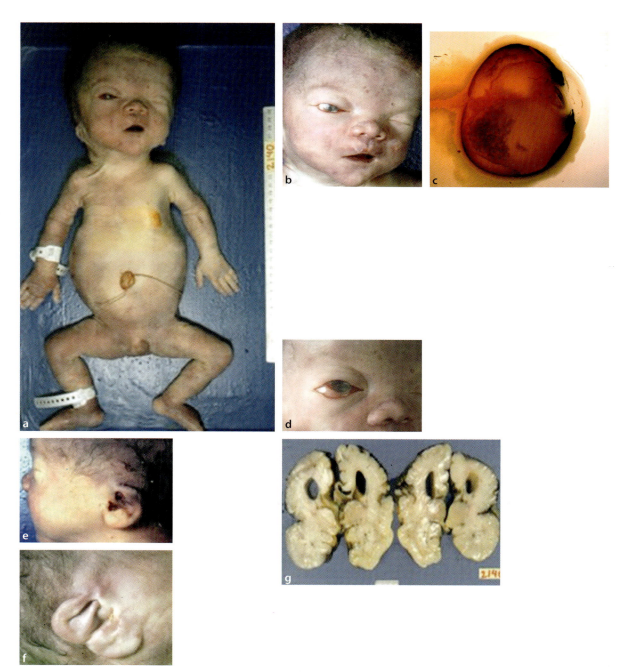

Fig. 25.3a–g Ocular manifestations of Norrie disease. Vascular anomalies in the posterior pole (**b, c**). Ocular anomalies (**d**). **e, f** Acoustic anomalies. **g** Cerebral anomalies

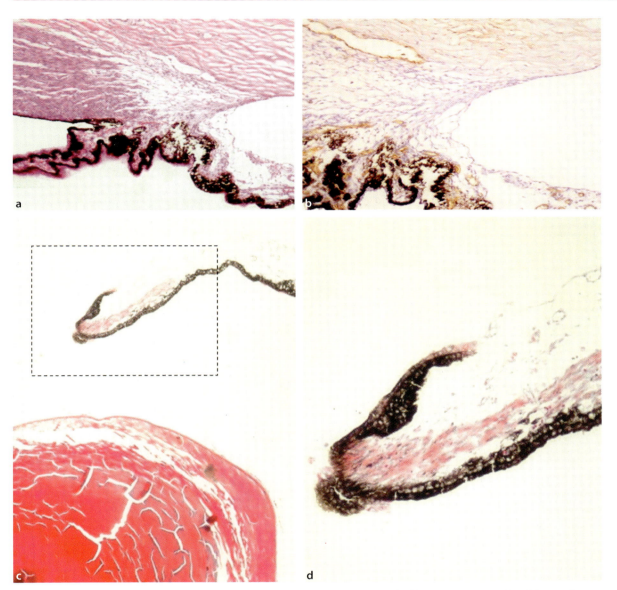

Fig. 25.4a–d Barkan's membrane in the angle of a newborn with Norrie disease (**a, b**). Constrictor muscle of the iris, hyperplastic (**c**). **d** Pigmentary uveal ectropion. Absent or hypoplastic dilator muscle

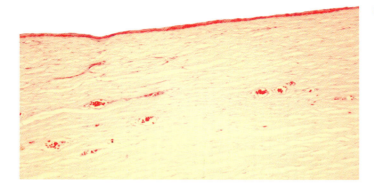

Fig. 25.5 Vascularized cornea

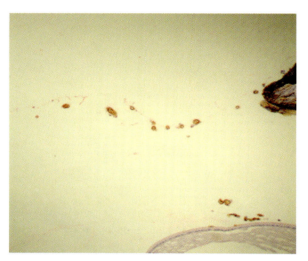

Fig. 25.6 Vascularized pupillary membrane with immunohistochemical staining for CD34 (vascular marker). The pupillary edge of the iris and the crystalline lens are also visible

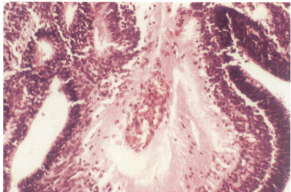

Fig. 25.7 Peripheral retina with dysplastic rosettes

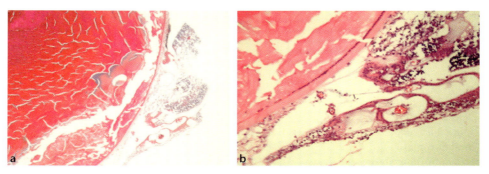

Fig. 25.8a,b Cataractous crystalline lens and dysplastic peripheral retina

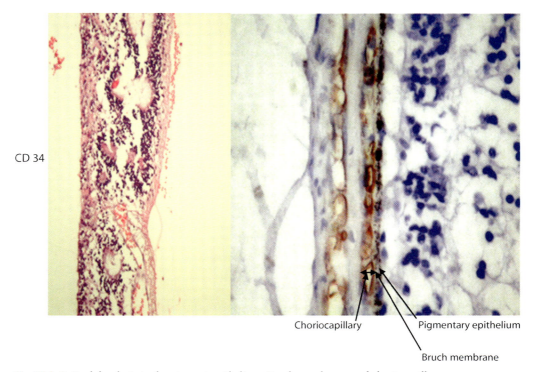

CD 34

Choriocapillary   Pigmentary epithelium

Bruch membrane

Fig. 25.9 Retinal dysplasia in the pigment epithelium, Bruck membrane, and choriocapillary

Secondary Pediatric Glaucomas

Retrolental Fibroplasia

In the United States in 1940, pediatricians began treating premature children with oxygen, because it was believed that their irregular breathing was due to anoxemia. In 1942, Terry [28] published the first paper on the relation between the premature child and retrolental fibroplasia. From then on, this disease was called retrolental fibroplasia and today it tends to be called retinopathy of prematurity. A total of 8,000 premature babies were recorded to be blind in the United States in 1953. This was the cause of blindness in 50% of the blind children under 7 years of age. The relationship between the use of oxygen at greater concentrations than in the air and retinopathy of prematurity was first established in 1958. It arises as a consequence of oxygen intoxication in premature children (800–1,000 g), placed in the incubator. It appears between 8 days and 8 months later. According to Owens [29], it has three phases: active, regressive, and cicatricial.

1. The active phase [30] is characterized by (a) arterial changes: narrow arteries, scarcity of blood vessels in the nasal hemiretina, lack of vascular ramifications, pale optic disc with pigment in the nasal area; (b) venous changes: tortuosity and dilation of the veins that can reach three or four times the normal size; (c) vascular neoformation at the retinal periphery; and (d) retinal alterations; with bluish edema, detached areas, hemorrhages, and fine white bands with vessels penetrating from the retina into the vitreous body.
2. The regressive phase in which the manifestations halt and regress.
3. The cicatricial phase, which is marked by areas of pigmented retina, retinal detachment on the temporal side, whitish retrolental mass, transparent crystalline lens, anterior and posterior synechiae, flat chamber, glaucoma, microphthalmos, and sometimes myopia.

The differential diagnosis of the disease must be made mainly with persistence of primary vitreous, metastatic endophthalmitis, and retinoblastoma.

It should be remembered that these three disorders are monocular, although retinoblastoma can be binocular. Consequently, the weight of the child at (premature) birth, whether or not it has been in an incubator, and bilaterality should all be considered.

It is important to know that only in severe cases does this disorder become pseudoglioma, that average cases show only vascular proliferation in and in front of the retina, and that the percentage of men and women is the same. In severe cases, when there is retrolental fibroplasia that leads to a membrane posterior to the crystalline lens, the lens is pushed forward so that the depth of the anterior chamber is greatly reduced. When the disorder produces a flat chamber, it is often complicated with angle-closure-type glaucoma. We have seen this complication, and according to Chandler and Grant [31], it appears between the 4th month of life and 22 years of age. When this occurs, the corneas are small. The glaucoma is always acute, with great pain, nausea, and vomiting, and it leads to iris stroma atrophy as seen in acute adult glaucoma. Although the chamber is flat, when the case has been developing for many years, the retraction of the retrolental membrane makes the anterior chamber form again, which can be very deep. Examination of the chamber angle reveals that it has no malformations and is normal. This is why the operation indicated in these cases is iridectomy.

In these cases, the decision for surgery requires knowing whether this angle is functionally narrow or anatomically narrow from previous synechiae. The pressure maneuver is performed with a contact lens (Fig. 25.10). If the narrow angle is functional, as seen in the figure, the angle will open. This can also be shown making the depression maneuver in the slit lamp OCT.

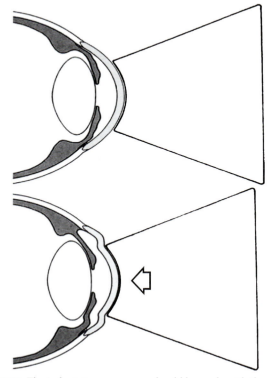

Fig. 25.10 The indentation maneuver should be made with the Sussman lens

Clinical History No. 3

This 10-month-old girl was placed in the incubator for 4 months because of premature birth. For the week preceding consultation, her parents had noted that she was troubled by light. This is why they consulted.

When examined under anesthesia with Penthrane, she presented:

1. Corneas, both eyes: 10.5 mm in diameter and bilateral athalamia; posterior synechia, slight corneal edema.
2. IOP: both eyes: 34 mmHg. The pupils did not dilate with mydriatics. Biomicroscopy showed an opaque greyish-white retrolental mass in both eyes.
3. Surgical intervention. Left eye: corneal incision half the circumference of the limbus. Transverse corneal folds appear: U suture. The incision was then widened to 180°: iridectomy in a broad area. The crystalline lens was transparent and through it a posterior whitish mass with three vascular loops. Total cryoextraction of the lens was done, which revealed a greyish-white mass with radiating fibers depressed in the center. Pulling this tissue with toothed tweezers, the ciliary processes were seen adhering to it. A piece of this tissue was extracted with toothed tweezers and scissors. It was closed with five silk sutures. Right eye: a linear extraction of the lens was done with sector iridectomy.

The child was examined under Penthrane anesthesia 6 days after surgery. In both eyes the cornea was clear, the anterior chamber well formed, the IOP with applanation was 9 mmHg in both eyes.

As the retrolental tissue was quite solid, a cavity remained behind the iris that filled with aqueous humor and reproduced the exact shape of the lens.

Clinical History No. 4

This 19-year-old man's maternal grandmother and paternal grandfather both had glaucoma. At birth, as he was premature, he was placed in an incubator with oxygen. After that, microcornea was found in the right eye. Later strabismus appeared and was operated. The ophthalmologist saw him at age 18 and found ocular hypertension in the right eye – 23 mmHg – and myopia. This eye had always helped him to read close up. When the ocular hypertension was confirmed, pilocarpine was administered, which kept the IOP at 18 mmHg. He then had two congestive attacks with pain and eccentric pupil. His IOP was 38 mmHg.

Currently he shows the following parameters:

	Right eye	Left eye
IOP	23 mmHg	10 mmHg
Visual acuity with correction	Sph. −10, good luminous projection: counts fingers	Sph. −1.50 and Cyl. +3 to 90°: 20/20
Radius of curvature	7.3° 46 D	7.5° 45 D
Corneal thickness	0.50 mm	0.54 mm
Depth of anterior chamber	1.9 mm	2.96 mm
Gonioscopy	Chamber angle in form of very narrow (narrow-flute)	Well open chamber angle, not pigmented, some vessel in the area of the root
Optic disc	With myopic alterations	Without alteration but with blurred edges
Visual field	Could not be done because of lack of fixation	Normal
Tonography C1.3-7	0.15	More than 0.45

Examining the fundus in the right eye with a Goldmann scleral depression lens, a ring-shaped white retrolental mass was seen extending from the ora serrata forward. This band was broken only between 1 and 3 o'clock. Each of the edges of this band was surrounded with areas of choroiditis with pigment dispersion. This change was seen both on the retinal and on the ciliary side. An opalescent filament came out of the 9 o'clock zone of this mass and continued as a translucent membrane, meeting immediately behind the lens. Diagnosis was partial retrolental fibroplasia occurring only in the microphthalmic eye. The differential diagnosis could be made only with a fetal pars planitis.

Clinical History No. 5

This male baby was born at 7 months gestation weighing 1.3 kg. He spent 1 month in the incubator with oxygen. The parents consulted when he was 15 months old, because he did not focus on objects. He was examined under anesthesia with Penthrane and presented bilateral leukocoria.

	Right eye	Left eye
Corneal diameter	9 mm; Absence of anterior chamber, posterior synechiae and white retrolental mass; blurred vitreous prevents him from seeing details	11 mm
IOP	4 mmHg	15 mmHg
Chamber angle	Closed; flat anterior chamber; leukocoria	Closed; flat anterior chamber; leukocoria

Provoking mild mydriasis, the left eye showed a greyish-white mass behind the crystalline lens. Actually, there were two masses moving toward the center of the eye, joined by a fibrous, vascular tissue with blood vessels passing in a corkscrew shape. The rest of the retina was detached with pigmented areas. The presence of neoformed blood vessels was seen in these two retrolental masses. The ciliary processes in the temporal zone were seen stretched and pulled toward the center of this greyish-white retrolental mass. There were the beginnings of aqueous imbibition of the posterior capsule of the lens and hazing.

Behind the ciliary processes dragged toward the posterior face of the lens in the area corresponding to the pars plana, there was a greyish-white cork making a prolapse (Fig. 25.11). The remains of the pupillary membrane can also be seen.

Clinical History No. 6

This 8-month old girl was born in the 7th month of gestation weighing 1 kg and spent 3 months in an incubator because of breathing problems. Sucking and pharyngeal reflexes were absent. She also had a respiratory difficulty syndrome, with bronchoalveolitis. She was brought for consultation at 8 months of age.

- Corneal diameter. Right eye: 9.5 mm; left eye: 9.5 mm.
- IOP: under anesthesia with Penthrane, 10 mmHg in both eyes.
- Funduscopy: a reduction was found in the nasal blood vessels and the presence of temporal blood vessels. In the temporal area, behind the ciliary processes, there is a band of grey tissue extending from the tail to the head of the ciliary processes and making contact at several points with the posterior face of the lens. In various areas, this caused a median traction of the ciliary processes.
- Chamber angle: all the elements were normal in both eyes; the ciliary body band is clearly seen, with obvious edema.
- Diagnosis: retrolental fibroplasia without glaucoma.

The age and the lack of knowledge of the history may lead to a false diagnosis of primary congenital glaucoma.

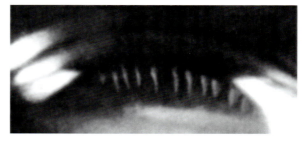

Fig. 25.11 Retrolental fibroplasias: ciliary processes dragged toward the posterior face of the lens

Pathological Anatomy in Retinopathy of Prematurity (Retrolental Fibroplasias)

The morphological changes seen in the retina as a consequence of the harmful effects of oxygen have two clearly characteristic phases: intraretinal and extraretinal. In the first phase, proliferative phenomena are seen in the nerve fiber layer of the retina, consisting of two types of cells: fusiform cells of probable fibroglial origin, also known as vanguard cells, and behind these, angioblastic or rearguard cells. Between these two groups there is a characteristic acellular space of great metabolic importance in the development of the definitive retinal vascular system.

In normal conditions this sequential development occurs through preformed channels and does not exceed 10% of the retinal thickness. In retinopathy of prematurity (ROP), this type of cell growth is hypertrophic. At first, the cells remain within the thickness of the fiber layer. At a later stage, as their numbers increase, they deform and raise the plane of the inner limiting membrane of the retina, clinically and microscopically forming the image of the so-called cord. If the injury continues, the vascular structures go beyond the limiting membrane, moving into the second extraretinal phase, in which the blood vessels are found in the vitreous.

As a consequence of this phenomenon, a traction mechanism is produced that later leads to detachment of the retina.

Figure 25.12a shows a perpendicular section of the retina, the first intraretinal phase with the fusiform or vanguard cells, the empty acellular space and the angioblastic cells within the normal thickness of the retina. Clinically, this gives the image of a line. Figure 25.12b, corresponding to a tangential section of the retina, shows the same phenomenon, only in the angioblastic type area.

Figure 25.13a shows the macroscopic image of the cord, i.e., the hump or elevation produced by the intense intraretinal proliferation both of fusiform and of angioblastic cells. This alteration can be clearly recognized in Fig. 25.13b, corresponding to the histopathology of this case.

Figure 25.14 represents the histopathology of the growth or extraretinal phase of the ROP, characterized by a vascular-type arborescent growth outside the retina, over the internal limiting membrane and within the vitreous.

These images correspond to the pathological phenomena most characteristic of this disease in its initial stages. Once the posterior detachment has occurred, retrolental fibroplasia sets in with the clinical image of leukocoria. The broken vertical line in Fig. 25.12a is a perpendicular tangential section from Fig. 25.12b.

Coats Disease

At the beginning of the last century, Coats described patients with leukocoria, strabismus, and poor vision [32]. He described this disease as a hemorrhagic and exudative external retinal disease, usually unilateral, in the juvenile population, and particularly in children between 2 and 16 years of age. Certainly more than 60% of all cases appear before the end of the first decade of life.

Because of the retinal vascular abnormalities, massive exudative detachments are present. Neovascular glaucoma may be a complication. The picture is one of retinal elevation due to massive amounts of yellow subretinal exudate. At the early stage, there are telangiectasias with intraretinal exudation, tortuous vasculature, with aneurysmal dilations and sheathings. Hemorrhages are often seen. At a later period, there is massive subretinal exudation with PAS-positive fluid in the outer retinal layers, lipid-laden macrophages and acicular cholesterol crystals (see Fig. 46.22a,b in [33]).

Enucleation in this disease is very infrequent in recent years because echographic and other new noninvasive methods make it possible to correct differential diagnoses with retinoblastoma and other leukocorias, such as hyperplastic primary vitreous, toxocariasis, ROP, toxoplasmosis, etc.

Gomez Morales [34] presented 22 cases, 14 (64%) with retinal detachment and seven (32%) with secondary glaucoma.

In the book *Ultrasonography in Ophthalmology 12* [35], Sampaolesi presented a variety of these lesions associated with secondary glaucoma and the importance of echograph tracings in its diagnosis.

Tumors

Intraocular tumors in children can give rise to a secondary glaucoma. The mechanism of this glaucoma is generally angle closure and it may pass unnoticed because of the severity of the case.

We attended a 5-month-old child who had had an intraocular tumor diagnosed. The retina almost touched the crystalline lens. The entire extent of the chamber angle was blocked, the anterior chamber was very flat, and the ocular pressure was 45 mmHg.

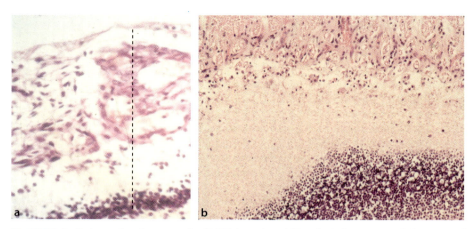

Fig. 25.12a,b Retinopathy of prematurity (ROP) (retrolental fibroplasias): intraretinal phase. **a** Hight power view. *Left* to *right* we can see fusocellular vanguard cells, acellular space and angioblastic retagular cells. **b** Panoramic view. Transversal section with angioblastic intraretinal proliferation

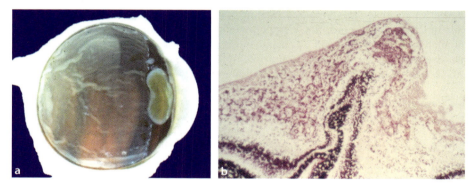

Fig. 25.13a,b Retinopathy of prematurity (ROP) (retrolental fibroplasias): intraretinal phase. **a** Gross appearence intraocular cordon lesion. This anterior formation is the macroscopic expression of **b**. **b** Cordon. Intraretinal elevated alteration.From *left* to *right*, fusocellular hiperplastic cells, acellular spaces and posterior angioblastic cells

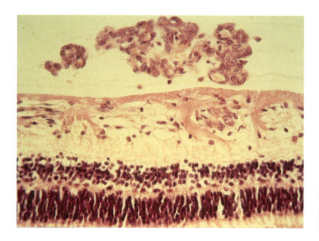

Fig. 25.14 Retinopathy of prematurity (ROP) (retrolental fibroplasias): extraretinal phase. Intermediate power view. Shows the important vascularization extraretinal into vitreous

Injuries

Contusion without perforation of the eyeball is very common in children. This generally causes a traumatic hyphema and in turn secondary hypertension. The hypertension may reach 70 or 80 mmHg. These cases require immediate surgery with a washing of the anterior chamber. The surgical maneuver is simple: while the assistant fixes the eye, for example the right eye at 11 and 3 o'clock, the surgeon simultaneously pierces the anterior chamber, 1 mm from the limbus, with two narrow Vessely-type probes, directly in the cornea at 8 and 2 o'clock. Generally the hyphema empties. If this does not occur, with a narrow Daviel curette half opening the corneal wound at 8 o'clock, the anterior chamber is irrigated with balanced saline solution through the other opening at 2 o'clock. Today we do the washing of the hyphema with a two-way cannula, and we use viscoelastic substances.

If the pressure is lower, 30 or 40 mmHg, we wait 1 or 2 days; most often the hyphema reabsorbs completely and the ocular hypertension disappears. The deadline for waiting before intervention, if the hyphema is not reabsorbed, is 8–10 days, but with careful monitoring with the slit-lamp and tonometer to avoid the hematic infiltration of the cornea. It should be remembered that for hematic infiltration to occur, ocular hypertension is needed as well as the hyphema.

If the injury has caused a small iridodialysis, it will again be a matter of waiting, just as in the previous case.

If the iridodialysis is large, an iridopexy should be done.

Often, after a physical injury, a child presents loss of vision from hemorrhage of the vitreous body. Examining the chamber angle shows no traumatic lesion (traumatic recession of the iris) nor hyphema. This is accompanied by ocular hypertension of 30–40 mmHg. If the hypertension does not recede, the therapy is vitrectomy, which not only restores all the function and the visual acuity but also definitively normalizes the intraocular pressure. As we were able to see in one of these cases, so-called ghost cells are found in the trabecular meshwork.

Clinical History No. 7

This 3-year-old girl came to the consultation 18 h after a contusion with a total hyphema in the left eye. The IOP, measured with general anesthesia and applanation, was 70 mmHg in the left eye and 12 mmHg in the right eye. We waited 12 h and, as neither the IOP nor the hyphema receded, a simultaneous double paracen-

tesis was performed. The chamber was left clean and reformed with balanced saline solution. After 6 days of good progress, the IOP was measured again with applanation, and 10 mmHg was found in the right eye and 9 mmHg in the left eye. Five months later, a check-up was made with general anesthesia. The IOP was 12 mmHg in both eyes, the corneal thickness was 0.65 mm in the right eye and 4 mm in the eye that had suffered the trauma. The gonioscopy showed a traumatic recession of the angle in the lower half of the circumference. In a check up 2 years later; the IOP remained normal.

Glaucomas Secondary to Congenital Cataract Surgery

It should be remembered that in every congenital cataract it is preferable to operate when the child is more than 6 months of age or even older. Before this, the chamber angle is in the middle of its development and is unable to reabsorb the crystalline masses. Moreover, before 6 months, the pupil does not dilate well.

After extracting the cataract, glaucoma generally occurs because of pupillary block, because the pupil sticks to the masses or to the posterior capsule. This can often be prevented with the frequent instilling of atropine over a long period. Some authors, in order to avoid this secondary glaucoma, advise sector iridectomy at 12 o'clock and small iridectomy at 6 o'clock.

When this glaucoma is not noticed and the ophthalmologist discovers it some years later, with serious damage to the optic nerve and the visual field, it is no longer a case of glaucoma from pupillary block, but rather chamber-angle-closure glaucoma, since the "tomato iris" caused by the pupillary block finally causes peripheral synechiae in the chamber angle. In this case, sector iridectomy may be used, cyclodialysis, and even filtering operations, but today a trabeculectomy is preferable.

There are cases in which a previously undiagnosed malformation of the chamber angle is combined with the cataract. Here there is always time for a new diagnosis; the surgical indications would be a goniotomy or a trabeculotomy.

Clinical History No. 8

This child, presenting at the age of 15 years, had been operated for bilateral congenital cataract at 10 months of age. The diagnosis was glaucoma secondary to congenital cataract surgery. At the time of the examination he presented:

	Right eye	Left eye
Visual acuity with correction	Finger counting with sph. + 10	0.1 With sph. + 9
IOP	24 mmHg	36 mmHg
Medication: acetazolamide 1 g daily		
Visual field	III	II
Corneal diameter	8.5 mm, Microphthalmia, nystagmus	8.5 mm, Microphthalmia, nystagmus
Chamber angle	Blockage from previous synechiae	Blockage from previous synechiae

A bilateral trabeculectomy was done with trabeculotomy in just one sector. At 3 months, visual acuity was maintained and ocular pressure was 16 mmHg in the right eye and 15 mmHg in the left eye.

Other Syndromes Associated with Glaucoma

Rubinstein–Taybi Syndrome

Rubinstein–Taybi syndrome [36] is characterized by mental deficiency, facial anomalies, and anomalies in the first digits of the hands and feet. Ophthalmologically, an antimongoloid palpebral fissure is seen, congenital cataract, optic atrophy, deep anterior chamber, and megalocornea. Manzitti et al. [37] studied three cases and found the presence of glaucoma in two of them. The appearance of the chamber angle in these patients was typical of congenital glaucoma.

Pierre Robin Syndrome

Pierre Robin syndrome [38] is characterized by the child's special birdlike facial appearance. Glossoptosis, micrognathia, microgenia, split palate, dental anomalies, anomalies of the fingers and toes, and cardiac anomalies complete the picture. Van der Helm [39] described three cases, two of which had glaucoma. Its heredity is dominant autosomal.

Summary

Nonhereditary Congenital Glaucomas

The embryopathies (rubella) and the fetopathies (persistence of hyperplastic primary vitreous; isolated, in the Patau syndrome, in Reese dysplasia, in Norrie disease) are accompanied by glaucoma, whose mechanism is generally secondary.

Secondary Pediatric Glaucomas

The following cause secondary pediatric glaucoma: retrolental fibroplasia (with flat chamber or athalamia with blockage of the angle), injuries, from the hyphema they cause, and some operated congenital cataracts, especially if they have been before the 6th month.

References

1. Beer GJ (1817) Lehre von den Augenkrankheiten. Wien 2:495

2. Reese AB (1955) Persistent hyperplastic primary vitreous. Am J Ophthal 40:317–331

3. Dolfus MA, Auvert A (1953) Le gliome de la rétine et les pseudo-gliomes. Bull Soc Fran Ophtalmol 42–87

4. Badtke G (1961) Die Missbildungen des menschlichen Auges. In: Der Augenarzt, Vol. IV. Georg Thieme, Leipzig, pp 428–431

5. Hamburg A (1963) Pseudoglioma. Ophthalmologica 146:355

6. Babel J (1964) Les malformations pseudotumorales du globe oculaire. Congr Eur Soc Ophthal Wien 2:79–90

7. Howard R (1856) Cited in: Heidenreich A (1959) Zur Pathogenese des Pseudoglioma. Klin Mbl Augenheilk 134:465

8. Manschot WA (1958) Persistent hyperplastic primary vitreous. Arch Ophthal 59:188–203

9. Friedenwald JS, Wilder HE et al (1952) Ophthalmic pathology: An atlas and textbook. Philadelphia, WB Saunders

10. Wätzhold, P.: Beitrag zur Pathologie der angeborenen Linsentrübungen. Min. Mbl. Augenheilk., 72:76-86 (1924).

11. von Hippel E (1931) Arteria hyaloidea persistens, Vol. 11. In: Henke F, Lubarsch O (eds) Springer, Berlin Heidelberg New York, pp 66–71

12. Sanders TE (1952) Pseudoglioma. Am J Ophthalmol 35:364–369

13. Jensen OA (1968) Persistent hyperplastic primary vitreous. Cases in Denmark 1942–1966. A mainly histopathological study. Acta Ophthal Kbh 46:418–429

14. Ullrich O (1951) Der Status Bonnevie-Ullrich im Rahmen anderes Dyscranio-Dysphalargien. Ergebn. Med Kinderheilk 2:457

15. Meyer-Schwickerath G, Grueterich E, Weyers H (1957) Mikrophthalmus-syndrome. Klin Mbl Augenheilk 131:18–88

16. Krause AC (1946) Congenital encephalo-ophthalmic dysplasia. Arch Ophthal 36:387–444

17. Reese AB, Blodi FC (1950) Retinal dysplasia. Ame J Ophthal 33:23–32

18. Reese AB, Straatsma BR (1958) Retinal dysplasia. Am J Ophthal 45:199–211

19. Zimmerman LE (1964) The contribution of pathology to clinical ophthalmology. Am J Ophthal 58:626–636

20. Hunter WS, Zimmerman LE (1965) Unilateral retinal dysplasia. Arch Ophthal 74:23–30

21. Norrie G (1927) Causes of blindness in children: twenty five years' experience of Danish Institutes for the Blind. Acta Ophthl Kbh5:357–386

22. Fradkin AH (1971) Norrie s Disease. Congenital progressive oculo-acoustico-cerebral degeneration. Am J Ophthalmol 72:947–948

23. Warburg M (1961) Norrie's disease. A new hereditary bilateral pseudotumour of the retina. Acta Ophthal Kbh 39:757–772

24. Warburg M (1966) Norrie s disease: a congenital progressive oculo-acoustico-cerebral degeneration. Acta Ophth Kbh 89 [Suppl]:1–47

25. Townes PL, Roca DP (1973) Norrie's disease. Hereditary oculo-acoustic-cerebral degeneration. Am J Ophthalmol 76:797–803

26. Richter M, Richter M, Gottanka J, May CA, Welge-Lüssen U, Berger W, Lütjen-Drecoll E (1998) Retinal vasculature changes in Norrie disease mice. Invest Ophthalmol Vis Sci 39:2450–2457

27. Zárate JO, Benavides S, Fuksman R. (1992) Retinopatía del prematuro. Cuadros típicos y atípicos. Patología (Mex) 36:309–315

28. Terry TL (1942) Fibroplastic overgrowth of persistent tunica vasculosa lentis in infants born prematurely. II. Studies in development and regression of hyaloid artery and tunica vasculosa lentis. Am J Ophthal 25:1409–1423

29. Owens WC (1953) Spontaneous regression in retrolental fibroplasia. Tr Am Ophth Soc 51:555–579

30. Bedrossian RH, Carmichael P, Ritter J (1954) Retinopathy of prematurity (retrolental fibroplasia) and oxygen. 1. Clinical study. II. Further observations in the disease. Ame J Ophthal 37:78–86

31. Chandler P, Grant WM (1965) Lectures on glaucoma. Lea and Febiger, Philadelphia

32. Coats G (1908) Forms of retinal disease with massive exudation. R Lond Ophthalmol Hosp Rev 17:440–525

33. Sampaolesi R (1991) Glaucoma, 2nd edn. Panamericana, Buenos Aires, p 537

34. Gomez Morales A (1965) Coats' disease. Natural history and results of treatment. Am J Ophthalmol 60:855–865

35. Sampaolesi R (ed) (1990) Ultrasonography in Ophthalmology, Documenta Ophthalmologica Proceedings Series 53, Kluwer, Dordrecht

36. Rubinstein JH, Taybi H (1963) Broad thumbs and toes and facial abnormalities. Am Dis Child 105:588–608

37. Manzitti E, Lavin JR, Prieto Díaz J (1969) Signos oftalmológicos del síndrome de Rubinstein-Taybi. Arch Oftal B Aires 44:228–230

38. Robin P (1929) La glossoptose, un grave danger pour nos enfants. Paris

39. Van der Helm GM (1963) Hydrophthalmia and its treatment. Bibl Ophthal 61:1–64

Anatomopathologic Evaluation in Pure Congenital Glaucoma

Contents

Pathological Anatomy of Pediatric Glaucomas

Pathology, associated with clinically correlated teamwork, has provided a large share of the pathogenic knowledge of pediatric glaucomas.

At first, ocular globes from autopsies or enucleation were studied. One of the problems arising from these observations was that in general, as the eyes had been affected by the disease for a prolonged time, the consequences of the glaucoma were seen more than the etiopathogenesis itself. Of course, this did not prevent great progress being made in the study of different dysgeneses or anterior segment anomalies involved in pediatric glaucomas, and even the particular modifications that the optic nerve showed in its papilla.

Beginning in the 1960s, different filtering operations in which a small surgical specimen was obtained, such as trabeculectomy, when done by experienced hands, enabled the early stages of lesions to be seen in surgical samples, allowing study of the aqueous humor drainage system.

In Argentina, I was the first to conduct these studies and send them for histopathological study. At the same time, French researchers also began to undertake these studies.

There are two fundamental points for proper evaluation: first, one should know exactly what is removed so as to know if any technical modification was needed to improve the results; second, the microscopic alterations in the early stages of the disease should be clarified.

From 1972 to today, we have studied more than 1,800 trabeculectomy specimens, and we can briefly note some general results. We have examined and classified the surgically extracted specimens in ideal, anterior, and posterior surgical limits.

They are called ideal surgical limits when the specimen consists of:

1. The corneoscleral flan;
2. A small fragment (200–300 µm) of the Descemet membrane;
3. The Schwalbe line;
4. The scleral spur;
5. A mall fragment of ciliary muscle (between 200 and 500 µm).

   It should be noted that we detect the corneal flap as it is covered by Descemet, and that inside the sclera we find collectors and veins in different proportions.
6. The corneoscleral and uveal trabecular meshwork;
7. The Schlemm canal.

When the trabeculectomy specimen has anterior surgical limits, we see abundant Descemet membrane (the surgeon previously cut more because it was a case of narrow-angle glaucoma), in general because of angle closure or some other technical difficulty related to the pathology in question. In these cases, it is common to find the trabecular meshwork and the Schlemm canal cut in their posterior part, and we have no spur or ciliary muscle.

When the sample has posterior surgical limits, the corneal structures cannot be recognized, and the vertex of the trabecular meshwork and the Schwalbe line are absent (the scleral flap, part of the trabecular meshwork and sometimes of the Schlemm, the spur and generally the ciliary muscle, which can be abundant, are visible). These three variants of trabeculectomy indicate indirectly the pathology to be found in the angle.

Over the years, we have had the opportunity to study specimens with generally ideal surgical limits and, if this is not the case, to discover the reason for the surgical difficulty.

We should keep in mind that this classification is important for the pathologist and for an accurate clinical and pathological correlation, and not for the filtering results, which in general are similar (Fig. 26.1).

Before analyzing the general and particular criteria of each structure mentioned and to complete the list of surgical material that enables the pathological study of the anterior segment in glaucoma, we must mention irido-cyclo-trabeculectomy, an operation described by Jorge Malbran, with more than 40 cases studied in the same period as the 1,800 trabeculectomies. Iridotrabeculectomy is actually a goniectomy, as the posterior cut of the specimen passes through the anterior ciliary furrow, and so the iris root is included within the specimen. This surgery, as we shall see later, is preferably indicated in neovascular glaucomas.

Recently, the so-called nonpenetrating deep sclerectomy has been added to the study of these tissues, where the two important structures to identify are (1) the second scleral flap, which, when well performed, should include the endothelial surface of the outer wall of the Schlemm canal, which we can easily identify with hematoxylin and eosin, and (2) in difficult cases CD34 or factor VIII, which are the endothelial markers studied by immunohistochemistry.

After this general panorama of the surgical and pathological technique, a detailed description of the technical methodology and the findings will be provided.

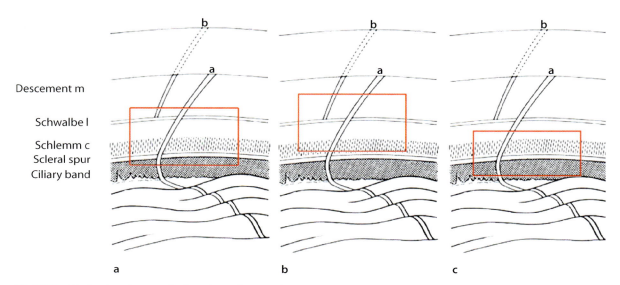

Fig. 26.1 a Ideal trabeculectomy. **b.** Anterior and **c** posterior

Requirements for Sending Glaucoma Pathology Samples

1. Biopsies. The samples obtained from biopsies (trabeculectomies, nonperforating deep sclerectomy, and irido-cyclo-trabeculectomies) must be fixed in 10% formaldehyde (except in cases where transmission electron microscopy is decided on from the start. In these cases, the fixative is glutaraldehyde, with its modifications). The quantity and quality of the fixative should be checked periodically. These specimens should be placed in small, transparent flasks so that they are permanently visible. The specimens are measured along their three axes: anteroposterior and transversal. The thickness is very difficult to measure and is done in the histological preparation. The specimens are photographed with a surface optical microscope, following a technique we have described, which will be explained below.
2. Surgical specimens. Enucleation or autopsy eye. just as in the biopsies, these are fixed in 10% formaldehyde, paying close attention to the volume of the container (glass or plastic bags). These should let the fixative liquid be approximately 20 times the volume of the specimen.
3. Anterior chamber cytologies. The best technique, which we always use in our laboratory, is to place any cytological material in preserving liquid, and then use the robot cytocentrifuge to perform the monolayer extended liquid technique, which enables the greatest cell concentration possible. To identify the materials, we recommend writing on the labels in pencil, since this prevents any liquid leakage. All material sent should be accompanied by the corresponding request for an examination with as much data as possible of all kinds, and photocopies or imaging studies made previously. These data are extremely important in making the best and most detailed histopathology report possible.

Macroscopic Study of the Specimens

As mentioned above, in all cases the macroscopic study of the specimens was made with surface optic microscopy, in a technique that we presented in 1990 in the 18th Congress of the International Academy of Pathology. This is based on two fundamental principles performed in the material inclusion process:

1. Transparency of the specimen when it is passed through Xylol;
2. Application of the Scheimpflug principle, which enables good-resolution documentation to be obtained of the different planes with great depth of focus.

Methodology of Trabeculectomy Structure Study

In all cases, a drawing of the specimen is made, which, together with the surface optical microscopy photo, enables the inclusion to be performed in the most suitable way, i.e., with the transversal axis of the specimen perpendicular to the histological cross-section, ensuring the classic anatomy of the chamber angle. Between 20 and 100 semiserial sections are made, depending on the size and interest of the material.

At least eight semiserial sections are placed in a holder, which sometimes makes it possible to detect the sequence, for example of a pigmentary thrombotic process.

Special techniques are used with the remaining sections:

- Masson's trichrome. This is useful because it marks out the fibroconnective tissues in blue and the muscle in red, which, in the case of an anterior surgical limit trabeculectomy, can be so scant that the hematoxylin-eosin does not show it.
- Gomori's reticulum. This technique is very useful to show the reticular fibers and procollagenase, present in the pretrabecular area of congenital glaucomas.
- PAS (periodic acid-Schiff). PAS stains the neutral mucopolysaccharides. This marker is useful to show the basal membranes.
- Alcian blue. This technique stains the acid mucopolysaccharides. Associated with trichrome and PAS, it defines certain characteristics in congenital glaucoma.

In the past 10 years, we have been using immunohistochemical techniques for cases requiring it, to make the structural alterations more evident. An example is the use of CD34 to mark small vessels that can pass unnoticed with hematoxylin and eosin and the use of desmin for muscular fibers, etc.

In some cases, we have performed transmission electron microscopy in material already included in paraffin. Even though the documentation is not the best, it can be useful in certain types of diagnoses.

Study of the Irido-cyclo-trabeculectomy

As with the trabeculectomies, surface optical microscopy photographs, a small prior sketch following the paraffin inclusion process are the basis for histological preparations with the smallest number of artifacts possible. In these specimens, great attention should be paid to the chamber angle and, as already specified, to detecting the vascular or fibrous membranes that may be found in this area with the use of conventional or special techniques. The data that can be provided by the iris root naturally adhering to the dried surgical specimen are very interesting. For the pathologist, this is, in this sense, the most significant specimen for panoramic and minute observation of all the structures related to the aqueous humor drainage system.

Study of Nonperforating Deep Sclerectomy

As regards the study of nonperforating deep sclerectomy (NPDS), we will go further into this in the study of nonpediatric glaucoma, but we will give a few useful rules related to what the pathologist is looking for in these specimens.

The biopsies are fixed in 10% formaldehyde. Then the biopsies are dehydrated in three consecutive 2-h steps, each in 96% alcohol and one 1-h step in 100% alcohol. They are then passed through xylol for 2–3 h. The material at this stage is placed in a holder under a magnifying glass to identify the corresponding zones, marking the endothelial structures, for their subsequent orientation in paraffin. The photographs are taken using the method described. The specimen is cut by freezing to confirm the position of the endothelium and is included. The third sample sent, consisting of the internal wall of the Schlemm canal and the outer half of the corneoscleral trabecular meshwork is very difficult to handle technically, because of its friability and size. We will devote a deeper study to this in nonpediatric glaucomas (Volume II: Primary Glaucomas, in preparation).

The following histological sections correspond to congenital, especially refractory, glaucomas, which were stained with the techniques described above.

Microscopy of Trabeculectomy Specimens

Surface Light and Electron Microscopy and Scanning Microscopy

When either goniotomy or trabeculectomy are the techniques used, no material can be obtained for pathological examination. Specimens for this purpose can only be obtained in trabeculectomies. It should be kept in mind that we use combined procedures (trabeculotomy + trabeculectomy) or only trabeculectomy in cases in which the axial length has already grown considerably, over 24 mm within the first 6 months of life, generally with corneas 13 mm or larger and endothelium and Descemet membrane tears. This means that anatomopathological evaluations can only be made in advanced cases.

Anatomopathologic results were presented for the first time in 1977 [1] and 1979 [2]. Numerous schools have also analyzed trabeculectomy specimens subsequently.

Material Collection

To obtain adequate specimens for analysis, we believe the surgical technique used should be very thorough and careful. During surgery, it is vital to use Minsky's transillumination for proper placement of the incision, opening the anterior chamber exactly at the corneal endothelium immediately beyond the Schwalbe line.

Using the Minsky technique, the cornea in the illuminated area can be 1 mm away from the light-darkness limit.

After careful dissection of a limbal-based scleral flap with a thickness half that of the corneoscleral thickness, two lateral incisions are marked perpendicular to the limbus. After opening the anterior chamber (third incision), these perpendicular incisions are completed with angled Vannas scissors. The trabeculectomy specimen is secured with a fine-toothed clamp for microsurgery, at half the thickness facing the external surface, in order to avoid damage to the fine trabecular structure. This is an open procedure and the surgeon can see the external wall of the chamber angle up to the spur. The final incision is made with the same Vannas scissors between the scleral spur and the ciliary body band. From the corneal incision to the last incision, the assistant should carefully and gently put saline drops on the specimen.

The specimen for light microscopy is kept in a bottle with 10% formol solution. After fixing it, it is embedded in paraffin and stained according to the following techniques: (1) hematoxylin-eosin, (2) Masson, (3) PAS, and (4) Gomori's and Del Rio Ortega's technique for reticulin determination. In each specimen, from 120 to 300 sections are made depending on size. The first 30 sections are stained with hematoxylin-eosin to determine whether the orientation of the sample is correct. Should this be the case, they are stained on three slides of 30 sections each with special techniques. If these stainings are incorrect, the rest are stained with hematoxylin. We have recently adopted fixation in 96°–100° alcohol, with the consequent addition of immunomarking techniques to the previous staining methods.

The specimen for electron microscopy is fixed immediately in the operating room, as explained above, by immersing it into 25% glutaraldehyde solution and a buffer solution (Millong's phosphate 0.1 M, with glucose, pH 7.4, for 24 h). Then it is washed with buffer isotonic solution for 15 min and fixed again in a solution of osmium peroxide 1% in a Millong's phosphate buffer with glucose, pH 7.4, for 2 h. After this, the specimen is dehydrated in acetone solutions of different degrees and dried according to the critical point method in CO_2, with the Sorvall system. Using this method, acetone is replaced by carbon dioxide in a high-pressure chamber. Once dried, the trabeculectomy specimen is placed on a device supporting it with the trabecular surface upward and it is covered with a fine coat of carbon and gold palladium, using a Geol vacuum unit. These specimens were examined with a scanning electron microscope, model T.S.M.-U.

Material Examined

The material examined is described in Table 26.1, where, in addition to age, gender, and intraocular pressure, echometric and corneal diameter values are reported, as well as whether there are endothelium or Descemet membrane tears reflecting the degree of disease progression.

In addition, four specimens obtained from young 15-year-old patients and one from a 32-year-old patient with late congenital glaucoma, have been studied.

Table 26.1 lists the most important clinical data of the first specimens studied. The clinical–pathologic correlation is the only way to advance the knowledge of the disease.

Table 26.2 lists the anatomopathologic findings in the first 13 cases. Furthermore, another 53 specimens were studied, but they were not included in the table for the sake of brevity.

Table 26.1 Anatomopathological findings

Case	Age	Sex	IOP RE	IOP LE	Corneal diameter RE	Corneal diameter LE	Descemet membrane tears RE	Descemet membrane tears LE	Right eye Total	Right eye v	Left eye Total	Left eye v
1	4 months	M	30	35	13	12.2	+	+	22.61	14.55	22.85	14.55
2	4 months	F	10	33	12	14	–	+	22.31	14.32	22.53	15.32
3	6 months	M	20	18	14.5	14.5	+	+	23.83	15.09	23.59	15.32
4	6 months	M	30	30	14	13.5	+	+	24.14	15.47	23.76	14.94
5	2 years	F	36	18	13.5	12	+	–	24.04	16.09	21.50	13.32
6	3 years	M	29	26	13.5	13.5	+	+	23.52	15.17	23.37	15.32
7	3 years	M	34	10	14	12	+	N	28.09	19.15	21.78	14.02
8	10 years	M	34	31	14	14.5	–	–	28.54	19.92	28.36	19.53
9	12 years	M	25	24	14	14	–	–	24.81	16.24	24.01	16.24
10	7 years	M	34	13			–	–	23.23		23.08	
11	14 years	M	32	52	12	12						
12	33 years	M	38	32	12	12	–	–				
13	32 years	F	26	16	12	12	–	–				

IOP intraocular pressure, *RE* right eye, *LE* left eye

Table 26.2 Anatomopathological findings of the first 13 cases

Gonioscopy, mesodermal remnants		Pathology, mesodermal remnants			Postop		Displaced pupil	
RE	LE	Diffuse	Ligamentous	Displaced CM	IOP	Follow-up	RE	LE
Diffuse ligament	Diffuse ligament	+	–	+	10; 10	3 years	–	–
–	–	–	–	–	10; 8	2 months	–	–
Diffuse aplasia	Diffuse aplasia	+	+	–	10; 11	3 years	–	–
Diffuse ligament	Diffuse ligament	+	+	+	8; 8	7 months	+	+
Diffuse ligament	Diffuse ligament	+	+	–	10; 12	2 years	+	–
Diffuse	–	+	+	+	9; 9	1 year	–	+
Diffuse	–	+	–	–	16; 14	14 months	–	–
Diffuse aplasia?	Aplasia	(Dense) +?	–	–	18; 18	1 year	–	–
Diffuse ligament	Diffuse ligament		+		18; 18	4 years	–	–
Diffuse ligament	Diffuse ligament	+	+		18; 14	2 years	–	–

Postop postoperative, *displaced CM* displaced ciliary muscle

Terminology

As already mentioned, in gonioscopy as well as in pathologic anatomy, there are many different terms to refer to the anomalous tissue located in the chamber angle. These terms were:

- Pectinate ligament. Given the similarity found by some authors with this anatomic formation exclusively belonging to ungulates (horses), at present we call them pathological mesodermal remnants.
- The Barkan membrane. This term is used to name a membrane discovered by Barkan, which is seen through the gonioscope and evidenced during surgery, because it is difficult to histologically demonstrate its presence. With electron microscopy, Jerndal demonstrated that it was a membrane covering the anomalous tissue formed by a layer of polygonal cells.
- Anterior insertion of the iris, high insertion of the iris. This term was coined by numerous authors, though it is an apparent image, since the iris root, only formed by its deep mesenchymal layer, always inserts in the same place: the ciliary body band, formed by the inner surface of this muscle. However, the anomalous tissue attaches to the actual insertion spot and always to the same place in the iris, and may reach as far as the spur; sometimes it extends to the trabecular meshwork and other structures. It can even cover the Schwalbe line by surpassing it, thus producing the appearance of an anterior or high insertion.
- Pathological mesodermal remnants. This is the terminology we currently prefer, as do other authors, since it is a mesodermal tissue remaining in the chamber angle that has failed to be resorbed before month 9 of gestation, in which reticulin fibers prevail, like the tissue which is normally located there in fetal life. In contrast, in normal mesodermal remnants, known as iridian processes, collagen fibers prevail and may be present in any subject.

The term used to name this tissue in the first edition of this book has thus been changed, since at that time the term "pectinate ligament" was used, following Busacca's concept.

Normal Mesodermal Remnants: Iridian Processes

Iridian processes are formed by a central collagen axis and a very small number of reticulin fibers with fibroblasts surrounded by numerous melanocytes. In other words, their structure is identical to that of the superficial mesodermal layer of the iris (Fig. 26.2).

The iridian processes extend from the inner wall of the chamber angle (iris) to the external wall (sclera and cornea). The iridian edge of these processes never reaches beyond the base of the last circular fold of the iris, i.e., they never originate in the iris root. The corneoscleral end may reach different heights of the external wall of the chamber angle: the corneoscleral trabecular meshwork, the scleral spur, the trabecular meshwork at the Schlemm canal or the Schwalbe line, but they never reach as far as the latter.

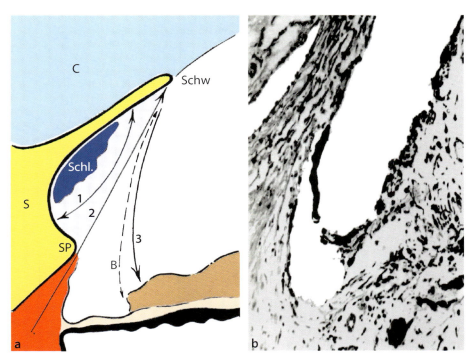

Fig. 26.2a,b   *1* corneoscleral trabecular meshwork, *2* tendon of the ciliary muscle, *3* Normal remnants: iridian process. *B* Iris root. *Schw* the Schwalbe line, *SP* scleral spur, *Schl* the Schlemm canal

Pathologic Mesodermal Remnants

Pathologic mesodermal remnants are found in pure congenital glaucoma, refractory congenital glaucoma, and late congenital glaucoma (goniodysgenesis) at 6–40 years of age.

As a primary concept, it should be stressed that there are pronounced differences in the pathologic anatomy of three types of glaucomas.

- In pure congenital glaucomas, these remnants are diffuse, in chamber angle type I and apparent high insertion of the iris in type II.
- In late congenital glaucomas, there are mesodermal pathological remnants from the scleral spur to the iris root. The ciliary band is not visible.

Diffuse Mesodermal Remnants: Pure Congenital Glaucoma

Diffuse mesodermal remnants in pure congenital glaucoma (70% of cases) have frequently been found in the chamber angle of pure congenital glaucoma specimens (Fig. 26.3).

In gonioscopy, they have the appearance of a tissue band that is seen around the entire circumference of the chamber angle, covering the structures of the external wall to different extents, from the roots of the iris, ciliary body band, the scleral spur, and sometimes in the trabecular meshwork.

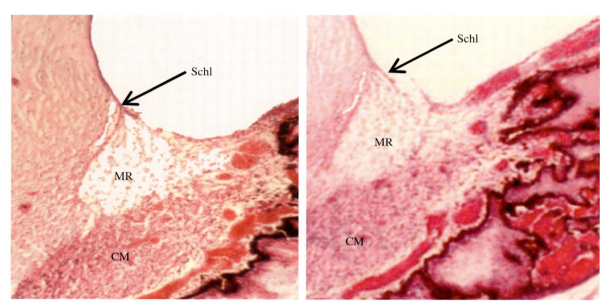

Fig. 26.3 *MR* Diffuse mesodermal remnants, *CM* ciliary muscle, *Schl* the Schlemm canal

Apparent High Insertion
of the Iris in Refractory Congenital Glaucoma

The mesodermal remnant advances to the Schwalbe line or a little higher (Fig. 26.4). The ophthalmologist had the impression of a high insertion of the iris and in fact the insertion is in the internal face of ciliary muscle.

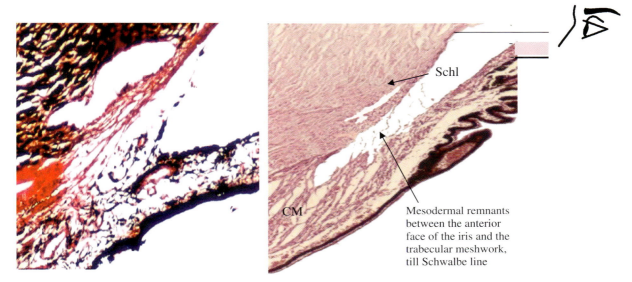

Schl

CM

Mesodermal remnants between the anterior face of the iris and the trabecular meshwork, till Schwalbe line

Fig. 26.4 Chamber angle in type II congenital glaucoma

Late Congenital Glaucoma

The mesodermal remnants extend to the scleral spur (gonioscopically absent from the ciliary band) (Fig. 26.5).

As revealed by light microscopy, the anatomopathologic section appears as a loose fibrillated mesh for the most part comprising reticulin fibers and a few collagen fibers. There are also endothelial cells and sometimes very fine pigment granules. It extends over as a mesh through the chamber angle from the iris up to the Schwalbe line. The characteristic of these diffuse pathologic remnants is that they are positive for argentic coloration (Gomori and Del Río Ortega staining) methods.

Reticulin fibers are very thin, with neither periodical striation nor determined arrangement. They evolve to become collagen fibers. The genesis of these fibers may be so altered that they may be present in abnormally smaller or larger numbers.

The most adequate expression for this pathology is the persistence of a marked reticulogenesis in cases of congenital glaucoma, which may be morphologically evidenced by the richness of these fibers in both ligamentous and diffuse remnants.

Table 26.3 is an outline of normal and pathologic mesodermal remnants.

The structures described above were differentiated according to two criteria:

a. Topographic: (1) gonioscopy; (2) analysis and photography of the trabeculectomy specimen under surgical microscopy and slit-lamp; (3) optical surface microscopy (Zarate's method), and (4) appraisal of the position of the elements of the chamber angle in magnified microscopy. Optical surface microscopy (Zarate's method) (Fig. 26.6).

1. The tissue specimen is immersed in different alcohol concentrations (50°, 96°, and 100°) for dehydration.
2. Then this material is immersed in a bath of xylene where it becomes highly transparent.
3. At this time, vital staining is used (toluidine or thionine).
4. The specimen is reviewed with light microscopy and the image is documented.

b. Structural morphology is according to the staining properties of the different tissues.
   – Hematoxylin-eosin can provide a topographic and morphologic criterion, but this technique is limited because it does not allow for differentiation between collagen and reticulin. This is the reason why other adequate additional techniques are used.
   – PAS can be useful for neutral mucopolysaccharides, in the intertrabecular spaces.
   – Masson's stain is very useful to accurately determine the position and length of the ciliary muscle (red) and the spur with a topographic criterion. Masson's stain is also useful for the differentiation of collagen structures, which acquire a blue coloration, as well as pathologic mesodermal remnants (diffuse or ligamentous), which stain in pink.
   – Gomori and Del Rio Ortega (reticulin method) use silver embedding exclusively for reticulin [2]. Diffuse mesodermal remnants are stained in black. With this technique, given the large quantity of reticulin fibers, the reticular fibers surrounding the fibers of the ciliary muscle are also stained (see Chap. 15, Fig. 15.34a–d).

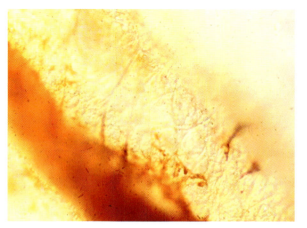

Fig. 26.5 The pathological mesodermal remnants extend to the scleral spur; gonioscopically it is not possible to see the ciliary band

Table 26.3 Further anatomopathological findings of the first 13 cases

Mesodermal tissue in the chamber angle	Normal	Corneoscleral trabecular meshwork, iris root	Collagen and reticulin
	Normal remnants	Iridian processes	
	Pathological remnants	Pure congenital glaucoma (diffuse)	Reticulin and collagen
		Refractory congenital glaucoma	
		Late CG (ligamentous)	

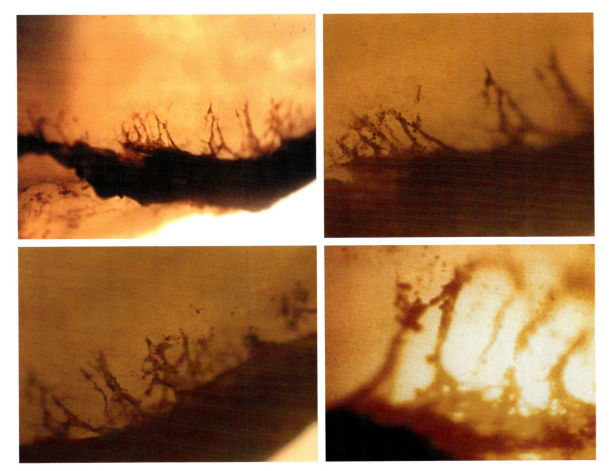

Fig. 26.6 Mesodermal pathological remnants seen with this technique

References

1. Sampaolesi R, Argento C (1977) Scanning electron micros-
    copy of the trabecular meshwork in normal and glaucoma-
    tous eyes. Invest Ophthalmol Vis Sci 16:302–314
2. Sampaolesi R, Zarate JO, Caruso R (1979) Congenital
    glaucoma: light and scanning electron microscopy of trab-
    eculectomy specimens. Glaucoma update. Springer, Berlin,
    pp 39–51

Contents

	Right eye	Left eye
IOP	13 mmHg	12 mmHg with applanation test
	13.1 mmHg	13.8 mmHg with Pascal test
Pachymetry	515 μm	517 μm
Refraction	20/20	20/20
Chamber angle	Normal	Normal (broad ciliary body band in both eyes)

In the past 4 years we have received 62 pediatric referrals asking for a second opinion: 49 children had a diagnosis of glaucoma, 46 with indications of unilateral or bilateral surgery, but 44 of these patients were normal and the surgical indication had to be cancelled. Forty-eight of the diagnoses were false-positives and the most common cause was megalopapilla. Six of these had been operated unilaterally or bilaterally even though they did not have the disease, and their optic nerves and visual fields were normal. It seems best to give a summary by presenting just four cases, two of Dr. Roberto Sampaolesi's and two of Dr. Juan Sampaolesi's.

Clinical History No. 1

Clinical history no. 1 was an 8-year-old boy who was brought by his parents, both of whom are pediatricians, with a diagnosis of congenital glaucoma and an indication to perform surgery immediately on both eyes.

The daily pressure curve (DPC) can be seen in Fig. 27.1. In this case, I had already operated three patients in this family: both the paternal grandparents and the child's father for open-angle glaucoma. The diagnosis for the child had been bilateral megalopapilla (false-positive) (Figs. 27.2, 27.3). I performed an iridencleisis on the grandfather in 1971, who maintained 20/20 vision in both eyes and visual field in stage II until 1996 when I operated him for cataract. He kept 20/20 vision and at the last appointment in 1998 I indicated an intraocular lens in the right eye. His visual field was unchanged and his vision was 20/20. I saw him last in 1999. When his wife was 66, I diagnosed her with glaucoma in both eyes with a visual field stage II, which was regulated with medical treatment. I attended their son as well, when he was 43, for open-angle glaucoma at a perimetric stage. The optic nerve was phase III in both eyes with normal visual field, and medical treatment regulated the pressure well.

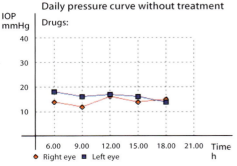

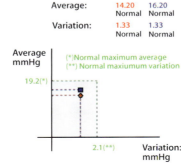

Fig. 27.1 Optic nerve and visual field

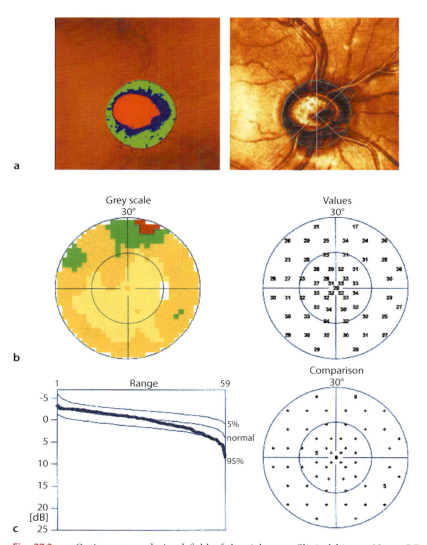

Fig. 27.2a–c Optic nerve and visual field of the right eye. Clinical history No. 1, RE: false positive bilateral glaucoma in a child of 8 years, the real diagnosis was bilateral megaopapilla

a HRT
b Octopus
c Bebie curve

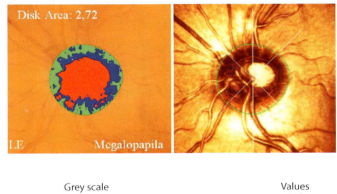

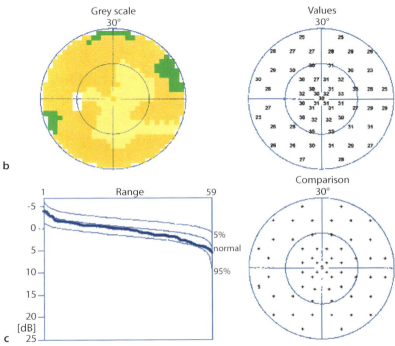

Fig. 27.3a–c Optic nerve and visual field of the left eye. Clinical history No. 1, RE: false positive bilateral glaucoma in a child of 8 years, the real diagnosis was bilateral megaopapilla

a HRT
b Octopus
c Bebie curve

Clinical History No. 2

Clinical history no. 2 was a 9-year-old boy. In the ophthalmological examination in 2002, his IOP was found to be 22 mmHg in the right eye and 24 mmHg in the left eye. No daily pressure curve was done. He was operated immediately with a diagnosis of congenital glaucoma. Trabeculotomy was performed in the right eye and in the same year trabeculotomy in the left eye. The left eye was reoperated in 2004 with a trabeculectomy. His 4-year-old brother was operated with trabeculotomy. The family history shows only one grandfather with glaucoma.

He was medicated with Alphagan. When the medication was suspended for 1 month, there was no increase of the IOP. The visual fields were repeated three times.

	Right eye	Left eye
IOP	15 mmHg	15 mmHg
Visual acuity	20/20	20/20
DPC	Normal	Normal
HRT(optic nerve)	Normal	Normal (Fig. 27.4)
Octopus visual field	Normal	Normal (Fig. 27.5)
FDT visual field	Normal	Normal (Fig. 27.5)
Pulsar visual field	Normal	Normal (Fig. 27.5)

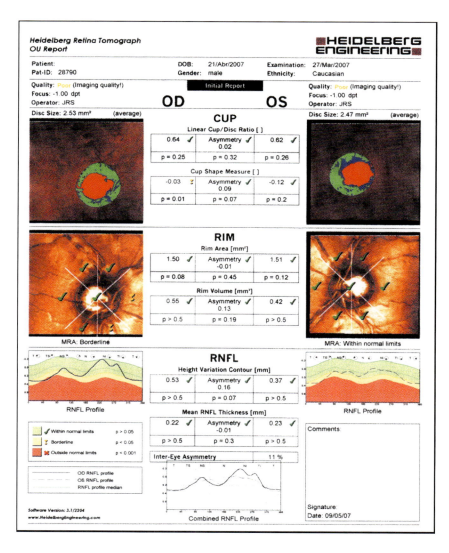

Fig. 27.4 HRT of the optic nerve of the right and left eye was normal

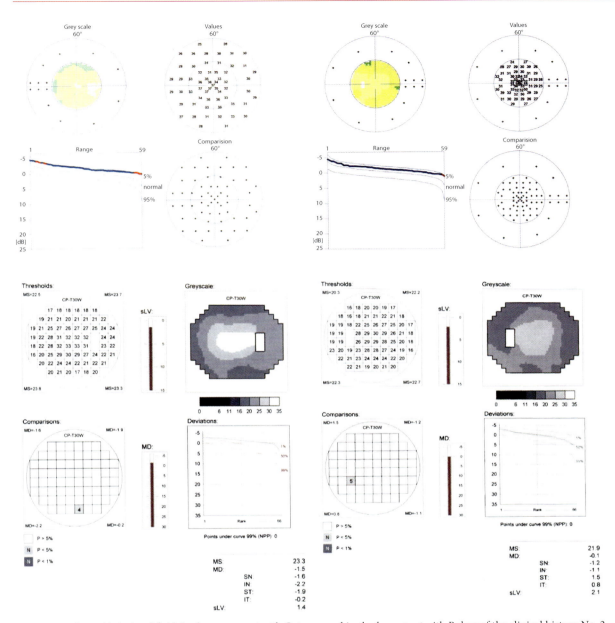

Fig. 27.5 Right and left visual field. in the *upper part* with Octopus and in the *lower part* with Pulsar of the clinical history No. 2 of false positive. Both visual fields were normal

Clinical History No. 3

Case history no. 3 was a female, aged 10 years. She had had a recent diagnosis of congenital glaucoma with an indication for glaucoma surgery in both eyes. She was treated with brimonidine tartrate (bid). Previous studies included CVF: level III (both eyes), HRT: phase III (both eyes). The child's family history was unknown (the patient had been adopted).

The visual fields that the patient presented, the two top images in Fig. 27.9, are known in campimetry as a clover-leaf visual field, and this is typical in children showing defects that do not really exist.

Five years later HRT and visual field are normal. Her definitive diagnosis is normal, false-positive glaucoma, for asymmetry of the papillary area (Fig. 27.10).

	Right eye	Left eye
IOP	12 mmHg	11 mmHg
Gonioscopy	Normal	Normal
Optic nerve	2/6	3/6, Papillary asymmetry (Fig. 27.6)
Ibopamine	Negative	Negative
DPC	Normal	Normal
HRT	Normal	Normal (Fig. 27.7, 27.8)
Visual field	Normal	Normal (Fig. 27.9)
Management	Washout 30 days and then DPC	

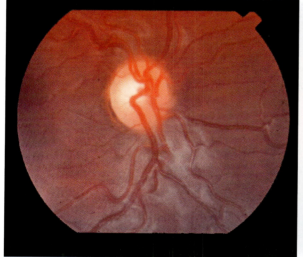 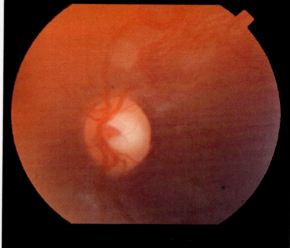

Fig. 27.6 Optic disc right and left eyes: papillary asymmetry

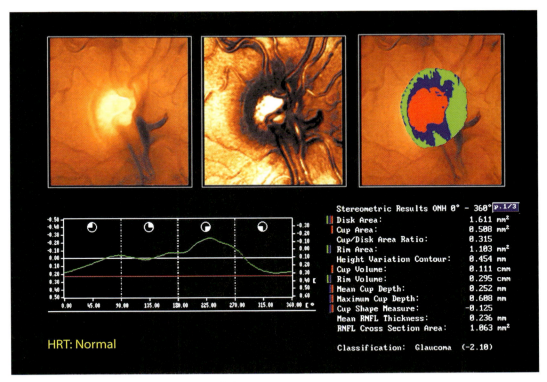

Fig. 27.7 HRT of the right and left eyes: megalodisc

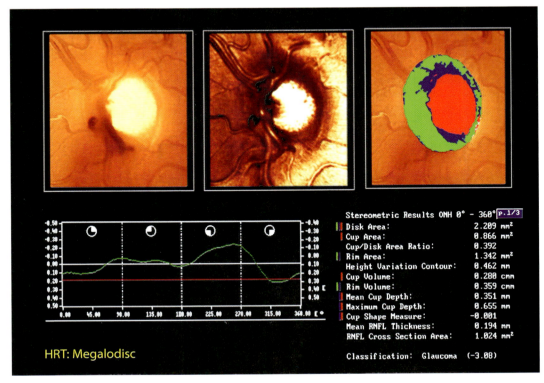

Fig. 27.8 HRT of the right and left eyes: megalodisc

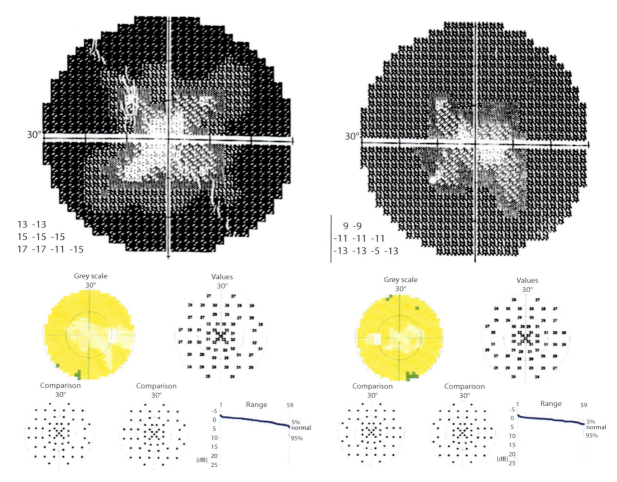

Fig. 27.9. Visual field of the right and left eyes. This visual field is known in campimetry as a clover leaf visual field; this is typical in children showing defects that do not really exist

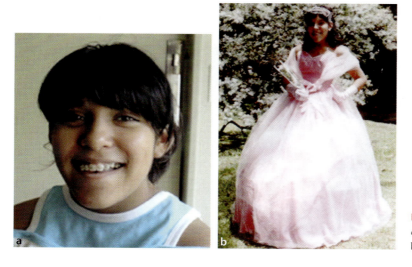

Fig. 27.10a,b Photograph of the girl of clinical history No. 3, **a** every day and **b** on her 15th birthday

Clinical History No. 4

Case history no. 4 was a young woman aged 18 years who had been diagnosed with normal pressure glaucoma. She was told that the prognosis was poor, as the optical nerve becomes damaged even with normal IOP. She wanted a second opinion. The family history included glaucoma in her mother treated with cortisone. She also had a personal history of migraine and headaches.

	Right eye	Left eye
IOP	10 mmHg	10 mmHg (Treated with prostaglandins)
Visual acuity	20/20	20/20
Gonioscopy	Normal	Normal
Optic nerve	Cupping 4/6	4/6 (Pink neuroretinal ring) (Fig. 27.11 and 27.12)
Computerized visual field SAP	Normal	Normal (Fig. 27.13)

Management: washout 40 days, then perform DPC without treatment

Daily pressure after washout: normal in both eyes

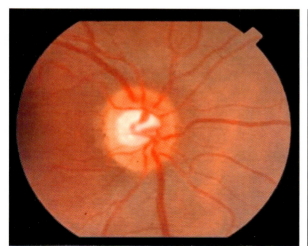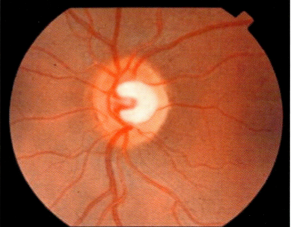

Fig. 27.11 Patient's optic disc

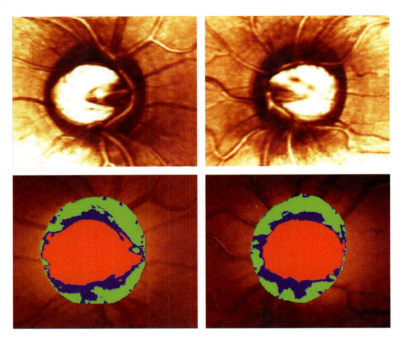

Fig. 27.12 Clinical history No. 4, RE and LE: Optic disc (HRT)

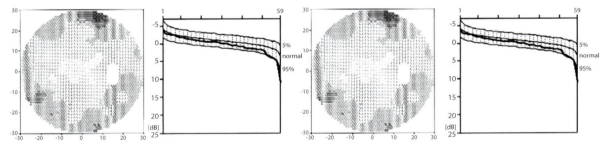

Fig. 27.13 HRT of the same patient. Visual field of the clinical history No. 4, normal in both eyes

Conclusion

This is a false positive glaucoma. The real diagnosis is congenital bilateral megalopapilla without glaucoma.

Epilog

The study of primary congenital glaucoma has shown that a congenital anomaly of the pretrabecular chamber angle leads to ocular hypertension. If its surgical treatment does not normalize the intraocular pressure it leads to glaucomatous optic neuropathy, identical to that found in adults, but with a much faster development and identical defects in the visual field. In the literature on congenital glaucomas, neither the risk factors nor the normal-tension glaucomas are described.

This simple summary should indicate that in the future, when 24-h IOP monitoring in open-angle glaucomas would be possible, the concept of glaucoma may change. Ocular pressure will not be seen as a risk factor, but rather the cause of glaucomatous optic neuropathy.

Currently, 24-h IOP monitoring is not possible, because it is very inconvenient for the doctor to take the pressure at 6 a.m. in the morning or because hospitals do not pay for DPC. In the near future, we will have a new automatic device that will enable such monitoring.

Printing and Binding: Stürtz GmbH, Würzburg